# Student Resources

Online Student Resources are **included** with this textbook.
Visit **http://nursing.pearsonhighered.com** for the following assets and activities:

- Learning Outcomes
- Chapter Review Questions
- Case Studies
- Appendices and additional content updates
- Weblinks
- Links to additional nursing resources

---

Additional resources available. For more information and purchasing options visit **nursing.pearsonhighered.com**

## CLASSROOM

## mynursinglab

- MyNursingLab provides you with a one-of-a-kind *guided learning path*. Its proven personalized study plan helps you to *synthesize vast amounts of information* with an engaging **REVIEW**, **REMEMBER**, and **APPLY** approach. Move *from memorization to true understanding* through application with:
  - Even more alternate-item format questions
  - More analysis and application level questions that gauge true understanding
  - An interactive eText (also available via iPad®) with multimedia resources built right in

## CLINICAL

### Pearson's Nurse's Drug Guide

- Published annually to be your current, comprehensive, and clinically relevant source for drug information

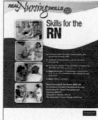

- Your complete mobile solution!

### Real Nursing Skills

- Video demonstrations of over 200 clinical nursing skills
- Each skill includes Purpose, Preparation, Procedure, Post-Procedure, Expected and Unexpected Outcomes, Documentation and References and Resources

## NCLEX®

- Concentrated review of core content
- Thousands of practice questions with comprehensive rationales

---

# PEARSON

ALWAYS LEARNING

# Instructor Resources—Redefined!

## PEARSON NURSING CLASS PREPARATION RESOURCES

### New and Unique!

- Use this preparation tool to find animations, videos, images, and other media resources that cross the nursing curriculum! Organized by topic and fully searchable by resource type and key word, this easy-to-use platform allows you to:
  - Search through the media library of assets
  - Upload your own resources
  - Export to PowerPoint™ or HTML pages

**Use this tool to find and review other unique instructor resources:**

### Correlation Guide to Nursing Standards

- Links learning outcomes of core textbooks to nursing standards such as the 2010 ANA Scope and Standards of Practice, QSEN Competencies, National Patient Safety Goals, AACN, Essentials of Baccalaureate Education and more!

### Pearson Nursing Lecture Series

- Highly visual, fully narrated and animated, these short lectures focus on topics that are traditionally difficult to teach and difficult for students to grasp
- All lectures accompanied by case studies and classroom response questions for greater interactivity within even the largest classroom
- Use as lecture tools, remediation material, homework assignments and more!

## MYTEST AND ONLINE TESTING

- Test questions even **more accessible** now with both pencil and paper (MyTest) and online delivery options (Online Testing)
- **NCLEX®-style** questions
- **All New!** Approximately 30% of all questions are in alternative-item format
- **Complete rationales** for correct and incorrect answers mapped to learning outcomes

## BOOK-SPECIFIC RESOURCES
### Also available to instructors:

- **Instructor's Manual and Resource Guide** organized by learning outcome
- Comprehensive **PowerPoint™** presentations integrating lecture notes and images
- **Image library**
- **Classroom Response Questions**
- **Online course management systems** complete with instructor tools and student activities

## mynursinglab

- **Proven Results:** Pearson's MyLab/Mastering platform has helped millions of students
- Provide your students with a one-of-a-kind guided learning path and personalized study plan! An engaging **REVIEW**, **REMEMBER**, and **APPLY** approach moves students from memorization to true understanding through application with:
  - Even more alternate-item format questions
  - More analysis and application level questions
  - An interactive eText (also available via iPad®) with multimedia resources built right in
- **Trusted Partner:** A network of customer experience managers and faculty advocates are available to help instructors maximize learning gains with MyNursingLab.

## REAL NURSING SIMULATIONS

- 25 simulation scenarios that span the nursing curriculum
- Consistent format includes learning objectives, case flow, set-up instructions, debriefing questions and more!
- Companion online course cartridge with student pre-and post-simulation activities, videos, skill checklists and reflective discussion questions

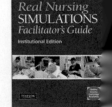

*Real Nursing* SIMULATIONS *Facilitator's Guide* Institutional Edition

# PEARSON

ALWAYS LEARNING

**Eighth Edition**

# Effective Leadership and Management in Nursing

**Eleanor J. Sullivan,** PhD, RN, FAAN

**PEARSON**

Boston   Columbus   Indianapolis   New York   San Francisco   Upper Saddle River
Amsterdam   Cape Town   Dubai   London   Madrid   Milan   Munich   Paris   Montréal   Toronto
Delhi   Mexico City   São Paulo   Sydney   Hong Kong   Seoul   Singapore   Taipei   Tokyo

Publisher: Julie Levin Alexander
Publisher's Assistant: Regina Bruno
Executive Acquisitions Editor: Pamela Fuller
Editorial Assistant: Cynthia Gates
Managing Production Editor: Central Publishing
Art Director: Christopher Weigand
Interior Designer: Black Horse Designs
Director of Marketing: David Gesell
Marketing Manager: Debi Doyle

Senior Marketing Manager: Phoenix Harvey
Marketing Specialist: Michael Sirinides
Media Product Manager: Travis Moses-Westphal
Assistant Editor for Media: Sarah Wrocklage
Media Project Managers: Rachel Collett and Leslie Brado
Production Manager: Fran Russello
Production Editor: Murugesh Rajkumar Namasivayam/PreMediaGlobal
Printer/Binder: R.R. Donnelley & Sons Company
Cover Printer: Lehigh Phoenix Color/Hagerstown

Notice: Care has been taken to confirm the accuracy of information presented in this book. The authors, editors, and the publisher, however, cannot accept any responsibility for errors or omissions or for consequences from application of the information in this book and make no warranty, express or implied, with respect to its contents.

The author and publisher have exerted every effort to ensure that drug selections and dosages set forth in this text are in accord with current recommendations and practice at time of publication. However, in view of ongoing research, changes in government regulations, and the constant flow of information relating to drug therapy and drug reactions, the reader is urged to check the package inserts of all drugs for any change in indications of dosage and for added warnings and precautions. This is particularly important when the recommended agent is a new and/or infrequently employed drug.

Copyright © **2013, 2009** by Pearson Education, Inc. All rights reserved. Manufactured in the United States of America. This publication is protected by Copyright, and permission should be obtained from the publisher prior to any prohibited reproduction, storage in a retrieval system, or transmission in any form or by any means, electronic, mechanical, photocopying, recording, or likewise. To obtain permission(s) to use material from this work, please submit a written request to Pearson Education, Inc., Permissions Department, One Lake Street, Upper Saddle River, New Jersey 07458, or you may fax your request to 201-236-3290.

**Library of Congress Cataloging-in-Publication Data**
Sullivan, Eleanor J.,
    Effective leadership and management in nursing / Eleanor J. Sullivan.—8th ed.
        p. ; cm.
    Includes bibliographical references and index.
    ISBN-13: 978-0-13-281454-6
    ISBN-10: 0-13-281454-4
I. Title.
    [DNLM: 1. Nurse Administrators. 2. Leadership. 3. Nursing Care—organization & administration. WY 105]
    LC Classification not assigned
    362.17'3068—dc23
                                                2012016912

10 9 8 7 6 5

**PEARSON**

ISBN-10: 0-13-281454-4
ISBN-13: 978-0-13-281454-6

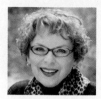 Eleanor J. Sullivan, PhD, RN, FAAN, is the former dean of the University of Kansas School of Nursing, past president of Sigma Theta Tau International, and previous editor of the *Journal of Professional Nursing*. She has served on the board of directors of the American Association of Colleges of Nursing, testified before the U.S. Senate, served on a National Institutes of Health council, presented papers to international audiences, been quoted in the *Chicago Tribune, St. Louis Post-Dispatch,* and *Rolling Stone Magazine*, and named to the "Who's Who in Health Care" by the *Kansas City Business Journal*. She earned nursing degrees from St. Louis Community College, St. Louis University, and Southern Illinois University and holds a PhD from St. Louis University.

Dr. Sullivan is known for her publications in nursing, including this award-winning textbook, *Effective Leadership & Management in Nursing*, and *Becoming Influential: A Guide for Nurses*, 2nd edition, from Prentice Hall. Other publications include *Creating Nursing's Future: Issues, Opportunities and Challenges* and *Nursing Care for Clients with Substance Abuse*.

Today, Dr. Sullivan is a mystery writer. Her first three (*Twice Dead, Deadly Diversion,* and *Assumed Dead*) feature nurse sleuth Monika Everhardt.

Her latest book, *Cover Her Body, A Singular Village Mystery*, is the first in a new series of historical mysteries featuring a 19th-century midwife and set in the Northern Ohio village of Dr. Sullivan's ancestors. Dr. Sullivan's blog posts, found at www.EleanorSullivan.com, reveal the history behind her historical fiction.

Connect with Dr. Sullivan at www.EleanorSullivan.com.

*This book is dedicated to my family*
*for their continuing love and support.*
*Eleanor J. Sullivan*

# THANK YOU

Our heartfelt thanks go out to our colleagues from schools of nursing across the country who have given their time generously to help us create this exciting new edition of our book. We have reaped the benefit of your collective experience as nurses and teachers and have made many improvements due to your efforts. Among those who gave us their encouragement and comments are:

## Reviewers

Theresa Ameri
Part-time/adjunct instructor,
Marymount University
Arlington, VA

Becky Brown, MSN, RN
Full-time instructor, College of Southern Idaho
Twin Falls, ID

Candace Burns, PhD, ARNP
Professor, University of South Florida College
of Nursing
Tampa, FL

Sandra Janashak Cadena, PhD, APRN, CNE
Professor, University of South Florida
Tampa, FL

Margaret Decker
Full-time instructor, Binghamton University
Binghamton, NY

Denise Eccles, MSN/Ed, RN
Professor, Miami Dade College
Miami, FL

Barb Gilbert, EdD, MSN, RN, CNE
Part-time/adjunct instructor, Excelsior College
Albany, NY

Karen Joris, MSN, RN
Assistant professor, Lorain County Community
College
Elyria, OH

Jean M. Klein, PhD, PMHCNS, BC
Associate professor, Widener University
Chester, PA

Jemimah Mitchell-Levy, MSN, ARNP
Professor, Miami Dade College
Miami, FL

Rorey Pritchard, EdS, MSN, RN, CNOR
Full-time instructor, Chippewa Valley Technical
College
Eau Claire, WI

Heather Saifman, MSN, RN, CCRN
Assistant professor, Nova Southeastern
University

Miami Kendall, FL
Linda Stone
Other
Cambridge, MA

Sandra Swearingen
Part-time/adjunct instructor, UCF
Orlando, FL

Diane Whitehead, EdD, RN, ANEF
Department chair, Nova Southeastern
University
Fort Lauderdale, FL

# PREFACE

Leading and managing are essential skills for all nurses in today's rapidly changing health care arena. New graduates find themselves managing unlicensed assistive personnel, and experienced nurses are managing groups of health care providers from a variety of disciplines and educational levels. Declining revenues, increasing costs, demands for safe care, and health care reform legislation mandate that every organization use its resources efficiently.

Nurses today are challenged to manage effectively with fewer resources. Never has the information presented in this textbook been needed more. *Effective Leadership & Management in Nursing*, eighth edition, can help both student nurses and those with practice experience acquire the skills needed to ensure success in today's dynamic health care environment.

## Features of the Eighth Edition

*Effective Leadership & Management in Nursing* has made a significant and lasting contribution to the education of nurses and nurse managers in its seven previous editions. Used worldwide, this award-winning textbook is now offered in an updated and revised edition to reflect changes in the current health care system and in response to suggestions from the book's users. The eighth edition builds upon the work of previous contributors to provide the most up-to-date and comprehensive learning package for today's busy students and professionals.

This book has been a success for many reasons. It combines practicality with conceptual understanding; is responsive to the needs of faculty, nurse managers, and students; and taps the expertise of contributors from a variety of disciplines, especially management professionals whose work has been adapted by nurses for current nursing practice. The expertise of management professors in schools of business and practicing nurse managers is seldom incorporated into nursing textbooks. This unique approach provides students with invaluable knowledge and skills and sets the book apart from others.

Features new or expanded in the eighth edition include:

- Information about the Patient Protection and Affordable Care Act
- An emphasis on quality initiatives, including Six Sigma, Lean Six Sigma, and DMAIC
- The use of Magnet-certified hospitals as examples of concepts

- The addition of emotional leadership concepts
- The use of social media in management
- An emphasis on multicratic leadership and interprofessional relationships
- Updated legal and legislative content
- Tips on how to deal with disruptive staff behaviors, including bullying
- Guidance on preparing for emergencies and mass casualty incidents
- Information on preventing workplace violence

## Student-Friendly Learning Tools

Designed with the adult learner in mind, the book focuses on the application of the content presented and offers specific guidelines on how to implement the skills included. To further illustrate and emphasize key points, each chapter in this edition includes these features:

- A chapter outline and preview
- New MediaLink boxes introduce readers to resources and activities on the Student Resources site through nursing.pearsonhighered.com.
- Key terms are defined in the glossary at the end of the book
- What You Know Now lists at the end of each chapter
- A list of "tools," or key behaviors, for using the skills presented in the chapter
- Questions to Challenge You to help students relate concepts to their experiences
- Up-to-date references and Web resources identified
- Case Studies with a Manager's Checklist to demonstrate application of content

## Organization

The text is organized into four sections that address the essential information and key skills that nurses must learn to succeed in today's volatile health care environment.

### Part 1. Understanding Nursing Management and Organizations.

Part 1 introduces the context for nursing management, with an emphasis on how organizations are designed, on ways that nursing care is delivered, on the concepts of leading and managing, on how to initiate and manage change, on providing quality care, and on using power and politics—all necessary for nurses to succeed and prosper in today's chaotic health care world.

### Part 2. Learning Key Skills in Nursing Management.

Part 2 delves into the essential skills for today's managers, including thinking critically, making decisions, solving problems, communicating with a variety of individuals and groups, delegating, working in teams, resolving conflicts, and managing time.

### Part 3. Managing Resources.

Knowing how to manage resources is vital for nurses today. They must be adept at budgeting fiscal resources; recruiting and selecting staff; handling staffing and scheduling; motivating and developing staff; evaluating staff performance; coaching, disciplining and terminating staff; managing absenteeism, reducing turnover, and retaining staff; and handling disruptive staff behaviors, including bullying. In addition, collective bargaining and preparing for emergencies and preventing workplace violence are included in Part 3.

### Part 4. Taking Care of Yourself.

Nurses are their own most valuable resource. Part 4 shows how to manage stress and to advance in a career.

## Resources for Teaching and Learning

Student and Instructor Resources can be accessed by registering or logging in at nursing.pearsonhighered.com.

## Acknowledgments

The success of previous editions of this book has been due to the expertise of many contributors. Nursing administrators, management professors, and faculty in schools of nursing all made significant contributions to earlier editions. I am enormously grateful to them for sharing their knowledge and experience to help nurses learn leadership and management skills. Without them, this book would not exist.

At Pearson Health Science, Acquisitions Editor Pamela Fuller and Development Editor Susan Geraghty guided this revision from start to finish. Editorial Assistant Cynthia Gates was also especially helpful.

Because health care continues to change, reviewers who are using the book in their management practice and in their classes provided invaluable comments and suggestions (see list on pages xi–xii).

I am especially grateful to experienced nurse manager and graduate student Rachel Pepper for her expert research assistance, ability to generate real-life examples, and expertise in creating case scenarios to exemplify the experience of nurses in management roles. She lent assistance throughout with ideas and suggestions. This book and *Becoming Influential: A Guide for Nurses*, 2nd edition, are better for her contributions.

To everyone who has contributed to this fine book over the years, I thank you.

*Eleanor J. Sullivan, PhD, RN, FAAN*
*www.EleanorSullivan.com*

# CONTENTS

# Introducing Nursing Management

Changes in Health Care

Paying for Health Care

HOW AMERICA PAYS
FOR HEALTH CARE

PAY FOR PERFORMANCE

Demand for Quality

QUALITY INITIATIVES

THE LEAPFROG GROUP

BENCHMARKING

EVIDENCE-BASED PRACTICE

MAGNET® CERTIFICATION

Evolving Technology

ELECTRONIC HEALTH
RECORDS

VIRTUAL CARE

ROBOTICS

COMMUNICATION
TECHNOLOGY

Cultural, Gender, and
Generational Differences

Violence Prevention
and Disaster Preparedness

Changes in Nursing's Future

EVEN MORE CHANGE . . .

CHALLENGES FACING NURSES
AND MANAGERS

## Learning Outcomes

*After completing this chapter, you will be able to:*

1. Describe the forces that are changing the health care system.
2. Discuss changes in paying for health care.
3. Explain how quality initiatives can reduce medical errors.
4. Describe how evidence-based practice is changing nursing.
5. Explain how to become a Magnet-certified hospital.
6. Explain what emerging technologies mean for nursing.
7. Describe how cultural, gender, and generational differences affect management.
8. Explain why preparation is the best defense against violence and disasters.
9. Discuss the changes and challenges that nurses face now and into the future.

## Key Terms

Benchmarking
Electronic health records
    (EHRs)
Evidence-based practice
Leapfrog Group

Magnet Recognition
    Program®
Patient Protection and
    Affordable Care Act
    (PPACA)

Quality initiatives
Robotics
Social media
Virtual care

Today, all nurses are managers. Whether you work in a freestanding clinic, an ambulatory surgical center, a critical unit in an acute care hospital, or in hospice care for a home care agency, you must deal with staff, including other nurses and unlicensed assistive personnel, who work with you and for you. At the same time, you must be vigilant about costs. To manage well, you must understand the health care system and the organizations where you work. You need to recognize what external forces affect your work and how to influence those forces. You need to know what motivates people and how you can help create an environment that inspires and sustains the individuals who work in it. You must be able to collaborate with others, as a leader, a follower, and a team member, in order to become confident in your ability to be a leader and a manager.

This book is designed to provide new graduates or novice managers with the information they need to become effective managers and leaders in health care. More than ever before, today's rapidly changing health care environment demands highly refined management skills and superb leadership.

## Changes in Health Care

Today's health care system is continuing to undergo significant changes. Costly lifesaving medicines, robotics, virtual care, and innovations in imaging technologies, noninvasive treatments, and surgical procedures have combined to produce the most sophisticated and effective health care ever—and the most expensive. Skyrocketing costs and inaccessibility to health care are ongoing concerns for employers, health care providers, policy makers, and the public at large. A number of factors are forcing change on the health care system.

## Paying for Health Care

### How America Pays for Health Care

The United States spends more money on health care than any other country, and health care spending continues to rise with costs of $2.5 trillion in 2009, consuming more than 17 percent of the country's gross domestic product (GDP) (CMS, 2011). With the goal of providing access to health care to most U.S. citizens and containing costs, Congress passed a health care reform bill known as the **Patient Protection and Affordable Care Act (PPACA)** that was signed into law March 23, 2010. While implementation of the bill is pending court challenges, the promise of providing adequate and affordable care to more Americans is on the horizon.

### Pay for Performance

In 1999, the Institute of Medicine (IOM, 1999) reported that 98,000 deaths occurred each year from preventable medical mistakes, such as falls, wrong site surgeries, avoidable infections, and pressure ulcers, among others. By 2008, researchers learned that "the effects of medical mistakes continue long after the patient leaves the hospital" (Encinosa & Hellinger, 2008, p. 2067). In spite of numerous efforts to prevent mistakes, the cost of medical errors has continued to climb. Recent estimates put such costs at $19.5 billion annually (Shreve et al., 2010).

In 2008, the Centers for Medicare and Medicaid Services, the agency that oversees government payments for care, tied payment to the quality of care by changing its reimbursement policy to no longer cover costs incurred by medical mistakes (Wachter, Foster, & Dudley, 2008). If medical mistakes occur, the hospital must absorb the costs. Thus, pay for performance became the norm, and performance is now measured by the quality of care (Milstein, 2009).

## Demand for Quality

### Quality Initiatives

In an effort to ameliorate medical mistakes, a number of **quality initiatives** have emerged. Quality management is a preventive approach designed to address problems before they become crises. The quality movement actually began in post–World War II Japan, when Japanese industries adopted a system that W. Edwards Deming designed to improve the quality of manufactured products. The philosophy of the system is that consumers' needs should be the focus and that employees should be empowered to evaluate and improve quality. In addition to businesses in the United States and elsewhere, the health care industry has adopted total quality management or variations on it.

Built into the system is a mechanism for continuous improvement of products and services through constant evaluation of how well consumers' needs are met and plans adjusted to perfect the process. Patient satisfaction surveys are one example of how health care organizations evaluate their customers' needs. Today, quality initiatives address all aspects of patient care and include government efforts as well as private sector endeavors.

Public reporting of heath care organizations has emerged as a strategy to improve quality (Christianson et al., 2010). To further that goal, the Agency for Healthcare Research and Quality (AHRQ)—whose mission is to improve the quality, safety, efficiency, and effectiveness of health care—funds projects that address three quality indicators: prevention, inpatient, quality, and patient safety (Dunton et al., 2011).

## The Leapfrog Group

Efforts by the **Leapfrog Group** constitute one private sector initiative to address quality. The Leapfrog Group is a consortium of public and private purchasers established to reduce preventable medical mistakes. The organization uses its mammoth purchasing power to leverage quality care for its consumers by rewarding health care organizations that demonstrate quality outcome measures. The quality indicators the group focuses on include ICU staffing, electronic medication ordering systems, and the use of higher performing hospitals for high-risk procedures. Leapfrog estimates that if these three patient safety practices were implemented, more than 57,000 lives could be saved, more than $12 billion dollars could be saved, and more than 3 million adverse drug events could be avoided (Binder, 2010).

## Benchmarking

In contrast to quality management strategies that compare internal measures across comparable units, such as the Leapfrog Group, **benchmarking** compares an organization's data with similar organizations. Outcome indicators are identified that can be used to compare performance across disciplines or organizations. Once the results are known, health care organizations can address areas of weakness and enhance areas of strength (Nolte, 2011). Interestingly, one study found that hospital size didn't affect the ability of institutions to compare results (Brown et al., 2010).

## Evidence-Based Practice

**Evidence-based practice** has emerged as a strategy to improve quality by using the best available knowledge integrated with clinical experience and the patient's values and preferences to provide care (Houser & Oman, 2010).

Similar to the nursing process, the steps in EBP are:

1. Identify the clinical question.

2. Acquire the evidence to answer the question.

3. Evaluate the evidence.

4. Apply the evidence.

5. Assess the outcome.

Research findings with conflicting results puzzle consumers daily, and nurses are no exception, especially when they search for practice evidence. Hader (2010) suggests that evidence falls into several categories:

- Anecdotal—derived from experience
- Testimonial—reported by an expert in the field

- Statistical—built from a scientific approach
- Case study—an in-depth analysis used to translate to other clinical situations
- Nonexperimental design research—gathering factors related to a clinical condition
- Quasi-experimental design research—a study limited to one group of subjects
- Randomized control trial—uses both experimental and control groups to determine the effectiveness of an intervention

While all forms of evidence are useful for clinical decision making, a randomized control design and statistical evidence are the most rigorous (Hader, 2010).

### Magnet® Certification

The **Magnet Recognition Program®** designates organizations that "recognize health care organizations that provide nursing excellence" (ANCC, 2011). To qualify for recognition as a magnet hospital the organization must demonstrate that they are:

- Promoting quality in a setting that supports professional practice
- Identifying excellence in the delivery of nursing services to patients/residents
- Disseminating "best practices" in nursing services.

Becoming a magnet hospital requires a significant investment of time and financial resources. Research shows, however, that patient safety is improved when nurse staffing meets Magnet standards (Lake et al., 2010).

Systems involving participatory management and shared governance create organizational environments that reward decision making, creativity, independence, and autonomy. These organizations retain and recruit independent, accountable professionals. Organizations that empower nurses to make decisions will better meet consumer requests. As the health care environment continues to evolve, more and more organizations are adopting consumer-sensitive cultures that require accountability and decision making from nurses.

Magnet hospitals are those institutions that have met the stringent guidelines for nurses and are credentialed by the American Nurses Credentialing Center. Characteristics common in magnet hospitals include:

- Higher ratios of nurses to patients
- Flexible schedules
- Decentralized administration
- Participatory management
- Autonomy in decision making
- Recognition
- Advancement opportunities

To retain the current workforce and attract other nurses, health care organizations can take from the magnet program characteristics to improve work-life conditions for nurses. Encouraging nurses to be full participants and to share a vested interest in the success of the organization can help alleviate the nursing shortage in those organizations and in the profession.

See Chapter 6 , Managing and Improving Quality, to learn more about improving quality in health care.

## Evolving Technology

Rapid changes in technology seem, at times, to overwhelm us. Hospital information systems (HIS); electronic health records (EHR); point-of-care data entry (POC); provider order entry; bar-code medication administration; dashboards to manage, report, and compare data across platforms; virtual care provided from a distance; and robotics—to name a few of the many evolving technologies—both fascinate and frighten us simultaneously. At the same time, communication technology—from smartphones to social media—continues to march into the future. It is no wonder that people who work in health care complain that they can't keep up! The rapidity of technological change promises, unfortunately, to continue unabated.

## Electronic Health Records

**Electronic health records (EHRs)** represent a technology destined for rapid expansion. While banks, retailers, airlines, and other industries began to rely on fully integrated systems to manage communication and reduce redundancies, health care was still continuing to rely on voluminous paper records duplicated in multiple locations. Keeping data safe continues to worry health care organizations, consumers, and policy makers, but the benefits of integrated systems outweigh the risks (Trossman, 2009a).

EHRs reduce redundancies, improve efficiency, decrease medical errors, and lower health care costs. Continuity of care, discharge planning and follow-up, ambulatory care collaboration, and patient safety are just a few of the additional advantages of EHRs. Furthermore, fully integrated systems allow for collective data analysis across clinical conditions, health care organizations, or worldwide and support evidence-based decision making. With the federal government funding health systems to upgrade to EHRs, the current 12 percent of hospitals with EHRs is expected to increase (Gomez, 2010).

## Virtual Care

**Virtual care**, previously known as telemedicine and now more commonly called telehealth, has evolved as technologies to assess, intervene, and monitor patients remotely improved. Both communication technology (i.e., audio and video) and improvements in mobile care technology contribute to the ability of health care professionals to provide care from a distance. Nurses, for example, can watch banks of video screens monitoring ICU patients' vitals signs miles away from the hospital. Electronic equipment, such as a stethoscope, can be accessed by a health care provider in a distant location. Such systems are especially useful in providing expert consultation for specialty care (Zapatochny-Rufo, 2010).

## Robotics

Another technological advance is **robotics**. In the hospital, supplies can be ordered electronically, and then laser-guided robots can fill the order in the pharmacy or central supply and deliver the requested supplies to nursing units via their own elevators more efficiently, accurately, and in less time than individuals can. Mobile robots can also monitor patients, report changes and conditions, and allow caregivers to communicate from a distance (Markoff, 2010) via a wireless connection to a laptop or a smart phone. Robot functionality will continue to expand, limited only by resources and ingenuity.

## Communication Technology

Just as rapidly as clinical and data technology are evolving, so are communication technologies, changing forever the ways people keep informed and interact (Sullivan, 2013). Information (accurate or inaccurate) is disseminated with lightening speed while smartphones capture real-time events and broadcast images instantaneously.

**Social media** has revolutionized communication beyond the realm of possibilities from just a few years ago (Kaplan & Haenlein, 2010). Social media connects diverse populations and encourages collaboration, the exchange of images, ideas, opinions, and preferences in networking Web sites, online forums, Web blogs, social blogs, wikis, podcasts, RSS feeds, photos, video content communities, social bookmarking, online chat rooms, microblogs, such as Twitter, and online communities, such as Facebook and LinkedIn (Sullivan, 2013).

Similar to other enterprises, most health care organizations have an online presence with a Web site and social media sites, such as Facebook, Twitter, and blogs. Units within the organization may have Facebook pages as well, with staff who post on those sites. These opportunities for information sharing and relationship building also come with risks (Raso, 2010; Trossman, 2010b). Patient confidentiality, the organization's reputation, and recruiting efforts can be enhanced or put in jeopardy by posts to the site (Sullivan, 2013).

## Cultural, Gender, and Generational Differences

According to the U.S. Census Bureau, the minority population in the U.S. increased from 31 to 36 percent from 2000 to 2010 (U.S. Census, 2011). The largest minority population is Hispanic, and that population increased to 50 million (16 percent of the total U.S. population) in 2010. The Asian population grew to 14 million (5 percent) in the same time period, and the African American population stands at 42 million (14 percent).

The cultural diversity seen in the general population is also reflected in nursing. The Health Resources and Services Administration (HRSA, 2011) reports that 16 percent of nurses are Asian, African American, Hispanic, or other ethnic minorities, an increase from 12 percent in 2004.

The gender mix found in nursing, however, differs from the general population, with men greatly outnumbered by women. Of the population of more than 3 million nurses in the U.S., only 6 percent are men, although changes suggest the ratio is improving. The proportion of men to women has risen to 1 in 10 in the decades since 1990 (HRSA, 2011). Both cultural diversity and gender diversity challenge the nurse manager to consider such differences when working with staff, colleagues, and administrators as well as mediating conflicts between individuals.

Generational differences in the nursing population is unprecedented, with four generational cohorts working together (Keepnews et al., 2010). Referred to as traditionals, baby boomers, Generation X, and Generation Y, each generational group has different expectations in the workplace. Traditionals value loyalty and respect authority. Baby boomers value professional and personal growth and expect that their work will make a difference.

Generation X members strive to balance work with family life and believe that they are not rewarded given their responsibilities (Keepnews et al., 2010). Generation Y (also called millenials) are technically savvy and expect immediate access to information electronically.

Similar to dealing with cultural and gender differences, the challenge for managers is to avoid stereotyping within the generations, to value the unique contributions of each generation, to encourage mutual respect for differences, and to leverage these differences to enhance team work (Chambers, 2010).

## Violence Prevention and Disaster Preparedness

Sadly, violence invades workplaces, and health care is no exception. Moreover, nearly 500,000 nurses are victims of workplace violence (Trossman, 2010c). In addition, recent disasters (e. g., the earthquake and tsunami in Japan, tornadoes in the U.S.) and the threats of terrorism and pandemics challenge health care organizations to prepare for the unthinkable.

Extensive staff training is required (AHRQ, 2011). Techniques include computer simulations, video demonstrations, disaster drills, and a clear understanding of communication systems and the incident command center. A natural disaster, an attack of terrorism, an epidemic, or other mass casualty events may, and probably will, occur at some time. All health care organizations must be prepared to care for a surge in casualties while reducing the impact on patients and staff.

## Changes in Nursing's Future

Nurses will face many changes in the future, including an increasing demand for nurses as the population ages, a worsening shortage as nurses age, and recommendations for changes to practice and education. The aging population is surviving previously fatal diseases and conditions due to ever-evolving health care technologies. These patients often require ongoing care for chronic illnesses as well as for acute episodes of illness.

Just as the population is aging and requiring more and more care, nurses too are growing older. The average age of the registered nurse is 46 years, although the number of RNs under age 30 is increasing at a faster pace than before (HRSA, 2011).

Slightly more than 3 million nurses are currently licensed as registered nurses in the U.S., and 85 percent of them practice full- or part-time in the profession (HRSA, 2011). Jobs for nurses, however, are expected to grow to 3.2 million by 2018, much faster than the average for all occupations (U.S. Department of Labor, 2011). Also, with implementation of health care reform, increases in the demand for nurses in primary care and acute care settings are expected.

The Institute of Medicine's report on the future of nursing makes sweeping recommendations for nursing's future, including that "nurses should be full partners, with physicians and other health care professionals, in redesigning health care in the United States" (IOM, 2010, p. 3). In addition, IOM posits that today's health care environment necessitates better-educated nurses and recommends that 80 percent of nurses be prepared at the baccaluareate or higher level by 2020.

At the same time, the Carnegie Foundation recommends radically transforming nursing education (Benner et al., 2009). Its recommendations include:

1. Focus on how to apply knowledge, not only acquire it.

2. Integrate clinical and classroom teaching, rather than separately.

3. Emphasize clinical reasoning, not only critical thinking.

4. Emphasize formation, rather than socialization and role taking (Benner et al., 2009).

## Even More Change . . .

What does the future hold for health care? Change is the one constant. Quality of care will continue to be monitored and reported with accompanying demands to tie pay to performance. Technology of care, communication, and data management will become more and more complex as computer processing power and storage capacity expand (Clancy, 2010) and equipment becomes smaller and more mobile. Access to care and how to pay for it will continue to drive policy and funding decisions. Everyone in health care must learn to live with ambiguity and be flexible enough to adapt to the changes it brings.

## Challenges Facing Nurses and Managers

Every nurse must be prepared to manage. Specific training in management skills is needed in nursing school as well as in the work setting. Most important, however, is that nurses be able to transfer their newly acquired skills to the job itself. Thus, nurse managers must be experienced in management themselves and be able to assist their staff in developing adequate management skills. Management training for nurses at all levels is essential for any organization to be efficient and effective in today's cost-conscious and competitive environment.

The challenge for nurse managers and administrators is how to manage in a constantly changing system. Working with teams of administrators and providers to deliver quality health care in the most cost-effective manner offers opportunity as well. Nurses' unique skills in communication, negotiation, and collaboration position them well for the system of today and for the future.

Nurse managers today are challenged to monitor and improve quality care, manage with limited resources, help design new systems of care, supervise teams of professionals and nonprofessionals from a variety of cultures, and, finally, teach personnel how to function well in the new system. This is no small task. It requires that nurses and their managers be committed, involved, enthusiastic, flexible, and innovative; above all else, it requires that they have good mental and physical health. Because the nurse manager of today is responsible for others' work, the nurse manager must also be a coach, a teacher, and a facilitator. The manager works through others to meet the goals of individuals, of the unit, and of the organization. Most of all, the manager must be a leader who can motivate and inspire.

Nurse managers must address the interests of administrators, colleagues in other disciplines, and employees. All want the same result—quality care. Administrators, however, must focus on cost and efficiency in order for the organization to compete and survive. Colleagues want collaborative and efficient systems of care. Employees want to be supported in their work with adequate staffing, supplies, equipment, and, most of all, time. Therein lies the conflict. Between all of them is the nurse manager, who must balance the needs of all. Being a nurse manager today is the most challenging opportunity in health care. This book is designed to prepare you to meet these challenges.

## What You Know Now

- Health care is radically changing and is expected to continue to change in the foreseeable future.
- The tension between providing adequate nursing care and paying for that care will continue to dominate health policy decisions.
- Reducing medical errors is the goal of quality initiatives.
- Cultural, gender, and generational diversity will continue to shape the nursing workforce.
- Evidence-based practice will guide nursing decisions into the future.
- Electronic health records, robotics, and virtual care are just a few of the many technologies continuing to evolve.
- Expansion in communication technologies will continue to offer opportunities and challenges to health care organizations.
- Threats of natural disasters, terrorism, and pandemics require all health care organizations to plan and prepare for mass casualties.
- The nurse manager is challenged to manage in a constantly changing environment.

## Questions to Challenge You

1. Name three changes that you would suggest to reduce the cost of health care without compromising patients' health and safety. Talk about how you could help make these changes.
2. What mechanisms could you suggest to improve and ensure the quality of care? (Don't just suggest adding nursing staff!)
3. How could you help reduce medical errors? What can you suggest that a health care organization could do?
4. Do your clinical decisions rely on evidence-based practice? If you answer no, why not?
5. What are some ways that nurses could take advantage of emerging technologies in health care and information systems? Think big.
6. Have you participated in a disaster drill? Did you notice ways to improve the organization's readiness for mass casualties? Name at least one.
7. What steps can you take to transfer the knowledge and skills you learn in this book into your work setting?

**Pearson Nursing Student Resources**

Find additional review materials at
**www.nursing.pearsonhighered.com**

Prepare for success with additional NCLEX®-style practice
questions, interactive assignments and activities, Web links,
animations and videos, and more!

## References

Agency for Healthcare Research and Quality. (2011). *AHRQ disaster response tools and resources.* Retrieved May 25, 2011 from http://www.ahrq.gov/research/altstand

American Nurses Credentialing Center (2011). *Magnet Recognition Program.* Retrieved April 27, 2011 from http://www.nursecredentialing.org/Magnet.aspx

Benner, P., Sutphen, M., Leonard, V., and Day, L. (2009). *Educating nurses: A call for radical transformation.* San Francisco: Jossey-Bass.

Binder, L. (2010). Leapfrog: Unique and salient measures of hospital quality and safety. *Prescriptions for Excellence in Health Care, 8,* 1–2.

Brown, D. S., Aydin, C. E., Donaldson, N., Fridman, M., & Sandhu, M. (2010). Benchmarking for small hospitals: Size didn't matter! *Journal of Healthcare Quality, 32*(4), 50–60.

Centers for Medicare and Medicaid Services (CMS) (2011). *National health expenditure data.* Retrieved April 25, 2011 from https://www.cms.gov/NationalHealthExpendData/25_NHE_Fact_Sheet.asp

Chambers, P. D. (2010). Tap the unique strengths of the millennial generation. *Nursing Management, 41*(3), 37–39.

Christianson, J. B., Volmar, K. M., Alexander, J., & Scanlon, D. P. (2010). A report card on provider report cards: Current status of the health care transparency movement. *Journal of General Internal Medicine, 25*(11), 1235–1241.

Clancy, T. R. (2010). Technology and complexity: Trouble brewing? *Journal of Nursing Administration, 40*(6), 247–249.

Dunton, N., Gonnerman, D., Montalvo, I., & Schumann, M. J. (2011). Incorporating nursing quality indicators in public reporting and value-based purchasing initiatives. *American Nurse Today, 6*(1), 14–18.

Encinosa, W. E., & Hellinger, F. J. (2008). The impact of medical errors on ninety-day costs and outcomes: An examination of surgical patients. *Health Services Research, 43*(6), 2067–2085.

Hader, R. (2010). The evident that isn't . . . interpreting research. *Nursing Management, 41*(9), 23–26.

Health Resources and Services Administration (HRSA) (2011). *The registered nurse population: Findings from the 2008 national sample survey of registered nurses.* Retrieved April 26, 2011 from http://bhpr.hrsa.gov/healthworkforce/rnsurvey2008.html

Houser, J., & Oman, K. S. (2010). *Evidence-based practice: An implementation guide for healthcare organizations.* Sudbury, MA: Jones & Bartlett.

Gomez, R. (2010). Automation: HER upgrade considerations. *Nursing Management, 41*(2), 35–37.

Institute of Medicine (1999). *To err is human: Building a safer health system.* Washington, DC: National Academy Press.

Institute of Medicine (2010). *The future of nursing: Leading change, advancing health.* Retrieved April 26, 2011 from http://www.thefutureofnursing.org/IOM-Report

Kaplan, A. M., & Haenlein, M. (2010). Users of the world, unite! The challenges and opportunities of social media. *Business Horizons, 53*(1), 59–68.

Keepnews, D. M., Brewer, C. S., Kovner, C. T., & Shin, J. H. (2010). Generational differences among newly licensed registered nurses. *Nursing Outlook, 58*(3), 155–163.

Lake, E. T., Shang, J., Klaus, S., & Dunton, N. E. (2010). Patient falls: Association with hospital magnet status and nursing unit staffing. *Research in*

*Nursing & Health, 33*(5), 413–425.

Markoff, J. (2010, September 4). *The boss is robotic, and rolling up behind you. New York Times.* Retrieved April 28, 2011 from http://www.nytimes.com/2010/09/05/science/05robots.html

Milstein, A. (2009). Encing extra payment for "never events"—Stronger incentives for patients' safety. *New England Journal of Medicine, 360*(23), 2388–2390.

Nolte, E. (2011). *International benchmarking of healthcare quality: A review of the literature.* The Rand Corporation. Retrieved April 26, 2011 from http://www.rand.org/pubs/technical_reports/TR738.html

Raso, R. (2010). Social media for nurse managers: What does it all mean? *Nursing Management, 41*(8), 23–25.

Shreve, J., Van Den Bos, J., Gray, T., Halford, M., Rustagi, K., & Ziemkiewicz, E. (2010). *The economic measurement of medical errors.* Society of Actuaries. Retrieved April 28, 2011 from http://www.soa.org/files/pdf/research-econ-measurement.pdf

Sullivan, E. J. (2013). *Becoming influential: A guide for nurses* (2nd ed.). Upper Saddle River, NJ: Prentice Hall Health.

Trossman, S. (2009a). Issues up close: No peeking allowed. *American Nurse Today, 4*(2), 31–32.

Trossman, S. (2010b). Sharing too much? Nurses nationwide need more information on social networking pitfalls. *American Nurse Today, 5*(11), 38–39.

Trossman, S. (2010c, November/December). Not "part of the job": Nurses seek an end to workplace violence. *The American Nurse,* p. 1, 6.

U.S. Census Bureau (2011, March 24). *2010 Census shows America's diversity.* Retrieved April 29, 2011 from http://2010.census.gov/news/releases/operations/cb11-cn125.html

U.S. Department of Labor. (2011). *Occupational outlook handbook, 2010–11 edition.* Retrieved April 26, 2011 from http://stats.bls.gov/oco/ocos083.htm#outlook

Wachter, R. M., Foster, N. E., & Dudley, R. A. (2008). Medicare's decision to withhold payment for hospital errors: The devil is in the details. *Joint Commission Journal on Quality and Patient Safety, 34*(2), 116–123.

Zapatochny-Rufo, R. J. (2010). Good-better-best: The virtual ICU and beyond. *Nursing Management, 41*(2), 38–41.

# Designing Organizations

## Learning Outcomes

*After completing this chapter, you will be able to:*

1. Discuss how organizational theories differ.
2. Describe the different types of health care organizations.
3. Explain how health care organizations are structured.
4. Discuss various ways that health care is provided.
5. Demonstrate how strategic planning guides the organization's future.
6. Discuss how the organizational environment and culture affect workplace conditions.

## Key Terms

Accountable care organization
Bureaucracy
Capitation
Chain of command
Diversification
Goals
Hawthorne effect
Horizontal integration
Integrated health care networks
Line authority

Logic model
Medical home
Mission
Objectives
Organization
Organizational culture
Organizational environment
Philosophy
Redesign
Retail medicine

Service-line structures
Shared governance
Span of control
Staff authority
Strategic planning
Strategies
Throughput
Values
Vertical integration
Vision statement

A n **organization** is a collection of people working together under a defined structure to achieve predetermined outcomes using financial, human, and material resources. The justification for developing organizations is both rational and economic. Coordinated efforts capture more information and knowledge, purchase more technology, and produce more goods, services, opportunities, and securities than individual efforts. This chapter discusses organizational theory, structures, and functions.

# Traditional Organizational Theories

The earliest recorded example of organizational thinking comes from the ancient Sumerian civilization, around 5000 B.C. The early Egyptians, Babylonians, Greeks, and Romans also gave thought to how groups were organized. Later, Machiavelli in the 1500s and Adam Smith in 1776 established the management principles we know as specialization and division of labor. Nevertheless, organizational theory remained largely unexplored until the Industrial Revolution during the late 1800s and early 1900s, when a number of approaches to the structure and management of organizations developed. The early philosophies are traditionally labeled classical theory and humanistic theory while later approaches include systems theory, contingency theory, chaos theory, and complexity theory.

## Classical Theory

The classical approach to organizations focuses almost exclusively on the structure of the formal organization. The main premise is efficiency through design. People are seen as operating most productively within a rational and well-defined task or organizational design. Therefore, one designs an organization by subdividing work, specifying tasks to be done, and only then fitting people into the plan. Classical theory is built around four elements: division and specialization of labor, organizational structure, chain of command, and span of control.

### Division and Specialization of Labor

Dividing the work reduces the number of tasks that each employee must carry out, thereby increasing efficiency and improving the organization's product. This concept lends itself to proficiency and specialization. Therefore, division of work and specialization are seen as economically beneficial. In addition, managers can standardize the work to be done, which in turn provides greater control.

### Organizational Structure

Organizational structure describes the arrangement of the work group. It is a rational approach for designing an effective organization. Classical theorists developed the concept of departmentalization as a means to maintain command, reinforce authority, and provide a formal system for communication. The design of the organization is intended to foster the organization's survival and success.

Characteristically, the structure takes shape as a set of differentiated but interrelated functions. Max Weber (1958) proposed the term **bureaucracy** to define the ideal, intentionally rational, most efficient form of organization. Today this word has a negative connotation, suggesting long waits, inefficiency, and red tape.

### Chain of Command

The **chain of command** is the hierarchy of authority and responsibility within the organization. Authority is the right or power to direct activity, whereas responsibility is the obligation to attain objectives or perform certain functions. Both are derived from one's position within the organization and define accountability. The line of authority is such that higher levels of management delegate work to those below them in the organization.

One type of authority is **line authority**, the linear hierarchy through which activity is directed. Another type is **staff authority**, an advisory relationship; recommendations and advice

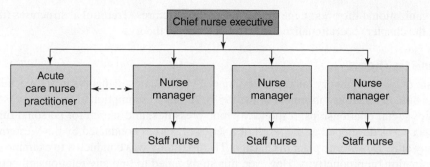

**Figure 2-1** ●
Chain of authority.

are offered, but responsibility for the work is assigned to others. In Figure 2-1, the relationships among the chief nurse executive, nurse manager, and staff nurse are examples of line authority. The relationship between the acute care nurse practitioner and the nurse manager illustrates staff authority. Neither the acute care nurse practitioner nor the nurse manager is responsible for the work of the other; instead, they collaborate to improve the efficiency and productivity of the unit for which the nurse manager is responsible.

## Span of Control

**Span of control** addresses the pragmatic concern of how many employees a manager can effectively supervise. Complex organizations usually have numerous departments that are highly specialized and differentiated; authority is centralized, resulting in a tall organizational structure with many small work groups. Less complex organizations have flat structures; authority is decentralized, with several managers supervising large work groups. Figure 2-2 depicts the differences.

In the professional bureaucracy, the operating core of professionals is the dominant feature. Decision making is usually decentralized, and the technostructure is underdeveloped. The support staff, however, is well developed. Most hospitals are professional bureaucracies.

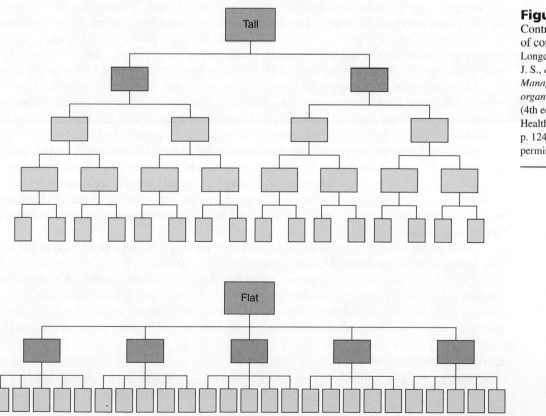

**Figure 2-2** ●
Contrasting spans of control. From Longest, B. B., Rakich, J. S., & Darr, K. (2000). *Managing health services organizations and systems* (4th ed.). Baltimore: Health Professions Press, p. 124. Reprinted by permission.

Organizational theories suggest organizational structures. Traditional structures (described later in the chapter) operationalize the tenets of classical theory.

## Humanistic Theory

Criticism of classical theory led to the development of humanistic theory, an approach identified with the human relations movement of the 1930s. A major assumption of this theory is that people desire social relationships, respond to group pressures, and search for personal fulfillment. This theory was developed as the result of a series of studies conducted by the Western Electric Company at its Hawthorne plant in Chicago. The first study was conducted to examine the effect of illumination on productivity. However, this study failed to find any relationship between the two. In most groups, productivity varied at random, and in one study productivity actually rose as illumination levels declined. The researchers concluded that unforeseen psychological factors were responsible for the findings.

Further studies of working conditions, such as rest breaks and the length of the workweek, still failed to reveal a relationship to productivity. The researchers concluded that the social setting created by the research itself—that is, the special attention given to workers as part of the research—enhanced productivity. This tendency for people to perform as expected because of special attention became known as the **Hawthorne effect**.

Although the findings are controversial, they led organizational theorists to focus on the social aspects of work and organizational design. (See Chapter 17 for a description of motivational theories.) One important assertion of this school of thought was that individuals cannot be coerced or bribed to do things they consider unreasonable; formal authority does not work without willing participants.

## Systems Theory

Organizational theorists who maintain a systems perspective view productivity as a function of the interplay among structure, people, technology, and environment. Like nursing theories based on systems theory (such as those of Roy and Neuman), organizational theory defines system as a set of interrelated parts arranged in a unified whole. Systems can be closed or open. Closed systems are self-contained and usually can be found only in the physical sciences. An open system, in contrast, interacts both internally and with its environment, much like a living organism.

An organization is a complex, sociotechnical, open system. This theory provides a framework by which the interrelated parts of the system and their functions can be studied. Resources, or input, such as employees, patients, materials, money, and equipment, are imported from the environment. Within the organization, energy and resources are utilized and transformed; work, a process called throughput, is performed to produce a product. The product, or output, is then exported to the environment. An organization, then, is a recurrent cycle of input, throughput, and output. Each health care organization—whether a hospital, ambulatory surgical center, or a home care agency, and so on—requires human, financial, and material resources. Each also provides a variety of services to treat illness, restore function, provide rehabilitation, and protect or promote wellness.

**Throughput** today is commonly associated with moving patients into and out of the system. Hospitals everywhere are focused on throughput of patients, such as if emergency departments are on diversion, how long a patient has to wait for a bed, and the number of readmissions (Handel et al., 2010). Using information technology, bed management systems have emerged as a strategy to identify bed availability in real time (Gamble, 2009). Joint Commission accreditation standards now require hospitals to show data "throughput" statistics (Joint Commission, 2011).

## Contingency Theory

Contingency theory posits that organizational performance can be enhanced by matching an organization's structure to its environment. The environment is defined as the people, objects, and ideas outside the organization that influence the organization. The environment of a health care organization includes patients and potential patients; third-party payers, including the government; regulators; competitors; and suppliers of physical facilities, personnel (such as schools of nursing and medicine), equipment, and pharmaceuticals.

Health care organizations are unique with respect to the kinds of products and services they offer. However, like all other organizations, health care organizations are shaped by external and internal forces. These forces stem from the economic and social environment, the technologies used in patient care, organizational size, and the abilities and limitations of the personnel involved in the delivery of health care, including nurses, physicians, technicians, administrators, and, of course, patients.

Given the variety of health care services and patients served today, it should come as no surprise that organizations differ with respect to the environments they face, the levels of training and skills of their caregivers, and the emotional and physical needs of patients. It is naive to think that the form of organization best for one type of patient in one type of environment is appropriate for another type of patient in a completely different environment. Think about the differences in the environment of a substance abuse treatment center compared to a women's health clinic. Thus, the optimal form of the organization is contingent on the circumstances faced by that organization.

### Chaos Theory

Chaos theory, which was inspired by the finding of quantum mechanics, challenges us to look at organizations and the nature of relationships and proposes that nature's work does not follow a straight line. The elements of nature often move in a circular, ebbing fashion; a stream destined for the ocean, for example, never takes a straight path. In fact, very little in life operates as a straight line; people's relationships to each other and to their work certainly do not. This notion challenges traditional thinking regarding the design of organizations. Organizations are living, self-organizing systems that are complex and self-adaptive.

The life cycle of an organization is fully dependent on its adaptability and response to changes in its environment. The tendency is for the organization to grow. When it becomes a large entity, it tends to stabilize and develop more formal standards. From that point, however, the organization tends to lose its adaptability and responsiveness to its environment.

Chaos theory suggests that the drive to create permanent organizational structures is doomed to fail. The set of rules that guided the industrial notions of organizational function and integrity must be discarded, and newer principles that ensure flexibility, fluidity, speed of adaptability, and cultural sensitivity must emerge. The role of leadership in these changing organizations is to build resilience in the midst of change and to maintain a balance between tension and order, which promotes creativity and prevents instability. This theory requires us to abandon our attachment to any particular model of design and to reflect instead on creative and flexible formats that can be quickly adjusted and changed as the organization's realities shift.

### Complexity Theory

Complexity theory originated in the computational sciences when scientists noted that random events interfered with expectations. The theory is useful in health care because the environment is rife with randomness and complex tasks. Patients' conditions change in an instant; necessary staff are not available; or equipment fails, all without warning. Tasks involve intricate interactions between and among staff, patients, and the environment. Managing in such ambiguous circumstances requires considering every aspect of the system as it interacts and adapts to changes. Complexity theory explains why health care organizations, in spite of concerted efforts, struggle with patient safety.

# Traditional Organizational Structures

The optimal organizational structure integrates organizational goals, size, technology, and environment. Various organizational structures have been utilized over time. Examples include functional structures, hybrid structures, matrix structures, and parallel structures.

### Functional Structure

In functional structures, employees are grouped in departments by specialty, with similar tasks being performed by the same group, similar groups operating out of the same department, and similar departments reporting to the same manager. In a functional structure, all nursing tasks fall under nursing service; the same is true of other functional areas. Functional structures tend to centralize decision making because the functions converge at the top of the organization.

Functional structures have several weaknesses. Coordination across functions is poor. Decision-making responsibilities can pile up at the top and overload senior managers, who may be uninformed regarding day-to-day operations. Responses to the external environment that require coordination across functions are slow. General management training is limited because most employees move up the organization within functional departments. Functional structures are uncommon in today's rapidly changing health care environment.

### Hybrid Structure

When an organization grows, it typically organizes both self-contained units and functional units; the result is a hybrid organization. The hybrid structure can provide simultaneous coordination within product divisions, can improve alignment between corporate and service or product goals, and foster adaptation to the environment while still maintaining efficiency.

The weakness of hybrid structures is conflict between top administration and managers. Managers often resent administrators' intrusions into what they see as their own area of responsibility. Over time, organizations tend to accumulate large corporate staffs to oversee divisions in an attempt to provide functional coordination across service or product structures.

### Matrix Structure

The matrix structure is unique and complex; it integrates both product and functional structures into one overlapping structure. In a matrix structure, different managers are responsible for function and product. For example, the nurse manager for the oncology clinic may report to the vice president for nursing as well as the vice president for outpatient services.

Matrices tend to develop where there are strong outside pressures for a dual organizational focus on product and function. The matrix is appropriate in a highly uncertain environment that changes frequently but also requires organizational expertise.

A major weakness of the matrix structure is its dual authority, which can be frustrating and confusing for departmental managers and employees. Excellent interpersonal skills are required from the managers involved. A matrix organization is time-consuming because frequent meetings are required to resolve problems and conflicts; the structure will not work unless participants can see beyond their own functional area to the big organizational picture. Finally, if one side of the matrix is more closely aligned with organizational objectives, that side may become dominant.

### Parallel Structure

Parallel structure is a structure unique to health care. It is the result of complex relationships that exist between the formal authority of the health care organization and the authority of its medical staff. In a parallel structure, the medical staff is separate and autonomous from the organization. The result is an organizational dilemma: two lines of authority. One line extends from the governing body to the chief executive officer and then to the managerial structure; the other line extends from the governing body to the medical staff. These two intersect in departments such as nursing because decision making involves both managerial and clinical elements.

Parallel structures are found in health care institutions with a functional structure and separate medical governance structure. Parallel structures are becoming less successful as health care organizations integrate into newer models that incorporate physician practice under the organizational umbrella.

## Service-Line Structures

More common in health care organizations today are **service-line structures** (Nugent et al., 2008). Service-line structures also are called product-line or service-integrated structures. In a service-line structure, clinical services are organized around patients with specific conditions (Figure 2-3).

Integrated structures are preferred in large and complex organizations because the same activity (for example, hiring) is assigned to several self-contained units, which can respond rapidly to the unit's immediate needs. This is appropriate when environmental uncertainty is high and the organization requires frequent adaptation and innovation.

One of the strengths of the service-line structure is its potential for rapid change in a changing environment. Because each division is specialized and its outputs can be tailored to the situation, client satisfaction is high. Coordination across function (nursing, dietary, pharmacy, and so on) occurs easily; work partners identify with their own service and can compromise or collaborate with other service functions to meet service goals and reduce conflict. Service goals receive priority under this organizational structure because employees see the service outcomes as the primary purpose of their organization.

The major weaknesses of service-integrated structures include possible duplication of resources (such as ads for new positions) and lack of in-depth technical training and specialization. Coordination across service categories (oncology, cardiology, and the burn unit, for example) is difficult; services operate independently and often compete. Each service category, which is independent and autonomous, has separate and often duplicate staff and competes with other service areas for resources. In addition, some service lines (e. g., pediatrics, obstetrics, bariatric surgery, and transplant centers) present special challenges due to low usage or the need for specialized personnel (Page, 2010).

Service-line structures are the most common structures found in Magnet-certified organizations (Kaplow & Reed, 2008). Such structures, however, present a challenge to nursing administrators and managers to maintain nursing standards across service lines (Hill, 2009). Armstrong, Laschinger, and Wong (2009) found improved patient safety in Magnet hospitals was related to nurses' perception of empowerment. This can be explained, possibly, by Magnet standards that encourage staff participation in decision making.

## Shared Governance

**Shared governance** is a process for empowering nurses in the practice setting. It is based on a philosophy that nursing practice is best determined by nurses. Participative decision making is the hallmark of shared governance and a standard for Magnet certification. Interdependence and

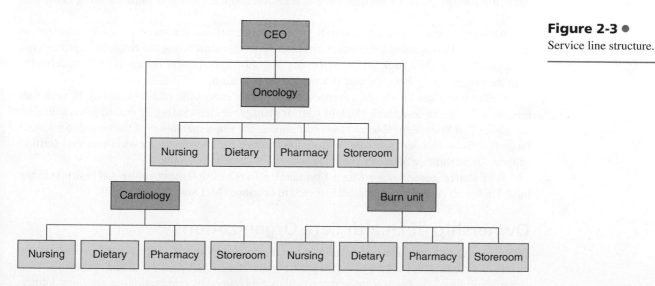

**Figure 2-3 ●**
Service line structure.

**Figure 2-4** ●

Shared governance model. Adapted from McDowell, J. B., Williams, R. L., Kautz, D. D., Madden, P., Heilig, A., & Thompson, A. (2010). Shared governance: 10 years later. *Nursing Management,* *41*(7), 32–37.

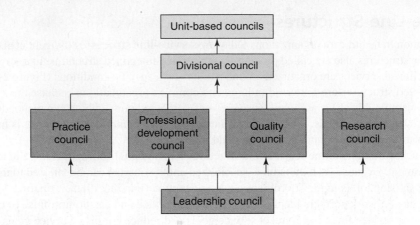

accountability are the basis for constructing a network of making nursing practice decisions in a decentralized environment. As a result, nurses gain significant control over their practice, efficiency and accountability are improved, and feelings of powerlessness are mitigated.

The ultimate outcome of shared governance is that nurses participate in an accountable forum to control their own practice within the health care organization. The assumption is that nursing staffs, like medical staffs, will predetermine the clinical skills of staff nurses and monitor the work of each through peer review while deciding on other practice issues through accountable forums or councils.

Shared governance allows staff nurses significant control over major decisions about nursing practice. Most shared governance systems are similar to and reflect the principles often found in academic or medical governance models. As shown in the example in Figure 2-4, nurses participate in unit-based councils that interface with divisional councils, specialty councils, and a leadership council, consisting of nurse managers and administrators.

Decisions are made by consensus, rather than by the manager's order or majority rule, a process that allows staff nurses an active voice in the decision. In the example in Figure 2-4, unit councils make decisions that directly affect the unit, divisional councils address issues that affect more than one unit, and a hospital-wide council determines overall issues.

The hospital-wide council consists of specific councils that address particular issues. The practice council, for example, is responsible for patient care standards. The professional development council maintains educational standards and competency assessments. The quality council monitors patient care quality. The research council assists in implementing evidence-based practice.

Although nursing practice councils have been operational for several decades, changes in health care and in organizational structures often require restructuring the councils, a process not without difficulty (Moore & Wells, 2010). Staffing shortages, patient demands and unfamiliarity with the process or its benefits may discourage participation.

Furthermore, not all shared governance models are successful (Ballard, 2010). Human factors, such as lack of leadership, lack of staff or manager understanding of shared governance, or the absence of knowledgeable mentors, can impede the implementation of the model. Structural factors, such as a known structure for decision making, time available for meetings, and staffing support for attendance also can affect the success of shared governance.

With shared governance a Magnet standard, efforts to implement, refine and restructure the model in health care organizations is expected to continue (McDowell et al., 2010).

## Ownership of Health Care Organizations

Today's health care organizations differ in ownership, role, activity, and size. Ownership can be either private or government, voluntary (not for profit) or investor-owned (for profit), and sectarian or nonsectarian (Figure 2-5). Private organizations are usually owned by corporations or religious entities,

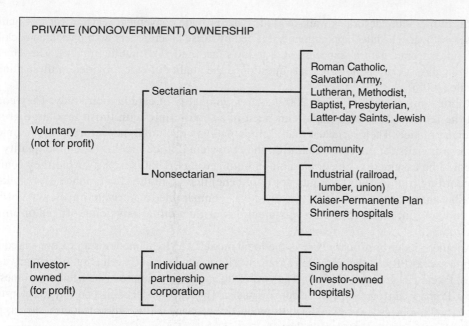

**Figure 2-5** ● Types of ownership in health care organizations. From Longest, B. S., Rakich, J. S., & Darr, K. (2000). *Managing Health Services Organizations and Systems* (4th ed.). Baltimore: Health Professions Press, p. 173. Reprinted by permission.

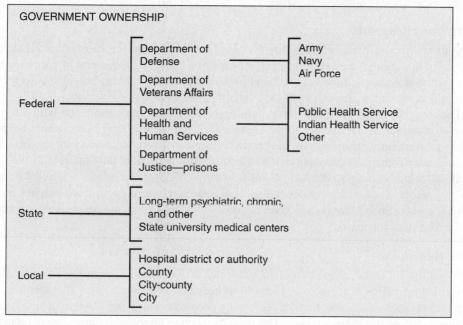

whereas government organizations are operated by city, county, state, or federal entities, such as the Indian Health Service. Voluntary organizations are usually not for profit, meaning that surplus monies are reinvested into the organization. Investor-owned, or for-profit corporations, distribute surplus monies back to the investors, who expect a profit. Sectarian agencies have religious affiliations.

# Health Care Settings

Organizations are further divided by the setting in which they deliver care. These include primary care, acute care hospitals, home health care, and long-term care organizations.

## Primary Care

Primary care is considered the patient's first encounter with the health care system. Primary care is delivered in physician's offices, emergency rooms, public health clinics, and in sites known as retail medicine.

**Retail medicine** describes walk-in clinics that provide convenient services for low-acuity illnesses without scheduled appointments. Staffed by nurse practitioners with physician backup, these clinics seem a natural expectation of today's fast food, 24/7 public mindset. The American Medical Association, however, has questioned the quality of care provided in these clinics (Costello, 2008).

Rohrer, Angstman, and Furst (2009) addressed quality of care in their study. They compared the reutilization rates of patients seen in a retail clinic with those in a large group physician practice. They surmised that if clinic patients had no higher return visits or emergency room visits for the same condition than physician office patients, then the quality of care could be assumed to be comparable in both settings. That is exactly what they found. So, according to this study, patients not only benefitted from the convenience of a walk-in clinic, but the quality of care they received was comparable to a private physician's office visit. In addition, the cost of care was much lower than either physician offices or emergency rooms.

Another model of primary care is the **logic model**. The logic model is a practice-based research network (PBRN) that provides a framework for planning and evaluation of primary care (Hayes, Parchman, & Howard, 2011). The goal of this model is to improve the health outcomes of patients. Primary care outcomes are seldom evaluated. The logic model offers one way to determine if efforts and resources are used in the most productive way and if subjective outcomes, such as patient satisfaction and easy access are achieved.

## Acute Care Hospitals

Hospitals are frequently classified by length of stay and type of service. Most hospitals are acute (short-term or episodic) care facilities, and they may be classified as general or special care facilities, such as pediatric, rehabilitative, and psychiatric facilities. Many hospitals also serve as teaching institutions for nurses, physicians, and other health care professionals.

The term "teaching hospital" commonly designates a hospital associated with a medical school that maintains a house staff of residents on call 24 hours a day. Nonteaching hospitals, in contrast, have only private physicians on staff. Because private physicians are less accessible than house staff, the medical supervision of patient care differs, as may the role of the nurse. This designation is changing dramatically as new forms of physician groups and allied practices emerge in partnerships with hospitals and medical schools. Some organizations hire hospitalists, physicians who provide care only to hospital inpatients; those who care for patients in intensive care are known as intensivists.

## Home Health Care

Home health care is the intermittent, temporary delivery of health care in the home by skilled or unskilled providers. With shortened lengths of hospital stay, more acutely ill patients are discharged to recuperate at home. Furthermore, more people are surviving life-threatening illnesses or trauma and require extended care. The primary service provided by home care agencies is nursing care; however, larger home care agencies also offer other professional services, such as physical or occupational therapy, and durable medical equipment, such as ventilators, hospital beds, home oxygen equipment, and other medical supplies. Hospice care for the final days of a patient's terminal illness may be provided by a home care agency or a hospital.

An outgrowth of the home health care industry is the temporary service agency. These agencies provide nurses and other health care workers to hospitals that are temporarily short-staffed; they also provide private duty nurses to individual patients either at home or in the hospital.

## Long-Term Care

Long-term care facilities provide professional nursing care and rehabilitative services. They may be freestanding, part of a hospital, or affiliated with a health care organization. Usually, length of

stay is limited. Residential care facilities, also known as nursing homes, are sheltered environments in which long-term care is provided by nursing assistants with supervision from licensed
professional or registered nurses.

As the population ages and the frail elderly account for more and more of the nation's citi-
zens, care in long-term care facilities is growing (Weaver et al., 2008). These organizations pose
different problems for staff. Ageism and infantilism permeate many settings (Ryvicker, 2009).
In addition, patients often transition between the nursing home and the hospital, and that care
may be fragmented and lead to poor outcomes (Naylor, Kurtzman, & Pauly, 2009). Challenges
in providing care to the elderly include addressing the tendency to stigmatize older, frail adults
and to provide continuity of care across settings.

# Complex Health Care Arrangements

## Health Care Networks

**Integrated health care networks** emerged as organizations struggled to find ways to survive in
today's cost-conscious environment. Integrated systems encompass a variety of model organizational structures, but certain characteristics are common. Network systems

- Deliver a continuum of care;
- Provide geographic coverage for the buyers of health care services; and
- Accept the risk inherent in taking a fixed payment in return for providing health care for
  all persons in the selected group, such as all employees of one company.

To provide such services, networks of providers evolved to encompass hospitals and physician practices. Most importantly, the focal point for care is primary care rather than the hospital.
The goal is to keep patients healthy by treating them in the setting that incurs the lowest cost and
thereby reducing expensive hospital treatments. The former goal—to keep hospital beds filled—
has been replaced with a new goal: to keep patients out of them!

A variety of other arrangements have emerged, varying from loose affiliations between hospitals to complete mergers of hospitals, clinics, and physician practices. These arrangements
continue to move and shift as alliances fail, return to separate entities, and form new affiliations.
Changes in health care payments offer possibilities for nurses to practice in expanding primary
care networks are anticipated.

## Interorganizational Relationships

With increased competition for resources and public and governmental pressures for better
efficiency and effectiveness, organizations have been forced to establish relationships with
one another for their continued survival. Multihospital systems and multiorganizational arrangements, both formal and informal, are mechanisms by which these relationships have
formed.

Arrangements between or among organizations that provide the same or similar services are
examples of **horizontal integration**. For instance, all hospitals in the network provide comparable services, as shown in Figure 2-6.

**Vertical integration**, in contrast, is an arrangement between or among dissimilar but related organizations to provide a continuum of services. An affiliation of a health maintenance
organization with a hospital, pharmacy, and nursing facility represents vertical integration
(see Figure 2-7).

Numerous arrangements using horizontal and vertical integration can be found, and these
models likely will become the common structure for delivery of health care. Examples of such
arrangements include affiliations, consortia, alliances, mergers, and consolidations. An assort-
ment of health care agencies under the umbrella of a corporate network is shown in the example
in Figure 2-8.

**Figure 2-6** ●
Horizontal integration.

**Figure 2-7** ●
Vertical integration.

**Figure 2-8** ●
Corporate health care
network.

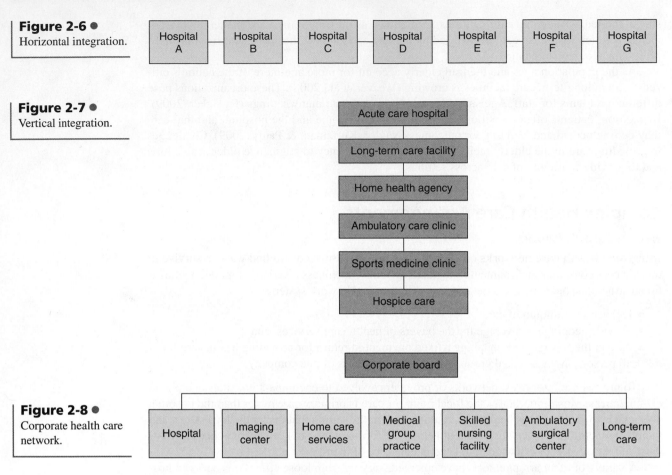

## Diversification

Diversification provides another strategy for survival in today's economy. **Diversification** is the expansion of an organization into new arenas. Two types of diversification are common: concentric and conglomerate.

*Concentric diversification* occurs when an organization complements its existing services by expanding into new markets or broadening the types of services it currently has available. For example, a children's hospital might open a day-care center for developmentally delayed children or offer drop-in facilities for sick child care.

*Conglomerate diversification* is the expansion into areas that differ from the original product or service. The purpose of conglomerate diversification is to obtain a source of income that will support the organization's product or service. For example, a long-term care facility might develop real estate or purchase a company that produces durable medical equipment.

Another type of diversification common to health care is the joint venture. A joint venture is a partnership in which each partner contributes different areas of expertise, resources, or services to create a new product or service. In one type of joint venture, one partner (general partner) finances and manages the venture, whereas the other partner (limited partner) provides a needed service. Joint ventures between health care organizations and physicians are becoming increasingly common. Integrated health care organizations, hospitals, and clinics seek physician and/or practitioner groups they can bond (capture) in order to obtain more referrals. The health care organization as financier and manager is the general partner, and physicians are limited partners.

## Managed Health Care Organizations

The managed health care organization is a system in which a group of providers is responsible for delivering services (that is, managing health care) through an organized arrangement with a group of individuals (for example, all employees of one company, all Medicaid patients in the state). Different types of managed-care organizations exist: health maintenance organizations (HMOs), preferred provider organizations (PPOs), and point-of-service plans (POS).

An HMO is a geographically organized system that provides an agreed-on package of health maintenance and treatment services provided to enrollees at a fixed monthly fee per enrollee, called **capitation**. Patients are required to choose providers within the network.

In a PPO, the managed-care organization contracts with independent practitioners to provide enrollees with established discounted rates. If an enrollee obtains services from a nonparticipating provider, significant copayments are usually required.

Point-of-service (POS) is considered to be an HMO–PPO hybrid. In a POS, enrollees may use the network of managed-care providers to go outside the network as they wish. However, use of a provider outside the network usually results in additional costs in copayments, deductibles, or premiums.

## Accountable Care Organizations

Effective January 2012, accountable care organizations have been able to contract with Medicare to provide care to a group of Medicare recipients (Ansel & Miller, 2010). Strong incentives to reduce cost, share information across networks and improve quality are included in the provisions for reimbursement.

An **accountable care organization** consists of a group of health care providers that provide care to a specified group of patients. Various structures can be used in accountable care organizations from loosely affiliated groups of providers to integrated delivery systems. An accountable care organization is more flexible than a HMO because consumers are free to choose providers from outside the network. Cognizant of the potential for Medicare contracts and, later, reimbursement by other third-party payers, health care providers and organizations are scrambling to establish collaborative arrangements and networks.

# Redesigning Health Care

Health care is a dynamic environment with multiple factors impinging on continuity and stability. Implementation of accountable care organizations, demands for safe, quality care, Magnet standards that promote decentralized organizational structures and an aging population with multiple chronic conditions are just two of the factors that make redesigning health care a reality today.

**Redesign** includes strategies to better provide safe, efficient, quality health care. Some examples of redesign strategies include adopting a patient-centered care model, focusing on specific service lines, applying lean thinking to the system, and establishing a flat, decentralized organizational structure.

The Institute of Medicine's 2001 report, *Crossing the Quality Chasm*, recommended ways to improve health care. One of those was to adopt a patient-centered care model (IOM, 2001). Success in implementing a patient- and family-centered care model has been reported in the literature (Zarubi, Reiley & McCarter, 2008).

Another patient-centered model is the **medical home** (Berenson et al., 2008). Centered by a primary care provider (primary care physician or nurse practitioner), a medical home links all care providers in the "home." The goal is to provide continuous, accessible, and comprehensive care. Challenges for coordinating care in a medical home include communication (e.g., absence of electronic medical records for all providers), the multiple needs of patients with chronic health problems, discomfort of patients and providers to use electronic communication of data and information, and compensation for primary care. To offset some of these challenges are several suggestions (Berenson et al., 2008). These include implementing electronic medical records using nurse practitioners to manage patients with chronic conditions, encouraging patients to self-manage chronic conditions, and persuading providers to use electronic communication with patients.

To meet both quality and cost-effective goals, the health care organization may decide to concentrate on specific service lines. Called big-dot focus areas, an organization selects a few major initiatives. They might, for example, put resources into building cardiology, cancer, and neuroscience while maintaining other services as is.

Another strategy is to adopt the quality concepts of lean thinking to redesign (Joosten, Bongers, & Janssen, 2009). Lean thinking focuses on the system rather than on individuals, concentrates on interventions that improve outcomes and disregards those that have little or no effect. A flat, decentralized organizational structure centers decision making closest to the problem. It promotes unit-based decision making and empowers staff to implement process improvements in a timely manner (Kramer, Schmalenberg, & Maguire, 2010). Furthermore, a decentralized structure encourages communication and collaboration and provides a quality improvement infrastructure.

Redesigning an organization presents numerous challenges. Staff may be concerned that their jobs will change or may disappear. Administrators may complain that loss of authority will result in poor performance. Everyone may worry that cost effective measures may diminish the quality of care. Significant stress is to be expected (Lavoie-Tremblay et al., 2010).

Nurse managers are key players in the redesign efforts. They are expected not only to initiate change while reducing costs, maintaining or improving quality of care, coaching and mentoring, and team building, but also to do so in an ever-changing environment full of ambiguities while their own responsibilities are expanded.

## Strategic Planning

Successful organizations know that they must focus their resources on their unique strengths, and health care is no exception. Organizations that focus on a few strategic initiatives, as discussed previously, do so after an intensive planning process. The competitive health care environment and limited resources require organizations to respond to public demands for safe, accessible quality health care.

This is a time-consuming and demanding process and should not be undertaken hurriedly. Put in use, however, a well-thought-out strategic plan guides the organization toward its goals, helps all the staff stay directed, and prevents the organization from responding to inappropriate requests.

A strategic plan projects the organization's goals and activities into the future, usually two to five years ahead (Schaffner, 2009). Based on the organization's philosophy and leaders' assessment of their organization and the environment, **strategic planning** guides the direction the organization is to take.

The **philosophy** is a written statement that reflects the organizational values, vision, and mission (Conway-Morana, 2009). **Values** are the beliefs or attitudes one has about people, ideas, objects, or actions that form a basis for behavior. Organizations use value statements to identify those beliefs or attitudes esteemed by the organizational leaders.

A **vision statement** describes the goal to which the organization aspires. The vision statement is designed to inspire and motivate employees to achieve a desired state of affairs. "Our vision is to be a regional integrated health care delivery system providing premier health care services, professional and community education, and health care research" is an example of a vision statement for a health care system.

The **mission** of an organization is a broad, general statement of the organization's reason for existence. Developing the mission is the necessary first step to designing a strategic plan. "Our mission is to improve the health of the people and communities we serve" is an example of a mission statement that guides decision making for the organization. Purchasing a medical equipment company, for example, might not be considered because it fails to meet the mission of improving the community's health.

The strategic plan is based on the organization's philosophy, vision, and mission. The first steps in strategic planning are:

- Appoint a strategic planning committee
- Interview key stakeholders
- Conduct a SWOT (strengths, weaknesses, opportunities, and threats) analysis
- Develop the plan
- Communicate the plan

People who are enthusiastic, experienced, and committed to the organization are the best representatives to serve on the planning committee. Naysayers can be included once some parts of the plan are formulated. Everyone in the organization must be involved even peripherally. "Buy-in" is critical to the plan's success.

Stakeholders include physicians, administrators, nurses, ancillary and support staff, and community representatives. They will have differing opinions about what the organization can and should do and provide valuable information unavailable elsewhere.

The SWOT analysis includes assessment of the external and internal environment (Kalisch & Curley, 2008). Data is collected from multiple sources, including stakeholder information.

To develop the plan:

- Determine goals, objectives and strategies
- Assess the projected costs
- Assign responsible units or individuals
- Identify outcome measures and expected dates of completion

**Goals** are specific statements of what outcome is to be achieved. Goals describe outcomes that are measurable and precise. "Every patient will be satisfied with his or her care" is an example of a goal.

Goals apply to the entire organization, whereas **objectives** are specific to an individual unit. A nursing objective to meet the above goal might be "Provide appropriate information and education to patients from preadmission to discharge." **Strategies** follow objectives and specify what actions will be taken. "Implement patient education classes for prenatal patients" is an example of a strategy to meet the patient satisfaction objective.

Other categories in a strategic plan include identifying the personnel responsible for each activity, determining the projected cost, establishing criteria to recognize that the goal has been met, and deciding the expected date of completion.

Strategic planning is an ongoing process, not an end in itself. It requires meticulous attention to how the organization is meeting its goals and, if goals are not met, what the reasons are for the variance. Maybe the goal needs to change, or possibly other personnel should be assigned to the task. Perhaps a change in the environment (reimbursement) or within the organization (shortage of key personnel) requires the goal to be abandoned. Continual evaluation will help the organization target its resources best.

## Organizational Environment and Culture

The terms **organizational environment** and **organizational culture** both describe internal conditions in the work setting. Organizational environment is the systemwide conditions that contribute to a positive or negative work setting. In 2005, the American Association of Critical-Care Nurses identified six characteristics of a healthy work environment, characteristics that the organization continues to promote (AACN, 2011 ). The characteristics are:

- Skilled communication
- True collaboration
- Effective decision making
- Appropriate staffing
- Meaningful recognition
- Authentic leadership.

One way to assess the organizational environment is to evaluate the qualities of those hired for key positions in the organization. An organization in which nursing leaders are innovative, creative, and energetic will tend to operate in a fast-moving, goal-oriented fashion. If humanistic, interpersonal skills are sought in candidates for leadership positions, the organization will focus on human resources, employees, and patient advocacy (Hersey, 2011).

Organizational culture, on the other hand, are the basic assumptions and values held by members of the organization (Sullivan, 2013). These are often known as the unstated "rules of the game." For example, who wears a lab coat? When is report given? To whom? Is tardiness tolerated? How late is acceptable?

Like environment, organizational culture varies from one institution to the next and subcultures and even countercultures, groups whose values and goals differ significantly from those of the dominant organization, may exist. A subculture is a group that has shared experiences or like interests and values. Nurses form a subculture within health care environments. They share a common language, rules, rituals, dress, and have their own unstated rules. Individual units also can become subcultures.

Systems involving participatory management and shared governance create organizational environments that reward decision making, creativity, independence, and autonomy (Kramer, Schmalenberg, & Maguire, 2010). These organizations retain and recruit independent, accountable professionals. Organizations that empower nurses to make decisions will better meet consumer requests. As the health care environment continues to evolve, more and more organizations are adopting consumer-sensitive cultures that require accountability and decision making from nurses.

## What You Know Now

- The schools of organizational theory include classical theory, humanistic theory, systems theory, contingency theory, chaos theory, and complexity theory.
- Organizations can be viewed as social systems consisting of people working in a predetermined pattern of relationships who strive toward a goal. The goal of health care organizations is to provide a particular mix of health services.
- Traditional organizational structures include functional, hybrid, matrix, and parallel structures.
- Service-line structures organize clinical services around specific patient conditions.
- Shared governance provides the framework for empowerment and partnership within the health care organization.
- Accountable care organizations are recent additions to health care design. They can contract with a payer to provide care to a specific group of patients.
- The medical home is one of the patient-centered models where all services are provided by a group of health care professionals.
- Strategic planning is a process used by organizations to focus their resources on a limited number of activities.
- Organizational environment and culture affect the internal conditions of the work setting.

## Questions to Challenge You

1. Secure a copy of the organizational chart from your employment or clinical site. Would you describe the organization the same way the chart depicts it? If not, redraw a chart to illustrate how you see the organization.
2. What organizational structure would you prefer? Think about how you might go about finding an organization that meets your criteria.
3. Organizational theories explain how organizations function. Which theory or theories describes your organization's functioning? Do you think it is the same theory your organization's administrators would use to describe it? Explain.

4. Have you been involved in strategic planning? If so, explain what happened and how well it worked in directing the organization's activities.

5. Using the six characteristics of a healthy work environment in the chapter, evaluate the organization where you work or have clinicals. How well does it rate? What changes would improve the environment?

**Pearson Nursing Student Resources**

Find additional review materials at

**www.nursing.pearsonhighered.com**

Prepare for success with additional NCLEX®-style practice questions, interactive assignments and activities, Web links, animations and videos, and more!

# References

American Association of Critical Care Nurses (AACN). (2011). *AACN standards for establishing and sustaining healthy work environments.* Retrieved May 5, 2011 from http://www.aacn.org/WD/HWE/Docs/HWEStandards.pdf

Ansel, T. C., & Miller, D. W. (2010). *Reviewing the landscape and defining the core competencies needed for a successful accountable care organization.* Louisville, KY: Healthcare Strategy Group.

Armstrong, K., Laschinger, H., & Wong, C. (2009). Workplace empowerment and Magnet hospital characteristics as predictors of patient safety climate. *Journal of Nursing Care Quality, 24*(1), 55–62.

Ballard, N. (2010). Factors associated with success and breakdown of shared governance. *Journal of Nursing Administration, 40*(10), 411–416.

Berenson, R. A., Hammons, T., Gans, D. H., Zuckerman, S., Merrell, K., Underwood, W. S., & Williams, A. F. (2008). A house is not a home: Keeping patients at the center of practice redesign. *Health Affairs, 27*(5), 1219–1230.

Conway-Morana, P. L. (2009). Nursing strategy: What's your plan? *Nursing Management, 40*(3), 25–29.

Costello, D. (2008). Report from the field: A checkup for retail medicine. *Health Affairs, 27*(5), 1299–1303.

Gamble, K. H. (2009). Connecting the dots: Patient flow systems are being leveraged to increase throughput, improve communication, and provide a more complete view of care. *Healthcare Informatics, 25*(13), 27–29.

Handel, D. A., Hilton, J. A., Ward, M. J., Rabin, E., Zwemer, F. L., & Pines, J. M. (2010). Emergency department throughput, crowding, and financial outcomes for hospitals. *Academic Emergency Medicine, 17*(8), 840–847.

Hayes, H., Parchman, M. L., & Howard, R. (2011). A logic model framework for evaluation and planning in a primary care practice-based research network (PBRN). *Journal of the American Board of Family Medicine, 24*(5), 576–582.

Hersey, P. H. (2011). *Management of organizational behavior* (10th ed.). Upper Saddle River, NJ: Prentice Hall.

Hill, K. S. (2009). Service line structures: Where does this leave nursing? *Journal of Nursing Administration, 39*(4), 147–148.

Institute of Medicine (2001). *Crossing the quality chasm: A new health system for the 21st century.* Retrieved October 24, 2011 from http://www.iom.edu/Reports/2001/Crossing-the-Quality-Chasm-A-New-Health-System-for-the-21st-Century.aspx

Joint Commission (2011). Edition standards. Retrieved May 12, 2011 from http://www.jcrinc.com/E-dition-Home/Joosten, T., Bongers, I., & Janssen, R. (2009). Application of lean thinking to health care: Issues and observations. *International Journal of Quality in Health Care, 21*(5), 341–347.

Kalisch, B. J., and Curley, M. (2008). Transforming a nursing organization. *Journal of Nursing Administration, 38*(2), 76–83.

Kaplow, R., & Reed, K. D. (2008). The AACN synergy model for patient care: A nursing model as a force of magnetism. *Nursing Economics, 26*(1), 17–25.

Kramer, M., Schmalenberg, C., & Maguire, P. (2010). Nine structures and leadership practices essential for a magnetic (healthy) work environment. *Nursing Administration Quarterly, 34*(1), 4–17.

Lavoie-Tremblay, M., Bonin, J. P., Lesage, A. D., Bonneville-Roussy, A., Lavigne, G. L., & Laroche, D. (2010). Contribution of the psychosocial work environment to psychological distress among health care professionals before and during a major organizational change. *The Health Care Manager, 29*(4), 293–304.

McDowell, J. B., Williams, R. L., Kautz, D. D., Madden, P., Heilig, A., & Thompson, A. (2010). Shared Governance: 10 years later. *Nursing Management, 41*(7), 32–37.

Moore, S. C., & Wells, N. J. (2010). Staff nurses lead the way for improvement to shared governance structure. *Journal of Nursing Administration, 40*(11), 477–482.

Naylor, M. D., Kurtzman, E. T., & Pauly, M. V. (2009). Transitions of elders between long-term care and hospitals. *Policy, Politics, & Nursing Practice, 10*(3), 187–194.

Nugent, M., Nolan, K. C., Brown, F., & Rogers, S. (2008, May 1). Seamless service line management: Service line organization is as important as market strategy if providers are to optimize their limited capital investment pool. *Healthcare Financial Management.* Retrieved May 3, 2011 from http://www.hfma.org/Templates/InteriorMaster.aspx?id=1523

Page, L. (2010). Challenges facing 10 hospital servicelines. Retrieved May 3, 2011 from www.beckershospitalreview.com/news-analysis/challenges-facing-10-hospital-service-lines.html

Rohrer, J. E., Angstman, K. B., & Furst, J. W. (2009). Impact of retail walk-in care on early return visits by adult primary care patients: Evaluation via triangulation. *Quality Management in Health Care, 18*(1), 19–24.

Ryvicker, M. (2009). Preservation of self in the nursing home: Contradictory practices within two models of care. *Journal of Aging Studies, 23*(1), 12–23.

Schaffner, J. (2009). Roadmap for success: The 10-step nursing strategic plan. *Journal of Nursing Administration, 39*(4), 152–155.

Sullivan, E. J. (2013). *Becoming influential: A guide for nurses* (2nd ed.). Upper Saddle River, NJ: Prentice Hall.

Weaver, F. M., Hickey, E. C., Hughes, S. L., Parker, V., Fortunato, D., Rose, J., Cohen, S., Robbins, L., Orr, W., Priefer, B., Wieland, D., & Baskins, J. (2008). Providing all-inclusive care for frail elderly veterans: Evaluation of three models of care. *Journal of the American Geriatric Society, 56*(2), 345–353.

Zarubi, K. L., Reiley, P. & McCarter, B. (2008). Putting patients and families at the center of care. *Journal of Nursing Administration, 38*(6), 275–281.

# CHAPTER 3

# Delivering Nursing Care

## Traditional Models of Care
FUNCTIONAL NURSING
TEAM NURSING
TOTAL PATIENT CARE
PRIMARY NURSING

## Integrated Models of Care
PRACTICE PARTNERSHIPS
CASE MANAGEMENT
CRITICAL PATHWAYS
DIFFERENTIATED PRACTICE

## Evolving Models of Care
PATIENT-CENTERED CARE
SYNERGY MODEL OF CARE
CLINICAL MICROSYSTEMS
CHRONIC CARE MODEL

## Learning Outcomes

*After completing this chapter, you will be able to:*

1. Describe how the delivery system structures nursing care

2. Describe what types of nursing care delivery systems exist.

3. Discuss the positive and negative aspects of different systems.

4. Describe evolving types of delivery systems that have emerged.

5. Explain characteristics of effective delivery systems.

## Key Terms

Chronic care model
Clinical microsystems

Critical pathways
Patient-centered care

Practice partnership
Synergy model of care

The core business of a health care organization is providing nursing care to patients. The purpose of a nursing care delivery system is to provide a structure that enables nurses to deliver nursing care to a specified group of patients. The delivery of care includes assessing care needs, formulating a plan of care, implementing the plan, and evaluating the patient's responses to interventions. This chapter describes how nursing care is organized to ensure quality care in an era of cost containment.

Since World War II, nursing care delivery systems have undergone continuous and significant changes (Box 3-1). Over the years, various nursing care delivery systems have been tried and critiqued. Debates regarding the pros and cons of each method have focused on identifying the perfect delivery system for providing nursing care to patients with varying degrees of need.

In addition, a delivery system must utilize specific nurses and groups of nurses, optimizing their knowledge and skills while at the same time ensuring that patients receive appropriate care. It's no small challenge. In fact, researchers have found that a better hospital environment for nurses is associated with lower mortality rates (Aiken et al., 2008) and nurse satisfaction (Spence-Laschinger, 2008).

## Traditional Models of Care

### Functional Nursing

Functional nursing, also called task nursing, began in hospitals in the mid-1940s in response to a national nursing shortage (see Figure 3-1). The number of registered nurses (RNs) serving in the armed forces during World War II depleted the supply of nurses at home. As a result of this loss of RNs, the composition of nursing staffs in hospitals changed. Staff that had been composed almost entirely of RNs gave way to the widespread use of licensed practical nurses (LPNs) and unlicensed assistive personnel (UAPs) to deliver nursing care.

In functional nursing, the needs of a group of patients are broken down into tasks that are assigned to RNs, LPNs, or UAPs so that the skill and licensure of each caregiver is used to his or her best advantage. Under this model an RN assesses patients whereas others give baths, make beds, take vital signs, administer treatments, and so forth. As a result, the staff become very efficient and effective at performing their regular assigned tasks.

---

**BOX 3-1** Job Description of a Floor Nurse (1887)

**Developed in 1887 and published in a magazine of Cleveland Lutheran Hospital.**

In addition to caring for your 50 patients, each nurse will follow these regulations:

1. Daily sweep and mop the floors of your ward, dust the patients' furniture and window sills.
2. Maintain an even temperature in your ward by bringing in a scuttle of coal for the day's business.
3. Light is important to observe the patient's condition. Therefore, each day fill kerosene lamps, clean chimneys, and trim wicks. Wash windows once a week.
4. The nurse's notes are important to aiding the physician's work. Make your pens carefully. You may whittle nibs to your individual taste.
5. Each nurse on day duty will report every day at 7 A.M. and leave at 8 P.M., except on the Sabbath, on which you will be off from 12 noon to 2 P.M.
6. Graduate nurses in good standing with the Director of Nurses will be given an evening off each week for courting purposes, or two evenings a week if you go regularly to church.
7. Each nurse should lay aside from each pay a goodly sum of her earnings for her benefits during her declining years, so that she will not become a burden. For example, if you earn $30 a month you should set aside $15.
8. Any nurse who smokes, uses liquor in any form, gets her hair done at a beauty shop, or frequents dance halls will give the Director of Nurses good reason to suspect her worth, intentions, and integrity.
9. The nurse who performs her labor, serves her patients and doctors faithfully and without fault for a period of five years will be given an increase by the hospital administration of five cents a day providing there are no hospital debts that are outstanding.

**Figure 3-1** ●
Functional nursing.

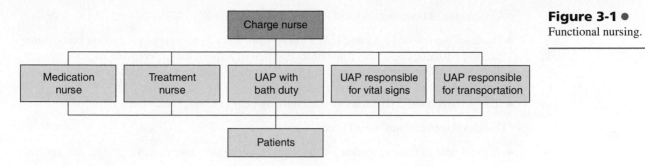

Disadvantages of functional nursing include:

- Uneven continuity
- Lack of holistic understanding of the patient
- Problems with follow-up

Because of these problems, functional nursing care is used infrequently in acute care facilities and only occasionally in long-term care facilities.

### Team Nursing

Team nursing (Figure 3-2) evolved from functional nursing and has remained popular since the middle to late 1940s. Under this system, a team of nursing personnel provides total patient care to a group of patients. In some instances, a team may be assigned a certain number of patients; in others, the assigned patients may be grouped by diagnoses or provider services.

The size of the team varies according to physical layout of the unit, patient acuity, and nursing skill mix. The team is led by an RN and may include other RNs, LPNs, and UAPs. Team members provide patient care under the direction of the team leader. The team, acting as a unified whole, has a holistic perspective of the needs of each patient. The team speaks for each patient through the team leader.

Typically, the team leader's time is spent in indirect patient care activities, such as:

- Developing or updating nursing care plans
- Resolving problems encountered by team members
- Conducting nursing care conferences
- Communicating with physicians and other health care personnel

With team nursing, the unit nurse manager consults with team leaders, supervises patient care teams, and may make rounds with all physicians. To be effective, team nursing requires that all team members have good communication skills. A key aspect of team nursing is the nursing care conference, where the team leader reviews with all team members each patient's plan of care and progress.

**Figure 3-2** ●
Team/modular nursing.

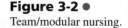

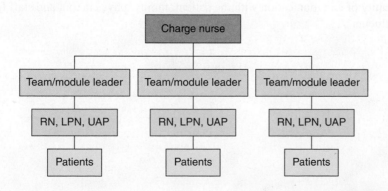

Advantages of team nursing are:

- It allows the use of LPNs and UAPs to carry out some functions (e.g., making beds, transporting patients, collecting some data) that do not require the expertise of an RN.
- It allows patient care needs requiring more than one staff member, such as patient transfers from bed to chair, to be easily coordinated.
- The geographical boundaries of team nursing help save steps and time.

Disadvantages of team nursing are:

- A great deal of time is needed for the team leader to communicate, supervise, and coordinate team members.
- Continuity of care may suffer due to changes in team members, leaders, and patient assignments.
- No one person considers the total patient.
- There may be role confusion and resentment against the team leader, who staff may view as more focused on paperwork and less directed at the physical or real needs of the patient.
- Nurses have less control over their assignments due to the geographical boundaries of the unit.
- Assignments may not be equal if they are based on patient acuity or may be monotonous if nurses continuously care for patients with similar conditions (e.g., all patients with hip replacements).

Skills in delegating, communicating, and problem solving are essential for a team leader to be effective. Open communication between team leaders and the nurse manager is also important to avoid duplication of effort, overriding of delegated assignments, or competition for control or power. Problems in delegation and communication are the most common reasons why team nursing is less effective than it theoretically could be.

## Total Patient Care

The original model of nursing care delivery was total patient care, also called case method (Figure 3-3), in which a registered nurse was responsible for all aspects of the care of one or more patients. During the 1920s, total patient care was the typical nursing care delivery system. Student nurses often staffed hospitals, whereas RNs provided total care to the patient at home. In total patient care, RNs work directly with the patient, family, physician, and other health care staff in implementing a plan of care.

The goal of this delivery system is to have one nurse give all care to the same patient(s) for the entire shift. Total patient care delivery systems are typically used in areas requiring a high level of nursing expertise, such as in critical care units or postanesthesia recovery areas.

The advantages of a total patient care system include:

- Continuous, holistic, expert nursing care
- Total accountability for the nursing care of the assigned patient(s) for that shift
- Continuity of communication with the patient, family, physician(s), and staff from other departments

**Figure 3-3 ●**
Total patient care.

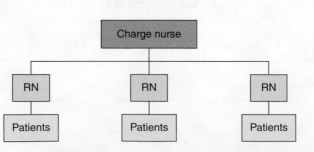

The disadvantage of this system is that RNs spend some time doing tasks that could be done more cost-effectively by less skilled persons. This inefficiency adds to the expense of using a total patient care delivery system.

### Primary Nursing

Conceptualized by Marie Manthey and implemented during the late 1960s after two decades of team nursing, primary nursing (Figure 3-4) was designed to place the registered nurse back at the patient's bedside (Manthey, 1980). Decentralized decision making by staff nurses is the core principle of primary nursing, with responsibility and authority for nursing care allocated to staff nurses at the bedside. Primary nursing recognized that nursing was a knowledge-based professional practice, not just a task-focused activity.

In primary nursing, the RN maintains a patient load of primary patients. A primary nurse designs, implements, and is accountable for the nursing care of patients in the patient load for the duration of the patient's stay on the unit. Actual care is given by the primary nurse and/or associate nurses (other RNs).

Primary nursing advanced the professional practice of nursing significantly because it provided:

- A knowledge-based practice model
- Decentralization of nursing care decisions, authority, and responsibility to the staff nurse
- 24-hour accountability for nursing care activities by one nurse
- Improved continuity and coordination of care
- Increased nurse, patient, and physician satisfaction.

Primary nursing also has some disadvantages, including:

- It requires excellent communication between the primary nurse and associate nurses.
- Primary nurses must be able to hold associate nurses accountable for implementing the nursing care as prescribed.
- Because of transfers to different units, critically ill patients may have several primary care nurses, disrupting the continuity of care inherent in the model.
- Staff nurses are neither compensated nor legally responsible for patient care outside their hours of work.
- Associates may be unwilling to take direction from the primary nurse.

Although the concept of 24-hour accountability is worthwhile, it is a fallacy. When primary nursing was first implemented, many organizations perceived that it required an all–RN staff. This practice was viewed as not only expensive but also ineffective because many tasks could be done by less skilled persons. As a result, many hospitals discontinued the use of primary nursing. Other hospitals successfully implemented primary nursing by identifying one nurse who was assigned to coordinate care and with whom the family and physician could communicate, and other nurses or unlicensed assistive personnel assisted this nurse in providing care.

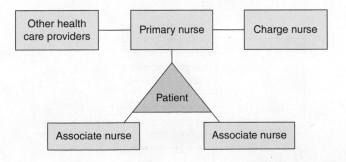

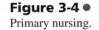

**Figure 3-4** ●
Primary nursing.

# Integrated Models of Care

## Practice Partnerships

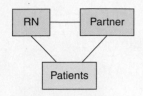

**Figure 3-5 ●**
Practice partnerships.

The **practice partnership** (Figure 3-5) was introduced by Marie Manthey in 1989 (Manthey, 1989). In the practice partnership model, an RN and an assistant—UAP, LPN, or less experienced RN—agree to be practice partners. The partners work together with the same schedule and the same group of patients. The senior RN partner directs the work of the junior partner within the limits of each partner's abilities and within limits of the state's nurse practice act.

The relationship between the senior and junior partner is designed to create synergistic energy as the two work in concert with patients. The senior partner performs selected patient care activities but delegates less specialized activities to the junior partner. When compared to team nursing, practice partnerships offer more continuity of care and accountability for patient care. When compared to total patient care or primary nursing, partnerships are less expensive for the organization and more satisfying professionally for the partners.

Disadvantages of this model are:

- Organizations tend to increase the number of UAPs and decrease the ratio of professional nurses to nonprofessional staff. If, for example, one UAP is assigned to more than one RN, the UAP must follow the instructions of several people, making a synergistic relationship with any one of them difficult.
- Another problem is the potential for the junior member of the team to assume more responsibility than appropriate. Senior partners must be careful not to delegate inappropriate tasks to junior partners.

Practice partnerships can be applied to primary nursing and used in other nursing care delivery systems, such as team nursing, modular nursing, and total patient care. As organizations restructured, practice partnerships offered an efficient way of using the skills of a mix of professional and nonprofessional staff with differing levels of expertise.

## Case Management

Following the introduction and impact of prospective payments, nursing case management, used for decades in community and psychiatric settings, was adopted for acute inpatient care. Nursing case management (Figure 3-6) is a model for identifying, coordinating, and monitoring the implementation of services needed to achieve desired patient care outcomes within a specified period of time. Nursing case management organizes patient care by major diagnoses or diagnosis-related groups (DRGs) and focuses on attaining predetermined patient outcomes within specific time frames and resources.

Nursing case management requires:

- Collaboration of all members of the health care team
- Identification of expected patient outcomes within specific time frames
- Use of principles of continuous quality improvement (CQI) and variance analysis
- Promotion of professional practice.

**Figure 3-6 ●**
Case management.

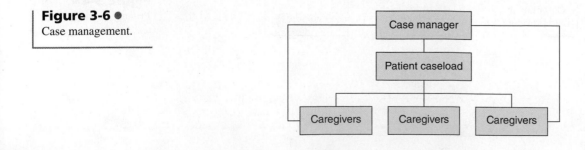

In an acute care setting, the case manager has a caseload of 10 to 15 patients and follows patients' progress through the system from admission to discharge, accounting for variances from expected progress. One or more nursing case managers on a patient care unit may coordinate, communicate, collaborate, problem solve, and facilitate patient care for a group of patients. Ideally, nursing case managers have advanced degrees and considerable experience in nursing.

After a specific patient population is selected to be "case managed," a collaborative practice team is established. The team, which includes clinical experts from appropriate disciplines (e.g., nursing, medicine, physical therapy) needed for the selected patient population, defines the expected outcomes of care for the patient population. Based on expected patient outcomes, each member of the team, using his or her discipline's contribution, helps determine appropriate interventions within a specified time frame.

To initiate case management, specific patient diagnoses that represent high-volume, high-cost, and high-risk cases are selected. High-volume cases are those that occur frequently, such as total hip replacements on an orthopedic floor. High-risk cases include patients or case types who have complications, stay in a critical care unit longer than two days, or require ventilatory support. Patients also may be selected because they are treated by one particular physician who supports case management.

Whatever patient population is selected, baseline data must be collected and analyzed first. These data provide the information necessary to measure the effectiveness of case management. Essential baseline data include length of stay, cost of care, and complication information.

Five elements are essential to successful implementation of case management:

- Support by key members of the organization (administrators, physicians, nurses)
- A qualified nurse case manager
- Collaborative practice teams
- A quality management system
- Established critical pathways (see next section)

In case management, all professionals are equal members of the team; thus, one group does not determine interventions for other disciplines. All members of the collaborative practice team agree on the final draft of the critical pathways, take ownership of patient outcomes, and accept responsibility and accountability for the interventions and patient outcomes associated with their discipline. The emphasis must be on managing interdisciplinary outcomes and building consensus with physicians. In addition, outcomes must be specified in measurable terms.

## Critical Pathways

Successful case management relies on **critical pathways** to guide care. The term *critical path,* also called a *care map,* refers to the expected outcomes and care strategies developed by the collaborative practice team. Again, interdisciplinary consensus must be reached and specific, and measurable outcomes determined.

Critical paths provide direction for managing the care of a specific patient during a specified time period. Critical paths are useful because they accommodate the unique characteristics of the patient and the patient's condition. Critical paths use resources appropriate to the care needed and, thus, reduce cost and length of stay. Critical paths are used in every setting where health care is delivered.

A critical path quickly orients the staff to the outcomes that should be achieved for the patient for that day. Nursing diagnoses identify the outcomes needed. If patient outcomes are not achieved, the case manager is notified and the situation analyzed to determine how to modify the critical path.

Altering time frames or interventions is categorized as a variance, and the case manager tracks all variances. After a time, the appropriate collaborative practice teams analyze the variances, note trends, and decide how to manage them. The critical pathway may need to be revised or additional data may be needed before changes are made.

Some features are included on all critical paths, such as specific medical diagnosis, the expected length of stay, patient identification data, appropriate time frames (in days, hours, minutes, or visits) for interventions, and patient outcomes. Interventions are presented in modality groups (medications, nursing activity, and so on). The critical path must include a means to identify variances easily and to determine whether the outcome has been met.

### Differentiated Practice

Differentiated practice is a method that maximizes nursing resources by focusing on the structure of roles and functions of nurses according to their education, experience, and competence. Differentiated practice is designed to identify distinct levels of nursing practice based on defined abilities that are incorporated into job descriptions.

In differentiated practice, the responsibilities of RNs (mainly those with bachelor's and associate degrees) differ according to the competence and training associated with the two education levels as well as the nurses' experience and preferences. The scope of nursing practice and level of responsibility are specifically defined for each level. Some organizations differentiate roles, responsibilities, and tasks for professional nurses, licensed practical nurses, and unlicensed assistive personnel, which are incorporated into their respective job descriptions.

## Evolving Models of Care

Recognizing the need for improving patient care, the Robert Wood Johnson Foundation and the Institute for Healthcare Improvement established a program titled Transforming Care at the Bedside (IHI, 2009). The goal was, and continues to be, to help hospitals achieve affordable and lasting improvements to care (Lavizzo-Mourey & Berwick, 2009). One of its premises is the use of a patient-centered care model.

### Patient-Centered Care

**Patient-centered care** is a model of nursing care delivery in which the role of the nurse is broadened to coordinate a team of multifunctional unit-based caregivers. In patient-centered care, all patient care services are unit-based, including admission and discharge, diagnostic and treatment services, and support services, such as environmental and nutrition services and medical records. The focus of patient-centered care is decentralization, the promotion of efficiency and quality, and cost control.

In this model of care, the number of caregivers at the bedside is reduced, but their responsibilities are increased so that service time and waiting time are decreased. A typical team in a unit providing patient-centered care consists of:

- Patient care coordinators (RNs)
- Patient care associates or technicians who are able to perform delegated patient care tasks
- Unit support assistants who provide environmental services and can assist with hygiene and ambulation needs
- Administrative support personnel who maintain patient records, transcribe orders, coordinate admission and discharge, and assist with general office duties

Success using a patient-centered care model continues to be reported in the literature (Miles & Vallish, 2010; Schneider & Fake, 2010). Furthermore, lower mortality in patients with acute myocardial infarctions has been found (Meterko et al., 2010). Patients with chronic conditions are appropriate candidates for patient-centered care approaches, including the use of complementary and alternative medicine therapies (Maizes, Rakel, & Niemiec, 2009).

The nurse manager's role in patient-centered care requires considerable time. No longer is the manager doing rounds and assisting with patient care. Instead, being responsible for a staff that is more diverse with fewer professional RN staff demands a strong leader proficient to interview, hire, train, and motivate staff. Some organizations share assistive staff between units, also increasing the need for more communication and coordination with other managers.

## Synergy Model of Care

Developed by the American Association of Critical Nurses, the **American Association of Critical Care Nurses** conceptualizes nursing practice based on the needs and characteristics of patients (AACN, 2011). These characteristics drive nurse competencies. Patient characteristics include:

- Resiliency
- Vulnerability
- Stability
- Complexity
- Resource availability
- Participation in care
- Participation in decision making
- Predictability

These characteristics are then matched with nurse competencies, including:

- Clinical judgment
- Advocacy and moral agency
- Caring practices
- Collaboration
- Systems thinking
- Response to diversity
- Facilitation of learning
- Clinical inquiry (AACN, 2011)

When patients' characteristics and nurses' competencies match, synergy is the outcome. The model is useful to nurses by delineating job descriptions, evaluation formats, and advancement criteria. Furthermore, a synergy model helps meet the standards for Magnet certification (Kaplow & Reed, 2008).

## Clinical Microsystems

**Clinical microsystems** are a recent addition to care delivery structures. Clinical microsystems evolved from the belief that decision making is best given to those involved in the smallest unit of care. Thus, a clinical microsystem is a small unit of care that maintains itself over time.

Clinical microsystems include the following elements:

- Core team of caregivers
- Defined population to receive care
- Informational system for both patients and caregivers
- Support staff, equipment and facilitative environment

The clinical microsystem model has been shown to be effective in neonatal intensive care units (Reis, Scott, & Rempel, 2009) and to increase quality improvement projects among medical residents (Tess et al., 2009). Additionally, using a clinical nurse leader improved quality outcomes in a hospital using a clinical microsystem model (Hix, McKeon, & Walters, 2009).

## Chronic Care Model

So far our discussion of delivery systems has focused on hospital nursing care. Increasingly, however, care is being delivered in ambulatory care environments. Additionally, most of the patients cared for in those environments suffer from chronic health conditions. The **chronic care model** addresses these concerns.

The goal of the chronic care model is not to manage a disease but to change how daily care is delivered by clinical teams (Coleman et al., 2009). Instead of reacting to changes in the patient's condition, the team provides proactive interventions. The model is systematic and requires six components. They are:

- Self-management support
- Decision support
- Delivery system design
- Clinical information systems
- Health care organization
- Community resources

Given that the population is aging and chronic conditions are expected to rise, the chronic care model is an appropriate one to consider for providing care to patients with chronic illnesses.

No delivery system is perfect. Or permanent. As health care adapts to changes in reimbursement, demands for quality, and technological advances, models for delivering care will continue to evolve.

## What You Know Now

- Nursing care delivery systems provide a structure for nursing care. Most organizations use a combination of nursing care delivery systems or modify one or more systems to meet their own needs.
- Traditional care models include functional nursing, team nursing, total patient care, and primary nursing.
- Integrated models of care include practice partnerships, case management, critical pathways, and differentiated practice.
- Evolving models of care include patient-centered care, a synergy model of care, clinical microsystems, and a chronic care model.
- Commonly used by Magnet-certified hospitals, the patient-centered care model provides care from admitting to discharge on the unit.
- The synergy model, developed by the American Association of Critical Care Nurses, matches patients' characteristics with nurses' competencies.
- Clinical microsystems use a structure that puts decision making in small units of those who provide the care.
- The chronic care model is a systemwide, proactive model designed to provide daily care to patients by clinical teams.
- As health care adapts to changes in reimbursement, demands for quality, and technological advances, models for delivering care will continue to evolve.

## Questions to Challenge You

1. Describe the patient care delivery system(s) at your place of work or clinical placement site. How well does it work? Can you suggest a better system?
2. Pretend that you are designing a new nursing care delivery system. Select the system or combination of systems you would use. Explain your rationale.
3. Why have different systems been used in earlier times? Would any of them be useful today? Explain what characteristics of the health care system today would make them appropriate or inappropriate to use.
4. As a manager, which system would you prefer? Why?
5. If you were a patient, which system do you think would provide you with the best care?

### Pearson Nursing Student Resources

Find additional review materials at

**www.nursing.pearsonhighered.com**

Prepare for success with additional NCLEX®-style practice questions, interactive assignments and activities, Web links, animations and videos, and more!

## References

Aiken, L. H., Clarke, S. P., Sloane, D. M., Lake, E. T., & Cheney, T. (2008). Effects of hospital care environment on patient mortality and nurse outcomes. *Journal of Nursing Administration, 38*(5), 223–229.

American Association of Critical Care Nurses (AACN) (2011). *The AACN synergy model for patient care.* Retrieved May 9, 2011 from http://www.aacn.org/WD/Certifications/Docs/SynergyModelforPatientCare.pdf

Coleman, K., Austin, B. T., Brach, C., & Wagner, E. H. (2009). Evidence on the chronic care model in the new millennium. *Health Affairs, 28*(1), 75–85.

Hix, C., McKeon, L., and Walters, S. (2009). Clinical nurse leader impact on clinical microsystems outcomes. *Journal of Nursing Administration, 39*(2), 71–76.

Institute for Healthcare Improvement (IHI) (2009). *IHI Collaborative: Transforming care at the bedside.* Retrieved May 9, 2011 from http://www.ihi.org/IHI/Programs/Collaboratives/TransformingCareattheBedside.htm.

Kaplow, R., & Reed, K. D. (2008). The AACN synergy model for patient care: A nursing model as a force of magnetism. *Nursing Economics, 26*(1), 17–25.

Lavisso-Mourey, R., & Berwick, D. M. (2009). Nurses transforming care. *American Journal of Nursing, 109*(11), 3.

Maizes, V., Rakel, D., & Niemiec, C. (2009). Integrative medicine and patient-centered care. *Explore: The Journal of Science & Healing, 5*(5), 277–289.

Manthey, M. (1980). *The practice of primary nursing.* St. Louis: Mosby.

Manthey, M. (1989). Practice partnerships: The newest concept in care delivery. *Journal of Nursing Association, 19*(2), 33–35.

Meterko, M., Wright, S., Lin, H., Lowy, E., & Cleary, P. D. (2010). Mortality among patients with acute myocardial infarction: The influences of patient-centered care and evidence-based medicine. *Health Services Research, 45*(5), 1188–1204.

Miles, K. S., & Vallish, R. (2010). Creating a personalized professional practice framework for nursing.

*Nursing Economics, 28*(3), 171–189.

Reis, M. D., Scott, S. D., & Rempel, G. R. (2009). Including parents in the evaluation of clinical microsystems in the neonatal intensive care unit. *Advances in Neonatal Care, 9*(4), 174–179.

Schneider, M. A., & Fake, P. (2010). Implementing a relationship-based care model on a large orthopaedic/neurosurgical hospital unit. *Orthopaedic Nursing, 29*(6), 374–378.

Spence-Laschinger, H. K. (2008). Effect of empowerment on professional practice environment, work satisfaction, and patient care quality: Further testing the nursing work life model. *Journal of Nursing Care Quality, 23*(4), 322–330.

Tess, A. V., Yang, J. J., Smith, C., Fawcett, C. M., Bates, C. K., & Reynolds, E. E. (2009). Combining clinical microsystems and an experiential quality improvement curriculum to improve residency education in internal medicine. *Academic Medicine, 84*(3), 326–334.

# Leading, Managing, Following

## Learning Outcomes

*After completing this chapter, you will be able to:*

1. Explain why every nurse is a manager and can be a leader.

2. Differentiate between leaders and managers.

3. Discuss how different theories explain leadership and management.

4. Describe what management roles nurses fill in practice.

5. Discuss how followership is essential to leadership.

6. Describe what makes a leader successful.

## Key Terms

Charge nurse
Clinical nurse leader
Controlling
Directing
Emotional intelligence
First-level manager

Followership
Formal [leadership]
Informal [leadership]
Leader
Manager
Organizing

Planning
Quantum leadership
Servant leadership
Shared leadership
Transactional leadership
Transformational leadership

M anagers are essential to any organization. A manager's functions are vital, complex, and frequently difficult. They must be directed toward balancing the needs of patients, the health care organization, employees, physicians, and self. Nurse managers need a body of knowledge and skills distinctly different from those needed for nursing practice, yet few nurses have the education or training necessary to be managers. Frequently, managers depend on experiences with former supervisors, who also learned supervisory techniques on the job. Often a gap exists between what managers know and what they need to know.

Today, all nurses are managers, not in the formal organizational sense but in practice. They direct the work of nonprofessionals and professionals in order to achieve desired outcomes in patient care. Acquiring the skills to be both a leader and a manager will help the nurse become more effective and successful in any position.

## Leaders and Managers

*Manager, leader, supervisor,* and *administrator* are often used interchangeably, yet they are not the same. A **leader** is anyone who uses interpersonal skills to influence others to accomplish a specific goal. The leader exerts influence by using a flexible repertoire of personal behaviors and strategies. The leader is important in forging links—creating connections—among an organization's members to promote high levels of performance and quality outcomes.

The functions of a leader are to achieve a consensus within the group about its goals, maintain a structure that facilitates accomplishing the goals, supply necessary information that helps provide direction and clarification, and maintain group satisfaction, cohesion, and performance.

A **manager**, in contrast, is an individual employed by an organization who is responsible and accountable for efficiently accomplishing the goals of the organization. Managers focus on coordinating and integrating resources, using the functions of planning, organizing, supervising, staffing, evaluating, negotiating, and representing. Interpersonal skill is important, but a manager also has authority, responsibility, accountability, and power defined by the organization. The manager's job is to:

- Clarify the organizational structure
- Choose the means by which to achieve goals
- Assign and coordinate tasks, developing and motivating as needed
- Evaluate outcomes and provide feedback

All good managers are also good leaders—the two go hand in hand. However, one may be a good manager of resources and not be much of a leader of people. Likewise, a person who is a good leader may not manage well. Both roles can be learned; skills gained can enhance either role.

## Leadership

Leadership may be **formal** or informal. Leadership is formal when practiced by a nurse with legitimate authority conferred by the organization and described in a job description (e.g., nurse manager, supervisor, coordinator, case manager). Formal leadership also depends on personal skills, but it may be reinforced by organizational authority and position. Insightful formal leaders recognize the importance of their own informal leadership activities and the informal leadership of others who affect the work in their areas of responsibility.

Leadership is **informal** when exercised by a staff member who does not have a specified management role. A nurse whose thoughtful and convincing ideas substantially influence the efficiency of work flow is exercising leadership skills. Informal leadership depends primarily on one's knowledge, status (e.g., advanced practice nurse, quality improvement coordinator, education specialist, medical director), and personal skills in persuading and guiding others.

## Traditional Leadership Theories

Research on leadership has a long history, but the focus has shifted over time from personal traits to behavior and style, to the leadership situation, to change agency (the capacity to transform), and to other aspects of leadership. Each phase and focus of research has contributed to managers' insights and understandings about leadership and its development. Traditional leadership theories include trait theories, behavioral theories, and contingency theories.

In the earliest studies researchers sought to identify inborn traits of successful leaders. Although inconclusive, these early attempts to specify unique leadership traits provided benchmarks by which most leaders continue to be judged.

Research on leadership in the early 1930s focused on what leaders do. In the behavioral view of leadership, personal traits provide only a foundation for leadership; real leaders are made through education, training, and life experiences.

Contingency approaches suggest that managers adapt their leadership styles in relation to changing situations. According to contingency theory, leadership behaviors range from authoritarian to permissive and vary in relation to current needs and future probabilities. A nurse manager may use an authoritarian style when responding to an emergency situation such as a cardiac arrest but use a participative style to encourage development of a team strategy to care for patients with multiple system failure.

The most effective leadership style for a nurse manager is the one that best complements the organizational environment, the tasks to be accomplished, and the personal characteristics of the people involved in each situation.

## Contemporary Theories

Leaders in today's health care environment place increasing value on collaboration and teamwork in all aspects of the organization. They recognize that as health systems become more complex and require integration, personnel who perform the managerial and clinical work must cooperate, coordinate their efforts, and produce joint results. Leaders must use additional skills, especially group and political leadership skills, to create collegial work environments.

### Quantum Leadership

**Quantum leadership** is based on the concepts of chaos theory (see Chapter 2). Reality is constantly shifting, and levels of complexity are constantly changing. Movement in one part of the system reverberates throughout the system. Roles are fluid and outcome oriented. It matters little what you did; it only matters what outcome you produced. Within this framework, employees become directly involved in decision making as equitable and accountable partners, and managers assume more of an influential facilitative role, rather than one of control (Porter-O'Grady & Malloch, 2010).

Quantum leadership demands a different way of thinking about work and leadership. Change is expected. Informational power, previously the purview of the leader, is now available to all. Patients and staff alike can access untold amounts of information. The challenge, however, is to assist patients, uneducated about health care, how to evaluate and use the information they have. Because staff have access to information only the leader had in the past, leadership becomes a shared activity, requiring the leader to possess excellent interpersonal skills.

### Transactional Leadership

**Transactional leadership** is based on the principles of social exchange theory. The primary premise of social exchange theory is that individuals engage in social interactions expecting to give and receive social, political, and psychological benefits or rewards. The exchange process between leaders and followers is viewed as essentially economic. Once initiated, a sequence of exchange behavior continues until one or both parties finds that the exchange of performance and rewards is no longer valuable.

The nature of these transactions is determined by the participating parties' assessments of what is in their best interests; for example, staff respond affirmatively to a nurse manager's request to work overtime in exchange for granting special requests for time off. Leaders are successful to the extent that they understand and meet the needs of followers and use incentives to enhance employee loyalty and performance. Transactional leadership is aimed at maintaining equilibrium, or the status quo, by performing work according to policy and procedures, maximizing self-interests and personal rewards, emphasizing interpersonal dependence, and routinizing performance (Weston, 2008).

## Transformational Leadership

**Transformational leadership** goes beyond transactional leadership to inspire and motivate followers (Marshall, 2010). Transformational leadership emphasizes the importance of interpersonal relationships. Transformational leadership is not concerned with the status quo, but with effecting revolutionary change in organizations and human service. Whereas traditional views of leadership emphasize the differences between employees and managers, transformational leadership focuses on merging the motives, desires, values, and goals of leaders and followers into a common cause. The goal of the transformational leader is to generate employees' commitment to the vision or ideal rather than to themselves.

Transformational leaders appeal to individuals' better selves rather than these individuals' self-interests. They foster followers' inborn desires to pursue higher values, humanitarian ideals, moral missions, and causes. Transformational leaders also encourage others to exercise leadership. The transformational leader inspires followers and uses power to instill a belief that followers also have the ability to do exceptional things.

Transformational leadership may be a natural model for nursing managers, because nursing has traditionally been driven by its social mandate and its ethic of human service. In fact, Weberg (2010) found that transformational leadership reduced burnout among employees, and Grant et al., (2010) reports transformational leadership positively affected the practice environment in one medical center. Transformational leadership can be used effectively by nurses with clients or coworkers at the bedside, in the home, in the community health center, and in the health care organization.

## Shared Leadership

Reorganization, decentralization, and the increasing complexity of problem solving in health care have forced administrators to recognize the value of **shared leadership**, which is based on the empowerment principles of participative and transformational leadership (Everett & Sitterding, 2011). Essential elements of shared leadership are relationships, dialogues, partnerships, and understanding boundaries. The application of shared leadership assumes that a well-educated, highly professional, dedicated workforce is comprised of many leaders. It also assumes that the notion of a single nurse as the wise and heroic leader is unrealistic and that many individuals at various levels in the organization must be responsible for the organization's fate and performance.

Different issues call for different leaders, or experts, to guide the problem-solving process. A single leader is not expected always to have knowledge and ability beyond that of other members of the work group. Appropriate leadership emerges in relation to the current challenges of the work unit or the organization. Individuals in formal leadership positions and their colleagues are expected to participate in a pattern of reciprocal influence processes. Kramer, Schmalenberg, and Maguire (2010) and Watters (2009) found shared leadership common in Magnet-certified hospitals.

Examples of shared leadership in nursing include:

- *Self-directed work teams.* Work groups manage their own planning, organizing, scheduling, and day-to-day work activities.
- *Shared governance.* The nursing staff are formally organized at the service area and organizational levels to make key decisions about clinical practice standards, quality assurance

and improvement, staff development, professional development, aspects of unit operations, and research. Decision making is conducted by representatives of the nursing staff who have been authorized by the administrative hierarchy and their colleagues to make decisions about important matters.

- *Co-leadership.* Two people work together to execute a leadership role. This kind of leadership has become more common in service-line management, where the skills of both a clinical and an administrative leader are needed to successfully direct the operations of a multidisciplinary service. For example, a nurse manager provides administrative leadership in collaboration with a clinical nurse specialist, who provides clinical leadership. The development of co-leadership roles depends on the flexibility and maturity of both individuals, and such arrangements usually require a third party to provide ongoing consultation and guidance to the pair.

## Servant Leadership

Founded by Robert Greenleaf (Greenleaf, 1991), **servant leadership** is based on the premise that leadership originates from a desire to serve and that in the course of serving, one may be called to lead (Keith, 2008; The Greenleaf Center for Servant Leadership, 2011). Servant leaders embody three characteristics:

- Empathy
- Awareness
- Persuasion (Neill & Saunders, 2008)

Servant leadership appeals to nurses for two reasons. First, our profession is founded on principles of caring, service, and the growth and health of others (Anderson et al., 2010). Second, nurses serve many constituencies, often quite selflessly, and consequently bring about change in individuals, systems, and organizations.

## Emotional Leadership

Social intelligence (Goleman, 2007), including emotional intelligence (Bradberry & Greaves, 2009; Goleman, 2006), has gained acceptance in the business world and more recently in health care (Veronsesi, 2009). **Emotional intelligence** involves personal competence, which includes self-awareness and self-management, and social competence, which includes social awareness and relationship management that begins with authenticity. (See Table 4-1.)

Goleman (2007) asserts that attachment to others is an innate trait of human beings. Thus, emotions are "catching." Consider a person having a pleasant day. Then an otherwise innocuous event turns into a negative experience that spills over into future interactions. Or the reverse. A positive experience lightens the mood and affects the next encounter. When people feel good, they work more effectively.

Emotional intelligence has been linked with leadership (Antonakis, Ashkanasy, & Dasborough, 2009; Cote et al., 2010; Lucas, Spence-Laschinger, & Wong, 2008). One study, however, found no relationship between emotional intelligence and transformational leadership (Lindebaum & Cartwright, 2010).

Nurses, with their well-honed skills as compassionate caregivers, are aptly suited to this direction in leadership that emphasizes emotions and relationships with others as a primary attribute for success. These skills fit better with the more contemporary relationship-oriented theories as well. Thus, the workplace is a more complex and intricate environment than previously suggested. The following chapters show you how to put these skills to work.

Health care environments require innovations in care delivery and therefore innovative leadership approaches. Quantum, transactional, transformational, shared, servant, and emotional leadership make up a new generation of leadership styles that have emerged in response to the need to humanize working environments and improve organizational performance. In practice, leaders tap a variety of styles culled from diverse leadership theories.

**TABLE 4-1   AONE Five Areas of Competency**

AONE BELIEVES THAT MANAGERS AT ALL LEVELS MUST BE COMPETENT IN THE FOLLOWING:

COMMUNICATION AND RELATIONSHIPS-BUILDING COMPETENCIES INCLUDE:
- Effective communication
- Relationship management
- Influence of behaviors
- Ability to work with diversity
- Shared decision making
- Community involvement
- Medical staff relationships
- Academic relationships

KNOWLEDGE OF THE HEALTH CARE ENVIRONMENT INCLUDES:
- Clinical practice knowledge
- Patient care delivery models and work design knowledge
- Health care economics knowledge
- Health care policy knowledge
- Understanding of governance
- Understanding of evidence-based practice
- Outcome measurement
- Knowledge of and dedication to patient safety
- Understanding of utilization/case management
- Knowledge of quality improvement and metrics
- Knowledge of risk management

LEADERSHIP SKILLS INCLUDE:
- Foundational thinking skills
- Personal journey disciplines
- The ability to use systems thinking
- Succession planning
- Change management

PROFESSIONALISM INCLUDES:
- Personal and professional accountability
- Career planning
- Ethics
- Evidence-based clinical and management practice
- Advocacy for the clinical enterprise and for nursing practice
- Active membership in professional organizations

BUSINESS SKILLS INCLUDE:
- Understanding of health care financing
- Human resource management and development
- Strategic management
- Marketing
- Information management and technology

Copyright © 2005 by the American Organization of Nurse Executives. Address reprint permission requests to aone@aha.org.

# Traditional Management Functions

In 1916, French industrialist Henri Fayol first described the functions of management as planning, organizing, directing, and controlling. These are still relevant today, however, the complexity of today's health care systems make these functions more difficult and less certain (Clancy, 2008).

## Planning

**Planning** is a four-stage process to:

- Establish objectives (goals)
- Evaluate the present situation and predict future trends and events
- Formulate a planning statement (means)
- Convert the plan into an action statement

Planning is important on both an organizational and a personal level and may be an individual or group process that addresses the questions of what, why, where, when, how, and by whom. Decision making and problem solving are inherent in planning. Numerous computer software programs and databases are available to help facilitate planning.

Organization-level plans, such as determining organizational structure and staffing or operational budgets, evolve from the mission, philosophy, and goals of the organization. The nurse manager plans and develops specific goals and objectives for her or his area of responsibility.

*Antonio, the nurse manager of a home care agency, plans to establish an in-home phototherapy program, knowing that part of the agency's mission is to meet the health care needs of the child-rearing family. To effectively implement this program, he would need to address:*

- *How the program supports the organization's mission*
- *Why the service would benefit the community and the organization*
- *Who would be candidates for the program*
- *Who would provide the service*
- *How staffing would be accomplished*
- *How charges would be generated*
- *What those charges should be*

Planning can be contingent or strategic. Using contingency planning, the manager identifies and manages the many problems that interfere with getting work done. Contingency planning may be reactive, in response to a crisis, or proactive, in anticipation of problems or in response to opportunities.

What would you do if two registered nurses called in sick for the 12-hour night shift? What if you were a manager for a specialty unit and received a call for an admission, but had no more beds? Or what if you were a pediatric oncology clinic manager and a patient's sibling exposed a number of immunocompromised patients to chickenpox? Planning for crises such as these are examples of contingency planning.

Strategic planning refers to the process of continual assessment, planning, and evaluation to guide the future (Fairholm & Card, 2009). Its purpose is to create an image of the desired future and design ways to make those plans a reality. A nurse manager might be charged, for example, with developing a business plan to add a time-saving device to commonly used equipment, presenting the plan persuasively, and developing operational plans for implementation, such as acquiring devices and training staff.

## Organizing

**Organizing** is the process of coordinating the work to be done. Formally, it involves identifying the work of the organization, dividing the labor, developing the chain of command, and assigning authority. It is an ongoing process that systematically reviews the use of human and material resources. In health care, the mission, formal organizational structure, delivery systems, job descriptions, skill mix, and staffing patterns form the basis for the organization.

*In organizing the home phototherapy project, Antonio develops job descriptions and protocols, determines how many positions are required, selects a vendor, and orders supplies.*

## Directing

**Directing** is the process of getting the organization's work done. Power, authority, and leadership style are intimately related to a manager's ability to direct. Communication abilities, motivational techniques, and delegation skills also are important. In today's health care organization, professional staff are autonomous, requiring guidance rather than direction. The manager is more likely to sell the idea, proposal, or new project to staff rather than tell them what to do. The manager coaches and counsels to achieve the organization's objectives. In fact, it may be the nurse who assumes the traditional directing role when working with unlicensed personnel.

*In directing the home phototherapy project, Antonio assembles the team of nurses to provide the service, explains the purpose and constraints of the program, and allows the team to decide how they will staff the project, giving guidance and direction when needed.*

## Controlling

**Controlling** involves comparing actual results with projected results. This includes establishing standards of performance, determining the means to be used in measuring performance, evaluating performance, and providing feedback. The efficient manager constantly attempts to improve productivity by incorporating techniques of quality management, evaluating outcomes and performance, and instituting change as necessary.

Today, managers share many of the control functions with the staff. In organizations using a formal quality improvement process, such as continuous quality improvement (CQI), staff participate in and lead the teams. Some organizations use peer review to control quality of care.

*When Antonio introduces the home phototherapy program, the team of nurses involved in the program identify standards regarding phototherapy and their individual performances. A subgroup of the team routinely reviews monitors designed for the program and identifies ways to improve the program.*

Planning, organizing, directing, and controlling reflect a systematic, proactive approach to management. This approach is used widely in all types of organizations, health care included, but Clancy (2008) asserts that today's rapidly changing health care environment makes it more difficult to control events and predict outcomes.

# Nurse Managers in Practice

Putting nursing management into practice in the dynamic health care system of today is a challenge. Organizations are in flux, structures are changing, and roles and functions of nurse managers become moving targets.

Titles for nurse managers vary as widely as do their responsibilities. The first level manager may be titled first-line manager or unit manager. A middle manager might be deemed a department manager. The top-level nursing administrator could be named executive manager, chief nursing officer, or vice president of patient care. In addition, clinical titles might include professional practice leaders who are clinical nurse specialists or nurse practitioners. Regardless of their titles, all nurse managers must hold certain competencies.

## Nurse Manager Competencies

The American Organization of Nurse Executives (AONE), an organization for the top nursing administrators in health care, identified five areas of competency necessary for nurses at all levels of management (AONE, 2005). Nurse managers must be skilled communicators and relationship builders, have a knowledge of the health care environment, exhibit leadership skills, display professionalism, and demonstrate business skills (see Table 4-2). These characteristics intersect to provide a common core of leadership competencies (see Figure 4-1).

---

**TABLE 4-2    Emotional Intelligence Domains and Associated Competencies**

PERSONAL COMPETENCE: These capabilities determine how we manage ourselves.

| | |
|---|---|
| Self-Awareness | • *Emotional self-awareness:* Reading one's own emotions and recognizing their impact; using "gut sense" to guide decisions<br>• *Accurate self-assessment:* Knowing one's strengths and limits<br>• *Self-confidence:* A sound sense of one's self-worth and capabilities |
| Self-Management | • *Emotional self-control:* Keeping disruptive emotions and impulses under control<br>• *Transparency:* Displaying honesty and integrity; trustworthiness<br>• *Adaptability:* Flexibility in adapting to changing situations or overcoming obstacles<br>• *Achievement:* The drive to improve performance to meet inner standards of excellence<br>• *Initiative:* Readiness to act and seize opportunities<br>• *Optimism:* Seeing the upside in events |

SOCIAL COMPETENCE: These capabilities determine how we manage relationships.

| | |
|---|---|
| Social Awareness | • *Empathy:* Sensing others' emotions, understanding their perspective, and taking active interest in their concerns<br>• *Organizational awareness:* Reading the currents, decision networks, and politics at the organizational level<br>• *Service:* Recognizing and meeting follower, client, or customer needs |
| Relationship Management | • *Inspirational leadership:* Guiding and motivating with a compelling vision<br>• *Influence:* Wielding a range of tactics for persuasion<br>• *Developing others:* Bolstering others' abilities through feedback and guidance<br>• *Change catalyst:* Initiating, managing, and leading in a new direction<br>• *Conflict management:* Resolving disagreements<br>• *Building bonds:* Cultivating and maintaining a web of relationships<br>• *Teamwork and collaboration:* Cooperation and team building |

From Goleman, D., Boyatsis, R., & McKee, A. *Primal Leadership* (2002). Boston: Harvard Business School Press, 39. Copyright © 2002 by the Harvard Business School Publishing Corporation; all rights reserved.

### Staff Nurse

Although not formally a manager, the staff nurse supervises LPNs, other professionals, and assistive personnel and so is also a manager who needs management and leadership skills. Communication, delegation, and motivation skills are indispensable.

In some organizations, shared governance has been implemented and traditional management responsibilities are allocated to the work team. In this case, staff nurses have considerable involvement in managing the unit. More information about shared governance and other innovative management methods is provided in Chapter 2.

### First-Level Management

The **first-level manager** is responsible for supervising the work of nonmanagerial personnel and the day-to-day activities of a specific work unit or units. With primary responsibility for motivating the staff to achieve the organization's goals, the first-level manager represents staff to upper administration, and vice versa. Nurse managers have 24-hour accountability for the management of a unit(s) or area(s) within a health care organization. In the hospital setting, the first-level

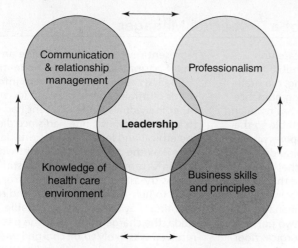

**Figure 4-1** ●
Core of leadership
competencies. *Source:*
Copyright © 2005 by the
American Organization of
Nurse Executives. Address
reprint permission
requests to aone@aha.org.

manager is usually the head nurse, nurse manager, or an assistant. In other settings, such as an ambulatory care clinic or a home health care agency, a first-level manager may be referred to as a coordinator. Box 4-1 describes a first-level manager's day.

## Charge Nurse

Another role that does not fit the traditional levels of management is the charge nurse. The **charge nurse** position is an expanded staff nurse role with increased responsibility. The charge nurse functions as a liaison to the nurse manager, assisting in shift-by-shift coordination and promotion of quality patient care as well as efficient use of resources. The charge nurse often troubleshoots problems and assists other staff members in decision making. Role modeling, mentoring, and educating are additional roles that the charge nurse often assumes. Therefore, the charge nurse usually has extensive experience, skills, and knowledge in clinical practice and is familiar with the organization's standards and practices.

The charge nurse's job differs, though, from that of the first-level manager. The charge nurse's responsibilities are confined to a specific shift or task, whereas the first-level manager has 24-hour responsibility and accountability for all unit activities. Also the charge nurse has limited authority; the charge nurse functions as an agent of the manager and is accountable to the manager for any actions taken or decisions made.

Although often involved in planning and organizing the work to be done, the charge nurse has a limited scope of responsibility, usually restricted to the unit for a specific time period. In the past, the charge nurse had limited involvement in the formal evaluation of performance, but in today's climate of efficiency, the charge nurse may be involved in evaluations as well. With the trend toward participative management, charge nurses are assuming more of the roles and functions traditionally reserved for the first-level manager.

In some organizations, the position may be permanent and assigned and thus a part of the formal management team; in other organizations, the job may be rotated among experienced staff. The charge nurse, who switches from serving as a manager one day and a staff nurse the next, is especially challenged to balance the rotating roles (Leary & Allen, 2005). In some organizations, a differential amount of compensation is paid to the person performing charge duties; in others, no differential is paid because the position is shared equally among staff or represents a higher rung of a career ladder (possibly the first rung of a management ladder).

The charge nurse is often key to a unit's successful functioning (Leary & Allen, 2005). A charge nurse usually has considerable influence with the staff and may actually have more informal power than the manager. Therefore, the charge nurse is an important leader and can benefit by developing the skills considered necessary for a manager. Acting as charge nurse is often the first step toward a formal management position.

## BOX 4-1   A Day in the Life of a First-Level Manager

As the manager for a surgical intensive care unit (SICU), Jamal Johnson is routinely responsible for supervising patient care, trouble shooting, maintaining compliance with standards, and giving guidance and direction as needed. In addition, he has fiscal and committee responsibilities and is accountable to the organization for maintaining its philosophies and objectives. The following exemplifies a typical day.

As Jamal came on duty, he learned that there had been a multiple vehicle accident and that three of the victims were currently in the operating room and destined for the unit. The assistant manager for nights had secured more staff for days: two part-time SICU nurses and a staff nurse from the surgical floor. However, she had not had time to arrange for two more patients to be moved out of the unit. From their assigned nurses, Jamal obtained an update on the patients who were candidates for transfer from the SICU to another floor and, in consultation with his assistant, made the appropriate arrangements for the transfers.

Other staffing problems were at hand: in addition to the nurse who had been pulled from the surgical floor, there were two orientees, and the staff needed to attend a safety in-service. As soon as the charge nurse came in, Jamal apprised her of the situation. Together, they reviewed the operating room schedule and identified staffing arrangements. Fortunately, Jamal had only one meeting today and would be available for backup staffing. In the meantime, he would work on evaluations.

After his discussions with the charge nurse, Jamal met with each of the night nurses to get an update on the status of the other patients. Then he went to his office to review his messages and plan his day. Tamera, an RN, had just learned she was pregnant but stated that she planned to work until delivery. Jamal learned that his budget hearing had been scheduled for the following Monday at 10 A.M. A pharmaceutical representative wanted to provide an in-service for the unit. Fortunately, there were no immediate crises.

Jamal called his supervisor to inform her of the status of affairs on the unit and learned that two other individuals in the accident had been transported to another hospital; one had since died. They discussed the ethical and legal ramifications. Jamal would need to review the policies on relations with the press and law enforcement and update his staff.

As the first patient returned from surgery, Jamal went to help admit the patient and receive a report. Learning that the patient was stable, he informed Lucinda, the charge nurse, that the patient they had just received was likely to be charged with manslaughter and reviewed media and legal policies with her. They also discussed how the staff were doing. There were some equipment problems in room 2110; Lucinda had temporarily placed the patient in that room on a transport monitor and was waiting for a biomedical technology staff member to check the monitor. Could Jamal follow up? Jamal agreed and commended Lucinda for her problem solving. She reminded Jamal they would need backup for lunch and in-services.

As Jamal returned to his office, he noted that the alarms were turned off on one of the patients. He pulled aside the nurse assigned to the patient and reminded her of the necessity to keep the alarms on at all times. Finally, back in his office, he called biomedical technology to ascertain their plans to check the monitor and made notes regarding the charge nurse's problem-solving abilities and the staff nurse's negligence.

He reviewed staffing for the next 24 hours and noted that an extra nurse was needed for both the evening and night shifts because of the increased workload. After finding staff, he was able to finish one evaluation before covering for the in-services and lunch and then attending the policy and procedure team meeting.

### Clinical Nurse Leader

The **clinical nurse leader** is not a manager, per se, but instead is a lateral integrator of care responsible for a specified group of clients within a microsystem of the health care setting (AACN, 2007). The CNL role is designed to respond more effectively to challenges in today's rapidly changing, complex technological environment (Harris & Roussel, 2009). Prepared at the master's level, the CNL coordinates care at the bedside and supervises the health care team, among other duties (Sherman, 2010).

Use of the clinical nurse leader positions in health care organizations has improved patient outcomes and reduced costs and is expected to expand as the demand for quality continues (Hix, McKeon, & Walters, 2009; Stanley et al., 2008). Problems have emerged, however, as CNLs transition into organizations. These include being drawn into direct patient care, explaining the role to other nurses and health care providers, and acceptance by the staff (Sherman, 2010).

Questions about the differences between a clinical nurse specialist and the CNL are also raised. While the CNS is assigned hospital-wide, the CNL is unit based. Ignatius (2010) suggests that hospitals are designed for the 19th century with little accommodation for the coordination of care needed in this century. CNLs can help bridge that gap.

## Followership: An Essential Component of Leadership

Leaders cannot lead without followers in much the same way that instructors need students to teach. Nor is anyone a leader all the time; everyone is a follower as well. Even the hospital CEO follows the board of directors' instructions.

**Followership** is interactive and complementary to leadership, and the follower is an active participant in the relationship with the leader. A skilled, self-directed, energetic staff member is an invaluable complement to the leader and to the group. Most leaders welcome active followers; they help leaders accomplish their goals and the team succeed.

Followers are powerful contributors to the relationship with their leaders. Followers can influence leaders in negative ways, as government cover-ups, Medicare fraud, and corporate law-breaking attest. The reverse is also true. Poor managers can undermine good followers by direct and indirect ways, such as criticizing, belittling, or ignoring positive contributions to the team (Arnold & Pulich, 2008). To counter such behaviors, you should note incidents that you experience, enlist others to help, and remain in control of yourself. (See Chapter 21 for more about handling difficult problems, such as bullying.)

Miller (2007) describes followership along two continuums: participative and thinking. Participation can vary from passive (ineffective follower) to active (successful follower). Thinking can fluctuate between dependent and uncritical to independent and critical. Courage to be active contributors to the team and to the leader characterizes the effective follower.

Followership is fluid in another way. The nurse may be a leader at one moment and become a follower soon afterward. In fact, the ability to move along the continuum of degrees of followership is a must for successful teamwork. The nurse is a leader with subordinate staff and a follower of the nurse manager, possibly at the same time.

A constructive follower has several positive characteristics:

- Self-directed
- Proactive
- Supportive
- Commitment
- Initiative

Many of these qualities are the same ones that make an excellent leader, discussed next.

## What Makes a Successful Leader?

Leadership success is an elusive quality. Some people seem to be natural leaders, and others struggle to attain leadership skills.

See how one nurse leader described her work:

*I believe that the most important role of a nurse leader is to live the life and exemplify at all times the qualities that every professional nurse leader should. I also believe the nurse leader/manager must be the person to set the bar high and perform at the highest levels in order to inspire their staff to achieve the same.*

*As a nurse manager, I at all times work to be an excellent communicator, compassionate, caring, vested in my job, willing to go above and beyond, and assist people with any task or issue they just need a little extra support on. I feel that by doing this, there is never a question what I expect from them and those around me. I verbally set expectations, but by living them as a role model.*

*For example, at shift change two nights ago, a physician wanted to do a bedside proce-
dure. I was actually planning on leaving soon after a long day. I knew it was shift change,
and didn't want the staff to be interrupted, so I volunteered to stay and do the procedure
so they could continue with report and the physician and patient were not kept waiting.
The staff were very appreciative, but more importantly, I think it set the right example of
teamwork, being flexible, being patient focused, etc.*

*I think it is important for the nurse leader to provide feedback at times other than evalu-
ations. The nurse leader should schedule time into the workweek to have informal conversations with staff on the floor about comments a patient or coworker has shared or to send
an e-mail to a staff member about feedback the leader has received. I think constructive
feedback needs to be timely and supportive and the need for improvement discussed long
before an evaluation.*

*I find having conversations about "What are your goals?" or "What can I help you
explore or do that you've been dreaming about to enhance your nursing career?" People
need to feel comfortable having these conversations with their trusted nurse leader. Building relationships with those you lead is important.*

Leaders are skilled in empowering others, creating meaning and facilitating learning,
developing knowledge, thinking reflectively, communicating, solving problems, making decisions, and working with others. Leaders generate excitement; they clearly define their purpose
and mission. Leaders understand people and their needs; they recognize and appreciate differences in people, individualizing their approach as needed.

## What You Know Now

- A leader employs specific behaviors and strategies to influence individuals and groups to attain goals.
- Managers are responsible for efficiently accomplishing the goals of the organization.
- Leadership approaches are not static; they can be adapted for different situations, tasks, individuals, and future expectations.
- Contemporary theorists assert that reality is fluid, complex, and interrelated and that interpersonal relationships are core to successful leadership.
- Traditional management functions include planning, organizing, directing, and controlling.
- Both leaders and followers contribute to the effectiveness of their relationship.
- Successful leaders inspire and empower others, generate excitement, and individualize their approach to differences in people.

## Tools for Leading, Managing, and Following

1. Pay attention to the context: Are you leading, managing, or following in this situation?
2. Recognize that each situation requires a specific skill set. Each is described in the chapter.
3. Notice others whose leadership style you admire and try to incorporate their behaviors in your own leadership if the situation is appropriate.
4. Evaluate yourself at regular opportunities in order to find ways to improve your abilities to lead, manage, and follow.

## Questions to Challenge You

1. Think about people you know in management positions. Are any of them leaders as well? Describe the characteristics that make them leaders.
2. Consider people you know who are not in management positions but are leaders nonetheless. What characteristics do they have that make them leaders?

3. Describe the manager to whom you report. (If you are not employed, use the first-level manager on a clinical placement site.) Evaluate this person using the management functions described in the chapter.
4. Imagine yourself as a manager whether you are in a management position or not. What skills do you possess that help you? What skills would you like to improve?
5. Evaluate yourself as a follower. Find at least one characteristic listed in the chapter that you would like to develop or improve. During the next week, try to find opportunities to practice that skill.
6. Assess yourself as a leader. How would you like to improve?

**Pearson Nursing Student Resources**

Find additional review materials at

**www.nursing.pearsonhighered.com**

Prepare for success with additional NCLEX®-style practice questions, interactive assignments and activities, Web links, animations and videos, and more!

# References

American Association of Colleges of Nursing (2007). *White paper on the education and role of the clinical nurse leader.* Retrieved May 20, 2011 from http://www.aacn.nche.edu/Publications/WhitePapers/ClinicalNurseLeader07.pdf

American Organization of Nurse Executives (2005). *Nurse executive competencies.* Retrieved May 20, 2011 from http://www.aone.org/aone/pdf/AONE_NEC.pdf

Anderson, B. J., Manno, M., O'Connor, P., & Gallagher, E. (2010). Listening to nursing leaders: Using national database of nursing quality indicators data to study excellence in nursing leadership. *Journal of Nursing Administration, 40*(4), 182–187.

Antonakis, J., Ashkanasy, N. M., & Dasborough, M. T. (2009). Does leadership need emotional intelligence? *The Leadership Quarterly, 20*(4), 247–261.

Arnold, E., & Pulich, M. (2008). Inappropriate selection of first-line managers can be hazardous to the health of organizations. *The Health Care Manager, 27*(3), 223–229.

Bradberry, T. & Greaves, J. (2009). *Emotional intelligence 2.0.* San Diego, CA: TalentSmart.

Clancy, T. R. (2008). Control: What we can learn from complex systems science. *Journal of Nursing Administration, 38*(6), 272–274.

Cote, S., Lopes, P. N., Salovey, P., & Miners, C. T. H. (2010). Emotional intelligence and leadership emergence in small groups. *The Leadership Quarterly, 21*(3), 496–508.

Everett, L. Q., & Sitterding, M. C. (2011). Transformational leadership required to design and sustain evidence-based practice: A system exemplar. *Western Journal of Nursing Research, 33*(3), 398–426.

Fairholm, M. R., & Card, M. (2009). Perspectives of strategic thinking: From controlling chaos to embracing it. *Journal of Management and Organization, 15*(1), 17–30.

Goleman, D. (2006). *Emotional intelligence: Why it can matter more than IQ.* New York: Bantam.

Goleman, D. (2007). *Social intelligence: The new science of human behavior.* New York: Bantam.

Grant, B., Colello, S., Riehle, M., & Dende, D. (2010). An evaluation of the nursing practice environment and successful change management using the new generation Magnet Model. *Journal of Nursing Management, 18*(3), 326–331.

Greenleaf, R. K. (1991). *The servant as leader.* Westfield, IN: Greenleaf Center for Servant Leadership.

Harris, J. D., & Roussel, L. (2009). *Initiating and sustaining the clinical nurse leader role: A practical guide.* Sudbury, MA: Jones & Bartlett Learning.

Hix, C., McKeon, L., & Walters, S. (2009). Clinical nurse leader impact on clinical microsystems outcomes. *Journal of Nursing Administration, 39*(2), 71–76.

Ignatious, A. Fixing healthcare. *Harvard Business Review, 88*(4), 49–73.

Keith, K. (2008). *The case for servant leadership*. Westfield, IN: Greenleaf Center for Servant Leadership.

Kramer, M., Schmalenberg, C., & Maguire, P. (2010). Nine structures and leadership practices essential for a magnetic (healthy) work environment. *Nursing Administration Quarterly, 34*(1), 4–17.

Leary, C., & Allen, S. (2005). *A charge nurse's guide: Navigating the path of leadership*. Cleveland, OH: Center for Leader Development.

Lindebaum, D., & Cartwright, S. (2010). A critical examination of the relationship between emotional intelligence and transformational leadership. *Journal of Management Studies, 47*(7), 1317–1342.

Lucas, V., Spence-Laschinger, H. K., & Wong, C. A. (2008). The impact of emotional intelligent leadership on staff nurse empowerment: The moderating effect of span of control. *Journal of Nursing Management, 16*(8), 964–973.

Marshall, E. (2010). *Transformational leadership in nursing: From expert clinician to influential leader*. New York: Springer.

Miller, L. A. (2007). Followership. *Journal of Perinatal & Neonatal Nursing, 21*(1), 76.

Neill, M. W., & Saunders, N. S. (2008). Servant leadership: Enhancing quality of care and staff satisfaction. *Journal of Nursing Administration, 38*(9), 395–400.

Porter-O'Grady, T., & Malloch, K. (2010). *Quantum leadership: Advancing information, transforming health care* (3rd ed.). Sudbury, MA: Jones & Bartlett.

Sherman, R. O. (2010). Lessons in innovation: Role transition experiences of clinical nurse leaders. *Journal of Nursing Administration, 40*(12), 547–554.

Stanley, J. M., Gannon, J., Gabuat, J., Hartranft, S., Adams, N., Mayes, C., Shouse, G. M., Edwards, B. A., & Burch, D. (2008). The clinical nurse leader: A catalyst for improving quality and patient safety. *Journal of Nursing Management, 16*(5), 614–622.

The Greenleaf Center for Servant Leadership (2011). Retrieved May 20, 2011 from http://www.greenleaf.org

Veronesi, J. F. (2009). Breaking news on social intelligence. *Journal of Nursing Administration, 39*(2), 57–59.

Watters, S. (2009). Shared leadership: Taking flight. *Journal of Nursing Administration, 39*(1), 26–29.

Weberg, D. (2010). Transformation leadership and staff retention: An evidence review with implications for healthcare systems. *Nursing Administration Quarterly, 34*(3), 246–258.

Weston, M. J. (2008). Transformational leadership at a national perspective. *Nurse Leader, 6*(4), 41–45.

# Initiating and Managing Change

## Learning Outcomes

*After completing this chapter, you will be able to:*

1. Explain why nurses have the opportunity to be change agents.
2. Describe how different theorists explain change.
3. Discuss how the change process is similar to the nursing process.
4. Differentiate among change strategies.
5. Discuss how to handle resistance to change.
6. Describe the nurse's role in change.

## Key Terms

Change
Change agent
Driving forces

Empirical–rational model
Normative–reeducative
   strategies

Power-coercive strategies
Restraining forces
Transitions

## Why Change?

Change is inevitable, if not always welcome. Organizational change is essential for adaptation; creative change is mandatory for growth (Heath & Heath, 2010). Change, though, is a continually unfolding process rather than an either/or event. The process begins with the present state, is disrupted, moves through a transition period, and ultimately comes to a desired state. Once the desired state has been reached, however, the process begins again.

Leading change is never needed more in today's rapidly evolving system of health care. Those who initiate and manage change often encounter resistance. Even when planned, it can be threatening and a source of conflict because **change** is the process of making something different from what it was. There is a sense of loss of the familiar, the status quo. This is particularly true when change is unplanned or beyond human control. Even when change is expected and valued, a grief reaction still may occur.

Although nurses should understand and anticipate these reactions to change, they need to develop and exude a different approach. They can view change as a challenge and encourage their colleagues to participate. They can become uncomfortable with the status quo and be willing to take risks.

This is a particular fortuitous time for the nursing profession (Nickitas, 2010). The Institute of Medicine's report on the future of nursing proposes radical change for the profession (IOM, 2010). Specifically, they propose:

- Nurses should practice to the full extent of their education and training.
- Nurses should achieve higher levels of education and training through an improved education system that promotes seamless academic progression.
- Nurses should be full partners with physicians and other health care professionals in redesigning health care in the United States.
- Effective workforce planning and policymaking require better data collection and an improved information infrastructure.

Furthermore, the IOM makes eight recommendations:

- Remove scope-of-practice barriers.
- Expand opportunities for nurses to lead and diffuse collaborative improvement efforts.
- Implement nurse residency programs.
- Increase the proportion of nurses with baccalaureate degrees to 80 percent by 2020.
- Ensure nurses engage in lifelong learning.
- Prepare and enable nurses to lead change to advance health.
- Build an infrastructure for the collection and analysis of interprofessional health care workforce data (IOM, 2010).

## The Nurse as Change Agent

A **change agent** is one who works to bring about a change. Being a change agent, however, is not easy. Although the end result of change may benefit nurses and patients alike, initially it requires time, effort, and energy, all in short supply in the high-stress environment of health care.

Several recent reports document nurses' roles in facilitating change. Holtrop et al. (2008) found that nurse consultants improved healthy behaviors in patients served by 10 primary care practices in two health care systems. Also, MacDavitt, Cieplincki, and Walker (2011) report that small changes in communication resulted in improved patient satisfaction on a pediatric inpatient unit. Finally, McMurray et al. (2010) found that nurse managers played a key role in implementing successful change in bedside handover in two hospitals.

Changes will continue at a rapid pace with or without nursing's expert guidance. Nurses, like organizations, cannot afford merely to survive changes. If they are to exist as a distinct profession that has expertise in helping individuals respond to actual or potential health problems, they must be proactive in shaping the future. Opportunities exist now for nurses, especially those in management positions, to change the system about which they so often complain.

## Change Theories

Because change occurs within the context of human behavior, understanding how change does (or doesn't) occur is helpful in learning how to initiate or manage change. Five theories explain the change process from a social–psychological viewpoint. See Table 5-1 for a comparison.

Lewin (1951) proposes a force-field model, shown in Figure 5-1. He sees behavior as a dynamic balance of forces working in opposing directions within a field (such as an organization). **Driving forces** facilitate change because they push participants in the desired direction. **Restraining forces** impede change because they push participants in the opposite direction.

To plan change, one must analyze these forces and shift the balance in the direction of change through a three-step process: unfreezing, moving, and refreezing. Change occurs by adding a new force, changing the direction of a force, or changing the magnitude of any one force. Basically, strategies for change are aimed at increasing driving forces, decreasing restraining forces, or both. The image of people's attitudes thawing and then refreezing is conceptually useful. This symbolism helps to keep theory and reality in mind simultaneously.

Lippitt and colleagues (1958) extended Lewin's theory to a seven-step process and focused more on what the change agent must do than on the evolution of change itself. (See Table 5-1.) They emphasized participation of key members of the target system throughout the change process, particularly during planning. Communication skills, rapport building, and problem-solving strategies underlie their phases.

Havelock (1973) described a six-step process, also a modification of Lewin's model. Havelock describes an active change agent as one who uses a participative approach.

Rogers (2003) takes a broader approach than Lewin, Lippitt, or Havelock (see Table 5-1). His five-step innovation–decision process details how an individual or decision-making unit

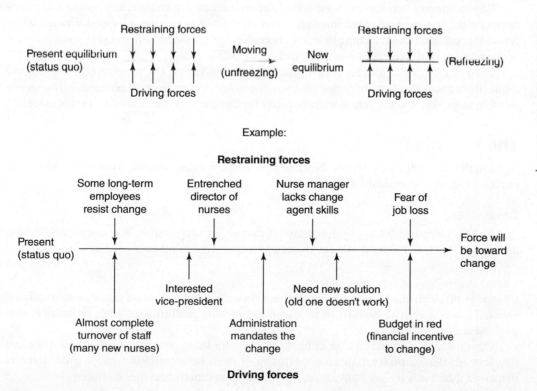

**Figure 5-1** •
Lewin's force-field model of change.
Adapted from *Resolving Social Conflicts and Field Theory in Social Science* by K. Lewin. Copyright © 1997, by the American Psychological Association. Adapted with permission.

| TABLE 5-1 | Comparison of Change Models | | | |
|---|---|---|---|---|
| Lewin | Lippitt | Havelock | Rogers | Prochaska & DiClemente |
| 1. Unfreezing<br>2. Moving<br>3. Refreezing | 1. Diagnose problem<br>2. Assess motivation<br>3. Assess change agent's motivations and resources<br>4. Select progressive change objects<br>5. Choose change agent role<br>6. Maintain change<br>7. Terminate helping relationships | 1. Building a relationship<br>2. Diagnosing the problem<br>3. Acquiring resources<br>4. Choosing the solution<br>5. Gaining acceptance<br>6. Stabilization and self-renewal | 1. Knowledge<br>2. Persuasion<br>3. Decision<br>4. Implementation<br>5. Confirmation | 1. Precontemplation<br>2. Contemplation<br>3. Preparation<br>4. Action<br>5. Maintenance |

passes from first knowledge of an innovation to confirmation of the decision to adopt or reject a new idea. His framework emphasizes the reversible nature of change: participants may initially adopt a proposal but later discontinue it, or the reverse—they may initially reject it but adopt it at a later time. This is a useful distinction. If the change agent is unsuccessful in achieving full implementation of a proposal, it should not be assumed the issue is dead. It can be resurrected, perhaps in an altered form or at a more opportune time.

Rogers stresses two important aspects of successful planned change: key people and policy makers must be interested in the innovation and committed to making it happen. Erwin (2009) found that organizational change in hospitals could only be successful and sustained if senior administrators were fully committed to the change.

Used primarily as a tool for patient teaching, Prochaska and DiClemente (2005) proposed a transtheoretical model of behavior change. Five stages characterize their model. The stages occur in sequence, and the person must be ready for change to occur, according to this model.

## The Change Process

Steps in the change process follow the same path as the nursing process: assessment, planning, implementation, and evaluation (see Table 5-2).

### Assessment

Emphasis is placed on the assessment phase of change for two reasons. Without data collection and analysis, planned change will not proceed past the "wouldn't it be a good idea if" stage.

#### Identify the Problem or the Opportunity

Change is often planned to close a discrepancy between the desired and actual state of affairs. Discrepancies may arise because of problems in reaching performance goals or because new goals have been created.

Opportunities demand change as much as (or more than) problems do, but they are often overlooked. Be it a problem or an opportunity, it must be identified clearly. If the issue is perceived differently by key individuals, the search for solutions becomes confused.

| **TABLE 5-2    Steps in the Change Process** |
| --- |

1.  Identify the problem or opportunity.
2.  Collect necessary data and information.
3.  Select and analyze data.
4.  Develop a plan for change, including time frame and resources.
5.  Identify supporters or opposers.
6.  Build a coalition of supporters.
7.  Help people prepare for change.
8.  Prepare to handle resistance.
9.  Provide a feedback mechanism to keep everyone informed of the progress of change.
10. Evaluate effectiveness of the change and, if successful, stabilize the change.

Start by asking the right questions, such as:

1.  Where are we now? What is unique about us? What should our business be?

2.  What can we do that is different from and better than what our competitors do?

3.  What is the driving stimulus in our organization? What determines how we make our final decisions?

4.  What prevents us from moving in the direction we wish to go?

5.  What kind of change is required?

This last question generates integrative thinking on the potential effect of change on the system. Organizational change involves modifications in the system's interacting components: technology, structure, and people.

Introducing new technology changes the structure of the organization. The physical plant may be altered if new services are added and then relationships among the people who work in the system change when the structure is changed. Surveillance cameras, cell phones, magnetic entry cards, bar codes, and communication technology, including social media, have altered the care environment as much as they've changed our personal world. New rules and regulations, new authority structures, and new budgeting methods may emerge. They, in turn, change staffing needs, requiring people with different skills, knowledge bases, attitudes, and motivations.

### Collect Data

Once the problem or opportunity has been clearly defined, the change agent collects data external and internal to the system. This step is crucial to the eventual success of the planned change. All driving and restraining forces are identified so the driving forces can be emphasized and the restraining forces reduced. It is imperative to assess the political pulse. Who will gain from this change? Who will lose? Who has more power and why? Can those power bases be altered? How?

Assess the political climate by examining the reasons for the present situation. Who in control may be benefiting now? Egos, commitment of the involved people, and personal likes and dislikes are as important to assess as the formal organizational structures and processes. The innovator has to gauge the potential for resistance.

The costs and benefits of the proposed change are obvious focal points. Also assess resources—especially those the manager can control. A manager who has the respect and support of an excellent nursing staff has access to a powerful resource in today's climate.

Analyze Data

The kinds, amounts, and sources of data collected are important, but they are useless unless they are analyzed. The change agent should focus more energy on analyzing and summarizing the data than on just collecting it. The point is to flush out resistance, identify potential solutions and strategies, begin to identify areas of consensus, and build a case for whichever option is selected.

*At a not-for-profit hospital in the process of seeking Magnet status, each service line is looking for opportunities to improve standards of care, efficiency, and patient safety. In the ambulatory surgery center, the process of providing preoperative services was often slow and inefficient. The surgery center nurses were charged with finding ways to improve efficiency.*

## Planning

Planning the who, how, and when of the change is a key step. What will be the target system for the change? Members from this system should be active participants in the planning stage. The more involved they are at this point, the less resistance there will be later. Lewin's unfreezing imagery is relevant here. Present attitudes, habits, and ways of thinking have to soften so members of the target system will be ready for new ways of thinking and behaving. Boundaries must melt before the system can shift and restructure.

This is the time to make people uncomfortable with the status quo. Plant the seeds of discontent by introducing information that may make people feel dissatisfied with the present and interested in something new. This information comes from the data collected (e.g., research findings, quantitative data, and patient satisfaction questionnaires or staff surveys). Couch the proposed change in comfortable terms as far as possible, and minimize anxiety about the new change.

Managers need to plan the resources required to make the change and establish feedback mechanisms to evaluate its progress and success. Establish control points with people who will provide the feedback and work with these people to set specific goals with time frames. Develop operational indicators that signal success or failure in terms of performance and satisfaction.

*Three surgery center nurses designed a flow chart of how the process could be improved. They took it to their administration and were put in charge of its implementation.*

## Implementation

The plans are put into motion (Lewin's moving stage). Interventions are designed to gain the necessary compliance. The change agent creates a supportive climate, acts as an energizer, obtains and provides feedback, and overcomes resistance. Managers are the key change-process actors. Some methods are directed toward changing individuals in an organization, whereas others are directed toward changing the group.

Methods to Change Individuals

The most common method used to change individuals' perceptions, attitudes, and values is information giving. Providing information is prerequisite to change implementation, but it is inadequate unless a lack of information is the only obstacle to effecting change. Providing information does not address the motivation to change.

Training is often considered a method to change individuals. Training combines information-giving with skill practice. Training typically shows people how they are to perform in a system, not how to change it. Therefore, it is a strategy to help make the transition to a planned change rather than a mechanism to initiate change.

Selecting and placing personnel or terminating key people often is used to alter the forces for or against change. When key supporters of the planned change are given the authority and accountability to make the change, their enthusiasm and legitimacy can be effective in leading others to support the change. Conversely, if those opposed to the change are transferred or leave the organization, the change is more likely to succeed.

### Methods to Change Groups

Some implementation tactics use groups rather than individuals to attain compliance to change. The power of an organizational group to influence its members depends on its authority to act on an issue and the significance of the issue itself. The greatest influence is achieved when group members discuss issues that are perceived as important and make relevant, binding decisions based on those discussions. Effectiveness in implementing organizational change is most likely when groups are composed of members who occupy closely related positions in the organization.

Individual and group implementation tactics can be combined. Whatever methods are used, participants should feel their input is valued and should be rewarded for their efforts. Some people are not always persuaded before a beneficial change is implemented. Sometimes behavior changes first, and attitudes are modified later to fit the behavior. In this case, the change agent should be aware of participants' conflicts and reward the desired behaviors. It may take some time for attitudes to catch up.

*The surgery center nurses worked with physician offices, insurance companies, and other hospital departments to implement the new process for preoperative services.*

## Evaluation

### Evaluate Effectiveness

At each control point, the operational indicators established are monitored. The change agent determines whether presumed benefits were achieved from a financial as well as a qualitative perspective, explaining the extent of success or failure. Unintended consequences and undesirable outcomes may have occurred.

### Stabilize the Change

The change is extended past the pilot stage, and the target system is refrozen. The change agent terminates the helping relationship by delegating responsibilities to target system members. The energizer role is still needed to reinforce new behaviors through positive feedback.

*Over the next three months, the preoperative services department was able to show a 90 percent decrease in duplicate test orders, a 50 percent decrease in patient waiting time, and an 80 percent increase in physician satisfaction with the process.*

# Change Strategies

Regardless of the setting or proposed change, the four-step change process should be followed. However, specific strategies can be used, depending on the amount of resistance anticipated and the degree of power the change agent possesses.

## Power-Coercive Strategies

**Power-coercive strategies** are based on the application of power by legitimate authority, economic sanctions, or political clout. Changes are made through law, policy, or financial appropriations. Those in control enforce changes by restricting budgets or creating policies. Those who are not in power may not even be aware of what is happening. Even if they are aware, they have little power to stop it. Health care reform legislation, is an example of power-coercive strategy by the federal government.

Power-coercive strategies are useful when a consensus is unlikely despite efforts to stimulate participation by those involved. When much resistance is anticipated, time is short, and the change is critical for organizational survival, power-coercive strategies may be necessary.

### Empirical–Rational Model

In the **empirical–rational model** of change strategies, the power ingredient is knowledge. The assumption is that people are rational and will follow their rational self-interest if that self-interest is made clear to them. It is also assumed that the change agent who has knowledge has the expert power to persuade people to accept a rationally justified change that will benefit them.

The flow of influence moves from those who know to those who do not know. New ideas are invented and communicated or diffused to all participants. Once enlightened, rational people will either accept or reject the idea based on its merits and consequences. Empirical–rational strategies are often effective when little resistance to the proposed change is expected and the change is perceived as reasonable.

Well-researched, cost-effective technology can be implemented using these strategies. Introducing a new technology that is easy to use, cuts nursing time, and improves quality of care might be accepted readily after in-service education and a trial use. Using bar codes to match medications to patients is another example.

The change agent can direct the change. There is little need for staff participation in the early steps of the change process, although input is useful for the evaluation and stabilization stages. The benefits of change for the staff and research documenting improved patient outcomes are the major driving forces.

### Normative–Reeducative Strategies

In contrast to the rational-empirical model, **normative–reeducative strategies** of change rest on the assumption that people act in accordance with social norms and values. Information and rational arguments are insufficient strategies to change people's patterns of actions; the change agent must focus on noncognitive determinants of behavior as well. People's roles and relationships, perceptual orientations, attitudes, and feelings will influence their acceptance of change.

In this mode, the power ingredient is not authority or knowledge, but skill in interpersonal relationships. The change agent does not use coercion or nonreciprocal influence, but collaboration. Members of the target system are involved throughout the change process. Value conflicts from all parts of the system are brought into the open and worked through so change can progress.

Normative–reeducative strategies are well suited to the creative problem solving needed in nursing and health care today. With their firm grasp of the behavioral sciences and communication skills, nurses are comfortable with this model. Changing from a traditional nursing system to self-governance or initiating a home follow-up service for hospitalized patients are examples of changes amenable to the normative–reeducative approach.

In most cases, the normative–reeducative approach to change will be effective in reducing resistance and stimulating personal and organizational creativity. The obvious drawback is the time required for group participation and conflict resolution throughout the change process. When there is adequate time or when group consensus is fundamental to successful adoption of the change, the manager is well advised to adopt this framework.

# Resistance to Change

Resistance to change is to be expected for a number of reasons: lack of trust, vested interest in the status quo, fear of failure, loss of status or income, misunderstanding, and belief that change is unnecessary or that it will not improve the situation (Yukl, 2009; Hellriegel, Jackson, & Slocum, 2007). In fact, if resistance does not surface, the change may not be significant enough.

Employees may resist change because they dislike or disapprove of the person responsible for implementing the change or they may distrust the change process. Regardless, managers continually deal with change—both the change that they themselves initiate and change initiated by the larger organization.

Resistance varies from ready acceptance to full-blown resistance. Rogers (2003) identified six responses to change:

- *Innovators* love change and thrive on it.
- Less radical, *early adopters* are still receptive to change.
- The *early majority* prefer the status quo, but eventually accept the change.
- The *late majority* are resistive, accepting change after most others have.
- *Laggards* dislike change and are openly antagonistic.
- *Rejecters* actively oppose and may even sabotage change.

The change agent should anticipate and look for resistance to change. It will be lurking somewhere, perhaps where least expected. It can be recognized in such statements as:

- We tried that before.
- It won't work.
- No one else does it like that.
- We've always done it this way.
- We can't afford it.
- We don't have the time.
- It will cause too much commotion.
- You'll never get it past the board.
- Let's wait awhile.
- Every new boss wants to do something different.
- Let's start a task force to look at it; put it on the agenda.

Expect resistance and listen carefully to who says what, when, and in what circumstances. Open resisters are easier to deal with than closet resisters. Look for nonverbal signs of resistance, such as poor work habits and lack of interest in the change.

Resistance prevents the unexpected. It forces the change agent to clarify information, keep interest level high, and establish why change is necessary. It draws attention to potential problems and encourages ideas to solve them. Resistance is a stimulant as much as it is a force to be overcome. It may even motivate the group to do better what it is doing now, so that it does not have to change.

On the other hand, resistance is not always beneficial, especially if it persists beyond the planning stage and well into the implementation phase. It can wear down supporters and redirect system energy from implementing the change to dealing with resisters. Morale can suffer.

To manage resistance, use the following guidelines:

1. Talk to those who oppose the change. Get to the root of their reasons for opposition.

2. Clarify information, and provide accurate feedback.

3. Be open to revisions but clear about what must remain.

4. Present the negative consequences of resistance (e.g., threats to organizational survival, compromised patient care).

5. Emphasize the positive consequences of the change and how the individual or group will benefit. However, do not spend too much energy on rational analysis of why the change is good and why the arguments against it do not hold up. People's resistance frequently flows from feelings that are not rational.

6. Keep resisters involved in face-to-face contact with supporters. Encourage proponents to empathize with opponents, recognize valid objections, and relieve unnecessary fears.

7. Maintain a climate of trust, support, and confidence.

8. Divert attention by creating a different disturbance. Energy can shift to a more important problem inside the system, thereby redirecting resistance. Alternatively, attention can be brought to an external threat to create a bully phenomenon. When members perceive a greater environmental threat (such as competition or restrictive governmental policies), they tend to unify internally.

# The Nurse's Role

### Initiating Change

Contrary to popular opinion, change often is not initiated by top-level management (Yukl, 2009), but rather emerges as new initiatives or problems are identified. Furthermore, Weiner, Amick, and Lee (2008) posit that organizational readiness is the key to initiating change.

Staff nurses often think that they are unable to initiate and create change, but that is not so.

*Home health nurses were often frustrated by not having appropriate supplies with them when seeing a patient for the first time. A team of nurses completed a chart audit to identify commonly used supplies and equipment that nurses were using on their home visits. Each nurse was then supplied with a small plastic container to keep in his or her car with these items. Frustration decreased and efficient use of nursing time was improved.*

The manager, as well, may resist leading change. Afraid of "rocking the boat," fearful that no one will join our efforts, recalling that past efforts at change had failed, or even the reluctance to become involved may prevent the nurse from initiating change.

Making change is not easy, but it is a mandatory skill for managers. Successful change agents demonstrate certain characteristics that can be cultivated and mastered with practice. These characteristics include:

- The ability to combine ideas from unconnected sources
- The ability to energize others by keeping the interest level up and demonstrating a high personal energy level
- Skill in human relations: well-developed interpersonal communication, group management, and problem-solving skills
- Integrative thinking: the ability to retain a big picture focus while dealing with each part of the system
- Sufficient flexibility to modify ideas when modifications will improve the change, but enough persistence to resist nonproductive tampering with the planned change
- Confidence and the tendency not to be easily discouraged
- Realistic thinking
- Trustworthiness: a track record of integrity and success with other changes
- The ability to articulate a vision through insights and versatile thinking
- The ability to handle resistance

Energy is needed to change a system. Power is the main source of that energy. Informational power, expertise, and possibly positional power can be used to persuade others.

To access optimum power, use the following strategies:

1. Analyze the organizational chart. Know the formal lines of authority. Identify informal lines as well.

2. Identify key persons who will be affected by the change. Pay attention to those immediately above and below the point of change.

3. Find out as much as possible about these key people. What are their "tickle points"? What interests them, gets them excited, turns them off? What is on their personal and organizational agendas? Who typically aligns with whom on important decisions?

4. Begin to build a coalition of support before you start the change process. Identify the key people who will be affected by the change. Talk informally with them to flush out possible objections to your idea and potential opponents. What will the costs and benefits be to them—especially in political terms? Can your idea be modified in ways that retain your objectives but appeals to more key people?

5. Follow the organizational chain of command in communicating with administrators. Don't bypass anyone to avoid having an excellent proposal undermined.

This information helps you develop the most sellable idea or at least pinpoint probable resistance. It is a broad beginning to the data-collection step of the change process and has to be fine-tuned once the idea is better defined. The astute manager keeps alert at all times to monitor power struggles.

Although a cardinal rule of change is, "Don't try to change too much too fast," the savvy manager develops a sense of exquisite timing by pacing the change process according to the political pulse. For example, the manager unfreezes the system during a period of coalition building and high interest, while resistance is low or at least unorganized.

You may decide to stall the project beyond a pilot stage if resistance solidifies or gains a powerful ally. In this case, do whatever you can to reduce resistance. If resistance continues, two options should be considered:

- The change is not workable and should be modified to meet the strongest objections (compromise).
- The change is fine-tuned sufficiently, but change must proceed now and resistance must be overcome.

## Implementing Change

In addition to initiating change, nurses and nurse managers are called on to assist with change in other ways. They may be involved in the planning stage, charged with sharing information with coworkers, or they may be asked to help manage the transition to planned change.

### Planning Change

One Magnet-recognized hospital engaged all its nurses in planning for the desired future of clinical nursing in its organization (Capuano et al., 2007). It held a series of group events to solicit ideas and opinions. Every nurse—executive, manager, or staff nurse—had an equal vote to approve or veto a proposed change. This process illustrates the normative–reeducative process of change.

### Managing Transitions to Change

**Transitions** are those periods of time between the current situation and the time when change is implemented (Bridges, 2009). They are the times ripe for a change agent to act. Just as initiating change is not easy, neither is transitioning to changed circumstances.

Letting go of long-term, comfortable activities is difficult. The tendency is to:

- Add new work to the old
- Make individual decisions about what to add and what to let go
- Toss out everything done before (Bridges, 2009)

Accepting loss and honoring the past with respect is essential. Passion for the work is based on results, not activities, regardless of their necessity or effectiveness.

*A large national for-profit health care system purchased a new hospital clinical information system. Because all paper charting would be eliminated, nurses would be directly*

## CASE STUDY 5-1

### ENCOURAGING CHANGE

Peter Beasley is the nurse manager of pediatric home care for a private home health care agency. Last year, the agency completed a pilot of wireless devices for use in documenting home visits. As nurses complete the documentation, charges for supplies and medical equipment are generated. The agency director informed the nurse managers that all nurses will be required to use the wireless devices within the next three months.

Charlene Ramirez has been a pediatric nurse for 18 years, working for the home health care agency for the past 5 years. Charlene has been active in updating the pediatric documentation and training staff when new paper-based documentation was implemented in the past. Although she was part of the pilot, Charlene is very opposed to using the new wireless devices. She complains that she can barely see the text. At a recent staff meeting, Charlene stated she would rather quit than learn to use the new wireless devices.

Peter empathizes with Charlene's reluctance to use the new technology. He also recognizes how much Charlene contributes in expertise and leadership to the department. However, he knows that the new performance standards require all employees to use the wireless devices. After three mandatory training sessions, Charlene repeatedly tells coworkers "We've tried things like this before, it never works. We'll be back on paper within six months, so why waste my time learning this stuff?" The program trainer reports that Charlene was disruptive during the class and failed her competency exam.

Peter meets privately with Charlene to discuss her resistance to the new technology. Charlene again states that she fails to see the need for wireless devices in delivering quality patient care. Peter reviews the new performance standards with Charlene, emphasizing the technology requirements. He asks Charlene if she has difficulty understanding the application or just in using the device. Charlene admits she cannot read the text on the screen and therefore cannot determine what exactly she is documenting. Peter informs Charlene that the agency's health benefits include vision exams and partial payment for corrective lenses. He suggests that she talk with an optometrist to see if special glasses would help her see the screen. Peter also makes a note to speak with the technology specialist to see if there are aids to help staff view data on the device.

### Manager's Checklist

The nurse manager is responsible for:

- Communicating openly and honestly with employees who oppose change.
- Understanding resistance to change.
- Maintaining support and confidence in staff even if they are resistive to change.
- Emphasizing the positive outcomes from initiating change.
- Finding solutions to problems that are obstacles to change.

---

*affected. Their participation could spell success or failure for the new system. To help the transition occur smoothly, nurses from each department met together for a demonstration of the new clinical information system and provided feedback to the IT department about nursing process and integrating patient care with the new system. Then a few nurses on each unit were selected to be trained as experts in the new technology, and they in turn trained other staff members, communicating with the IT department when concerns arose.*

A nurse manager in a home health care agency used change management strategies to overcome resistance, as shown in Case Study 5-1.

## Handling Constant Change

Change has always occurred; what's different today is both the pace of change and that an initial change causes a chain reaction of more and more change (Bridges, 2009). Change, rather than an occasional event, has become the norm.

Regardless of their position in an organization, nurses find themselves constantly dealing with change. Whether they thrive in such an atmosphere is a function of both their own personal resources and the environment in which change occurs.

If you don't like the current situation, you may look forward to change. As Midwesterners are fond of saying when asked about the weather: "If you don't like it today, just wait until tomorrow. It will change."

## What You Know Now

- In today's health care system, change is inevitable, necessary, and constant.
- With changes proposed for the nursing profession, nurses are in a pivotal position to initiate and participate in change.
- For change to be positive for nurses, they must develop change agent skills.
- Critical evaluation of change theories provides guidance and direction for initiating and managing change.
- The change process is similar to the nursing process and includes assessment, planning, implementation, and evaluation.
- Resistance to change is to be expected, and it can be a stimulant as well as a force to be overcome.
- The nurse may be involved in change by initiating it or participating in implementing change.
- Handling constant change is a challenge in today's health care environment.

## Tools for Initiating and Managing Change

1. Communicate openly and honestly with employees who oppose change.
2. Maintain support and confidence in staff even if they are resistive to change.
3. Emphasize the positive outcomes from the change.
4. Find solutions to problems that are obstacles to change.
5. Accept the constancy of change.

## Questions to Challenge You

1. Identify a needed change in the organization where you practice. Using the change process, outline the steps you would take to initiate change.
2. Consider your school or college. What change do you think is needed? Explain how you would change it to become a better place for learning.
3. Have you had an experience with change occurring in your organization? What was your initial reaction? Did that change? How well did the change process work? Was the change successful?
4. Do you have a behavior you would like to change? Using the steps in the change process, describe how you might effect that change.
5. How do you normally react to change? Choose from the following:
   a. I love new ideas, and I'm ready to try new things.
   b. I like to know that something will work out before I try it.
   c. I try to avoid change as much as possible.
6. Did your response to the above question alter how you would like to view change? Think about this the next time change is presented to you.
7. Think back to your first time on a clinical unit. How did you feel? Overwhelmed? Afraid of failing? That's the feeling that people have when facing change. Try to remember how you felt when you encounter resistance to change.

### Pearson Nursing Student Resources

Find additional review materials at
**www.nursing.pearsonhighered.com**

Prepare for success with additional NCLEX®-style practice questions, interactive assignments and activities, Web links, animations and videos, and more!

## Web Resources

Agency for Healthcare Research and Quality. http://www.ahrq.gov/
Institute of Medicine. http://www.iom.edu/

## References

Bridges, W. (2009). *Managing transitions: Making the most of change.* Cambridge, MA: Da Capo Press.

Capuano, T., Durishin, L. D., Millard, J. L., & Hitchings, K. S. (2007). The desired future of nursing doesn't just happen—engaged nurses create it. *Journal of Nursing Administration, 37*(2), 61–63.

Erwin, D. (2009). Changing organizational performance: Examining the change process. *Hospital Topics: Research and Perspectives on Healthcare, 87*(3), 28–40.

Havelock, R. (1973). *The change agent's guide to innovation in education.* Englewood Liffs, NJ: Educational Technology Publications.

Heath, C., & Heath, D. (2010). *Switch: How to change things when change is hard.* New York: Crown.

Hellriegel, D., Jackson, S. E., & Slocum, J. W. (2007). *Management: A competency-based approach* (11th ed.). Eagan, MN: South-Western.

Holtrop, J. S., Baumann, J., Arnold, A. K., & Torres, T. (2008). Nurses as practice change facilitators for healthy behaviors. *Journal of Nursing Care Quality, 23*(2), 123–131.

Institute of Medicine (2010). The future of nursing: Leading change, advancing health. Retrieved May 24, 2011 from http://www.iom.edu/Reports/2010/The-Future-of-Nursing-Leading-Change-Advancing-Health.aspx

Lewin, K. (1951). *Field theory in social science.* New York: Harper & Row.

Lippitt, R., Watson, J., & Westley, B. (1958). *The dynamics of planned change.* New York: Harcourt & Brace.

MacDavitt, K., Cieplinski, J. A., & Walker, V. (2011). Implementing small tests of change to improve patient satisfaction. *Journal of Nursing Administration, 41*(1), 5–9.

McMurray, A., Chaboyer, W., Wallis, M., & Fetherston, C. (2010). Implementing bedside handover: Strategies for change management. *Journal of Clinical Nursing, 19*(17–18), 2580–2589.

Nickitas, D. M. (2010). A vision for future health care: Where nurses lead the change. *Nursing Economics, 28*(6), 361, 385.

Prochaska, J. O. & DiClemente, C. C. (2005). The transtheoretical approach. In: Norcross, J. C., & Goldfried, M. R. (Eds.), *Handbook of psychotherapy integration* (2nd ed.). New York: Oxford University Press.

Rogers, E. (2003). *Diffusion of innovations* (5th ed.). New York: Free Press.

Sare, M. V., & Ogilvie, L. (2009). *Strategic planning for nurses: Change management in health care.* Sudbury, MA: Jones and Bartlett.

Weiner, B. J., Amick, H., & Lee, S. D. (2008). Conceptualization and measurement of organizational readiness for change: A review of the literature in health services research and other fields. *Medical Care Research and Review, 65*(4), 379–436.

Yukl, G. A. (2009). *Leadership in organizations* (7th ed.). Upper Saddle River, NJ: Prentice Hall.

# Managing and Improving Quality

## Quality Management

TOTAL QUALITY MANAGEMENT

CONTINUOUS QUALITY IMPROVEMENT

COMPONENTS OF QUALITY MANAGEMENT

SIX SIGMA

LEAN SIX SIGMA

DMAIC METHOD

## Improving the Quality of Care

NATIONAL INITIATIVES

HOW COST AFFECTS QUALITY

EVIDENCE-BASED PRACTICE

ELECTRONIC MEDICAL RECORDS

DASHBOARDS

NURSE STAFFING

REDUCING MEDICATION ERRORS

PEER REVIEW

## Risk Management

NURSING'S ROLE IN RISK MANAGEMENT

INCIDENT REPORTS

EXAMPLES OF RISK

ROOT CAUSE ANALYSIS

ROLE OF THE NURSE MANAGER

CREATING A BLAME-FREE ENVIRONMENT

## Learning Outcomes

*After completing this chapter, you will be able to:*

1. Describe how total quality management, continuous quality management, Six Sigma, Lean Six Sigma, and DMAIC address quality.

2. Describe national efforts to improve the quality of health care.

3. Explain how evidence-based practice, electronic medical records, and dashboards can improve quality.

4. Point out how nurses are involved in reducing risks.

5. Discuss how to create a blame-free environment.

## Key Terms

Continuous quality improvement (CQI)
Dashboards
DMAIC
Incident reports
Indicator
Just culture

Outcome standards
Lean Six Sigma
Peer review
Process standards
Quality management
Reportable incident
Risk management

Root cause analysis
Six Sigma
Standards
Structure standards
Total quality management (TQM)

In today's highly competitive health care environment, each member of the health care organization must be accountable for the quality and cost of health care. Concern about quality gained national attention after publication of the Institute of Medicine's (IOM) reports on medical errors in 1999 (IOM, 1999) and their later recommendations for health professionals' education (IOM, 2003). Additionally, concern about cost continues unabated. Both quality and cost containment are found in the concept of total quality management, which has evolved into a model of continuous quality improvement designed to improve system and process performance. Risk management is integrated within a quality management program.

# Quality Management

**Quality management** moved health care from a mode of identifying failed standards, problems, and problem people to a proactive organization in which problems are prevented and ways to improve care and quality of care are sought. This paradigm shift involves all in the organization and promotes problem solving and experimentation.

A quality management program is based on an integrated system of information and accountability. Clinical information systems can provide the data needed to enable organizations to track activities and outcomes. For example, data from clinical information systems can be used to track patient wait times from admitting to outpatient testing to admission in an inpatient care unit. Delays in the process can be identified so appropriate staff and resources are available at the right time to decrease delays and increase efficiency and patient satisfaction. Methods can be devised to discover problems in the system without blaming the "sharp end," the last individual in the chain to act (e.g., the nurse gives a wrong medication). The system must be accepted and used by the entire staff.

## Total Quality Management

**Total quality management (TQM)** is a management philosophy that emphasizes a commitment to excellence throughout the organization. The creation of Dr. W. Edwards Deming, TQM was adopted by the Japanese after World War II and helped transform their industrial development. Dr. Deming based his system on principles of quality management that were originally applied to improve quality and performance in the manufacturing industry. They are now widely used to improve quality and customer satisfaction in a number of service industries, including health care.

### TQM Characteristics

Four core characteristics of total quality management are:

- Customer/client focus
- Total organizational involvement
- Use of quality tools and statistics for measurement
- Key processes for improvement identified

**Customer/Client Focus.**   An important theme of quality management is to address the needs of both internal and external customers. Internal customers include employees and departments within the organization, such as the laboratory, admitting office, and environmental services. External customers of a health care organization include patients, visitors, physicians, managed-care organizations, insurance companies, and regulatory agencies, such as the Joint Commission, which accredits health care organizations, and public health departments.

Under the principles of TQM, nurses must know who the customers are and endeavor to meet their needs. Providing flexible schedules for employees, adjusting routines for A.M. care to meet the needs of patients, extending clinic hours beyond 5 P.M., and putting infant changing tables in restrooms are some examples. Putting the customer first requires creative and innovative methods to meet the ever-changing needs of internal and external customers.

**Total Organizational Involvement.**   The goal of total quality management is to involve all employees and empower them with the responsibility to make a difference in the quality of

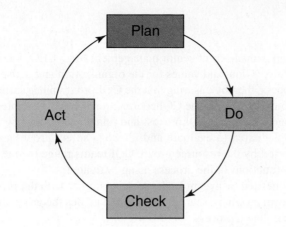

**Figure 6-1** ●
PDCA cycle.

service they provide. This means all employees must have knowledge of the TQM philosophy as it relates to their job and the overall goals and mission of the organization. Knowledge of the TQM process breaks down barriers between departments. The phrase "That's not my job" is eliminated. Departments work together as a team. On occasion, nursing personnel might clean a bed for a new admission from the emergency room or an administrator might transport a patient to the radiology department. Sharing processes across departments and patient care functions increases teamwork, productivity, and patient positive outcomes.

**Use of Quality Tools and Statistics for Measurement.**   A common management adage is, "You can't manage what you can't (or don't) measure." There are many tools, formats, and designs that can be used to build knowledge, make decisions, and improve quality. Tools for data analysis and display can be used to identify areas for process and quality improvement, and then to benchmark the progress of improvements. Deming applied the scientific method to the concept of TQM to develop a model he called the PDCA cycle (Plan, Do, Check, Act) depicted in Figure 6-1.

**Identification of Key Processes for Improvement.**   All activities performed in an organization can be described in terms of processes. Processes within a health care setting can be:

- Systems related (e.g., admitting, discharging, and transferring patients)
- Clinical (e.g., administering medications, managing pain)
- Managerial (e.g., risk management and performance evaluations).

   Processes can be very complex and involve multidisciplinary or interdepartmental actions. Processes involving multiple departments must be investigated in detail by members from each department involved in the activity so that they can proactively seek opportunities to reduce waste and inefficiencies and develop ways to improve performance and promote positive outcomes.

## Continuous Quality Improvement

TQM is the overall philosophy, whereas **continuous quality improvement (CQI)** is used to improve quality and performance. TQM and CQI often are used synonymously. In health care organizations, CQI is the process used to investigate systematically ways to improve patient care. As the name implies, continuous quality improvement is a never-ending endeavor (Hedges, 2006).

   CQI means more than just meeting standards and thresholds or solving problems. It involves evaluation, actions, and a mind-set to strive constantly for excellence. This concept is sometimes difficult to grasp because patient care involves the synchronization of activities in multiple departments. Therefore, the importance of developing and implementing a well-thought-out process is key to a successful CQI implementation.

   There are four major players in the CQI process:

- Resource group
- Coordinator

- Team leader
- Team

The resource group is made up of senior management (e.g., CEO, vice presidents). It establishes overall CQI policy, vision, and values for the organization and actively involves the board of directors in this process, thereby ensuring that the CQI program has sufficient emphasis and is provided with the resources needed. The CQI coordinator is often appointed by the CEO to provide day-to-day management of the CQI process and related activities (e.g., training programs).

CQI teams are designated to evaluate and improve select processes. They are formally established and supported by the resource group. CQI teams range in size from 5 to 10 people, representing all major functions of the process being evaluated.

Each CQI team is headed by a team leader who is familiar with the process being evaluated. The leader organizes team meetings, sets the agenda, and guides the group through the discussion, evaluation, and implementation process.

## Components of Quality Management

A comprehensive quality management program includes:

- *A comprehensive quality management plan.* A quality management plan is a systematic method to design, measure, assess, and improve organizational performance. Using a multidisciplinary approach, this plan identifies processes and systems that represent the goals and mission of the organization, identifies customers, and specifies opportunities for improvement. Critical paths, which are described in Chapter 3, are an example of a quality management plan. Critical paths identify expected outcomes within a specific time frame. Then variances are tracked and accounted for.
- *Set standards for benchmarking.* **Standards** are written statements that define a level of performance or a set of conditions determined to be acceptable by some authorities. Standards relate to three major dimensions of quality care:
  a. Structure
  b. Process
  c. Outcome

**Structure standards** relate to the physical environment, organization, and management of an organization. **Process standards** are those connected with the actual delivery of care. Outcome standards involve the end results of care that has been given.

An **indicator** is a tool used to measure the performance of structure, process, and outcome standards. It is measurable, objective, and based on current knowledge. Once indicators are identified, benchmarking, or comparing performance using identified quality indicators across institutions or disciplines, is the key to quality improvement.

In nursing, both generic and specific standards are available from the American Nurses Association and specialty organizations; however, each organization and each patient care area must designate standards specific to the patient population being served. These standards are the foundation on which all other measures of quality are based.

An example of a standard is, "Every patient will have a written care plan within 12 hours of admission."

- *Performance appraisals.* Based on requirements of the job, employees are evaluated on their performance. This feedback is essential for employees to be professionally accountable. (See Chapter 18 for more on performance appraisals.)
- *A focus on intradisciplinary assessment and improvement.* There will always be a need for groups to assess, analyze, and improve their own performance. Methods to assess performance should, however, focus on the CQI philosophy, which involves group or intradisciplinary performance. Peer review, discussed later in the chapter, is an example of intradisciplinary assessment.

- *A focus on interdisciplinary assessment and improvement.* Multidisciplinary, patient-focused teamwork emphasizing collaboration, communication, coordination, and integration of care is the core of CQI in health care. It is important not to disband departmental quality functions, such as patient satisfaction, utilization review, or infection control, but rather to refocus information on improving the process.

Resources are used to collect data, such as the number of postoperative infections or the number of return clinic visits, to guide the decision-making process. Throughout the evaluation and implementation process, the team's focus is the patient. Implementation is continually evaluated using a patient satisfaction survey, which is just one of the methods used to monitor nursing care. For example, some organizations follow up outpatient surgery clients with direct phone calls from nursing staff to ensure patients understand discharge instructions and that pain was controlled following discharge. Any potential complications are referred to the surgeon.

## Six Sigma

**Six Sigma** is another quality management program that uses, primarily, quantitative data to monitor progress. Six Sigma is a *measure*, a *goal*, and a *system of management*.

- *As a measure.* Sigma is the Greek letter—σ—for standard, meaning how much performance varies from a standard. This is similar to how CQI monitors results against an outcome measure.
- *As a goal.* One goal might be accuracy. How many times, for example, is the right medication given in the right amount, to the right patient, at the right time, by the right route?
- *As a management system.* Compared to other quality management systems, Six Sigma involves management to a greater extent in monitoring performance and ensuring favorable results.

The system has six themes:

- Customer (patient) focus
- Data driven
- Process emphasis
- Proactive management
- Boundaryless collaboration
- Aim for perfection; tolerate failure.

The first three themes are similar to other quality management programs. The focus is on the object of the service; in nursing's case, this is the patient. Data provide the evidence of results, and the emphasis is on the processes used in the system.

The latter three themes, however, differ from other programs. Management is actively involved and boundaries are breached (e.g., the disconnect between departments). More radically, Six Sigma tolerates failure (a necessary condition for creativity) while striving for perfection.

## Lean Six Sigma

**Lean Six Sigma** focuses on improving process flow and eliminating waste. Waste occurs when the organization provides more resources than are required. Data driven, Lean Six Sigma focuses on identifying steps that have little or no value to the care and cause unnecessary delays. Furthermore, the method strives to eliminate variations in care and improve efficiencies and effectiveness. Because the goal of Lean Six Sigma is to identify and reduce waste, it provides tools that can be used with a Six Sigma management system.

Studies have shown Lean Six Sigma to be effective in reducing inappropriate hospital stays, improving the quality of care and reducing costs at the same time (Yamamoto et al., 2010).

**Figure 6-2** ●
DMAIC: The Six Sigma Method. Adapted from DMAIC tools: Six Sigma training tools. Retrieved October 21, 2011, from www.dmaictools.com

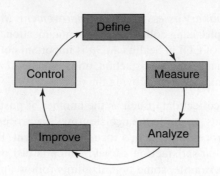

In addition, when the method was used in one hospital, researchers found that a collaborative effort improved the care of inpatient diabetic patients (Niemeijer et al., 2010).

### DMAIC Method

**DMAIC** is a Six-Sigma process improvement method (as shown in Figure 6-2). Steps in the method are:

- Define what measures will indicate success
- Measure baseline performance
- Analyze results
- Improve performance
- Control and sustain performance (DMAIC Tools: Six Sigma Training Tools, 2011)

TQM, CQI, Six Sigma, Lean Six Sigma, and DMAIC are quantifiable systems that measure performance against set standards. The goal is to improve the quality of health care. In addition, other efforts to improve the quality of care are ongoing.

## Improving the Quality of Care

### National Initiatives

The National Quality Forum is a nonprofit organization that strives to improve the quality of health care by building consensus on performance goals and standards for measuring and reporting them (National Quality Forum, 2011). Additionally, the Institute of Healthcare Improvement (IHI) offers programs to assist organizations in improving the quality of care they provide (IHI, 2011). Their goals are:

- No needless deaths
- No needless pain or suffering
- No helplessness in those served or serving
- No unwanted waiting
- No waste

Joint Commission, hospitals' accrediting body, has adopted mandatory national patient safety goals (Joint Commission, 2011). They charge hospitals to:

- Identify patients correctly
- Improve staff communication
- Use medicines safely
- Prevent infection
- Check patient medicines
- Identify patient safety risks
- Prevent mistakes in surgery

Joint Commission collects data on 57 inpatient measures; 31 of these are currently made public with others scheduled to be publicly reported soon (Chassin et al., 2010). The focus is now on maximizing health benefits to patients. They recommend that quality measures be based on four criteria:

1. The measure must be based on research that shows improved outcomes. More than one research study is required for documentation.

2. Reports document that evidence-based practice has been given. Aspirin following an acute myocardial infarction is an example.

3. The process documents desired outcome. Appropriately administering medications is an example.

4. The process has minimal or no unintended adverse effects (Chassin et al., 2010)

Measured standards are used extensively in industrial settings to reveal errors. However, the same cannot be said when measuring human behavior, which can vary and still be effective. Also, if the organization embraces these systems to such an extent that all variance is discouraged, then innovation is also suppressed. Improvement in quality is sacrificed at the expense of innovative ideas and processes; organizations fail to allow input, become stagnant, and cease to be effective. This is the danger of all living systems that depend on outside input for survival. This is not to say that quality systems are not essential. They are. Organizations must find ways to foster creativity and innovation without compromising quality management.

## How Cost Affects Quality

Quality measures can also reduce costs. Wasted resources is an example. These include the time nurses spend looking for missing supplies or lab results, the costs of agency nurses because of unfilled positions, and delays in patient discharge due to a lack of coordination or an adverse event (e.g., medication error).

Using the Institute for Healthcare Improvement (2009) project, Transforming Care at the Bedside (TCAB), Unruh, Agrawal, and Hassmiller (2011) found that improving quality reduces costs. Specifically, the researchers report that in a three-year period, RN overtime was reduced, RN turnover was lowered, and fewer patients suffered falls.

## Evidence-Based Practice

Evidence-based practice (EBP) suggests that using research to decide on clinical treatments would improve quality of care, and that might be the case. Barriers, however, prevent EBP from being widely used by nurses. Such barriers, consistent across settings, include lack of time, autonomy over their practice, ability to find and assess evidence, and support from administration (Brown et al., 2008).

Furthermore, EBP is most reliable when the research study includes a rigorous design (Hader, 2010), and when more than one study has confirmed the results (Chassin et al., 2010). These are not easily surmountable hurdles due to the fast-paced clinical environment and the barriers mentioned above.

## Electronic Medical Records

Similar to the argument that EBP improves quality, electronic medical records (EMR) should do so as well. Instant access to identical records should improve accuracy and speed communication among care providers. Kazley and Ozcan (2008), however, found limited correlation between the use of EMR and 10 quality indicators in their study of more than 4,000 hospitals in the U.S. In a review of the literature, Chan, Fowles, and Weiner (2010) could not link quality indicators and EMR. Cebul (2008), however, did find direct correlation between the use of EMR and the quality of care provided to diabetic patients. EMR use, is expected to expand and will provide more data for comparison with quality.

## Dashboards

**Dashboards** are electronic tools that can provide real-time data or retrospective data, known as a scorecard. Both are useful in assessing quality. Ease of access and the visual appearance of the dashboard make its use more likely. Dashboards may report on hospital census or patient satisfaction results, for example. Dashboards are also useful to guide staffing and match staffing with patient outcomes (Frith, Anderson, & Sewell, 2010) and to provide accurate financial data on nurse staffing and quality (Anderson, Frith, & Caspers, 2011). As technology advances, widespread use of dashboards to aggregate data and guide decision making is expected (Hyun et al., 2008).

## Nurse Staffing

Evidence is growing that increased nurse staffing results in better patient outcomes (Frith, Tseng, & Anderson, 2008; Anderson, Frith, & Caspers, 2011). Earlier studies found that a higher RN-to-patient ratio resulted in reduced patient mortality, fewer infections, and shortened lengths of stay (Reeves, 2007). Needleman (2008) agrees that increasing the level of nurse staffing improves quality, but asserts that higher staffing levels also increase costs.

## Reducing Medication Errors

Ever since Medicare discontinued payment for hospital-based errors, pressure has increased for hospitals to prevent costly errors. In 2009, the federal government passed the Health Information Technology for Economic and Clinical Health Act (HITECH). The purpose of HITECH is to stimulate technology use in health care, including improving technology for medication administration.

Studies have shown that when nurses are interrupted during medication preparation, a 25 percent rate of injury-causing errors are made (Westbrook et al., 2010). One strategy to alert others that a nurse should not be interrupted is the use of a sash or vest that the nurse dons to prepare medications (Heath & Heath, 2010).

Other strategies to reduce medication errors include computerized prescriber order entry (CPOE), electronic medication administration record (eMAR), remote order review by pharmacists, automated dispensing at the bedside, bar code administration, smart pumps, and unit doses ready to be administered (Federico, 2010). Future strategies include radio frequency identification and electronic reconciliation, both expensive technologies currently being tested (Federico, 2010).

## Peer Review

In addition to its value for self-evaluation and performance appraisal (Davis, Capozzoli, & Parks, 2009), **peer review** can be used to identify clinical standards of practice that improve the quality of care. Used for quality improvement, the peer review process is not intended to serve as a performance appraisal nor to be punitive. The purpose is to review the incident, determine if clinical standards were met or not, and to propose an action plan to prevent a future incident.

The peer review process is appropriate in the following situations:

- An adverse patient outcome has occurred.
- A serious risk or injury to a patient occurred.
- A failure to rescue incident occurred (Fujita et al., 2009).

A shared governance structure facilitates the peer review process, fostering peer-to-peer accountability (Fujita et al., 2009). Furthermore, the process can help determine if a breach in practice is an isolated incident or a trend occurring across a unit or throughout the organization. In a shared governance environment, unit councils or the nursing council can address unit-wide or system problems. To aggregate trends, peer review cases can be categorized as:

- Appropriate care with no adverse outcomes
- Appropriate care with adverse/unexpected outcomes
- Inappropriate care with no adverse outcomes
- Inappropriate care with adverse/unexpected outcomes (Hitchings et al., 2008)

# Risk Management

**Risk management** is a component of quality management, but its purpose is to identify, analyze, and evaluate risks and then to develop a plan for reducing the frequency and severity of accidents and injuries. Risk management is a continuous daily program of detection, education, and intervention.

A risk management program involves all departments of the organization. It must be an organization-wide program, with the board of directors' approval and input from all departments. The program must have high-level commitment, including that of the chief executive officer and the chief nurse.

A risk management program:

1. Identifies potential risks for accident, injury, or financial loss. Formal and informal communication with all organizational departments and inspection of facilities are essential to identifying problem areas.

2. Reviews current organization-wide monitoring systems (incident reports, audits, committee minutes, oral complaints, patient questionnaires), evaluates completeness, and determines additional systems needed to provide the factual data essential for risk management control.

3. Analyzes the frequency, severity, and causes of general categories and specific types of incidents causing injury or adverse outcomes to patients. To plan risk intervention strategies, it is necessary to estimate the outcomes associated with the various types of incidents.

4. Reviews and appraises safety and risk aspects of patient care procedures and new programs.

5. Monitors laws and codes related to patient safety, consent, and care.

6. Eliminates or reduces risks as much as possible.

7. Reviews the work of other committees to determine potential liability and recommend prevention or corrective action. Examples of such committees are infection, medical audit, safety/security, pharmacy, nursing audit, and productivity.

8. Identifies needs for patient, family, and personnel education suggested by all of the foregoing and implements the appropriate educational program.

9. Evaluates the results of a risk management program.

10. Provides periodic reports to administration, medical staff, and the board of directors.

## Nursing's Role in Risk Management

In the organizational setting, nursing is the one department involved in patient care 24 hours a day; nursing personnel are therefore critical to the success of a risk management program. The chief nursing administrator must be committed to the program. Her or his attitude will influence the staff and their participation. After all, it is the staff, with their daily patient contact, who actually implement a risk management program.

High-risk areas in health care fall into five general categories:

- Medication errors
- Complications from diagnostic or treatment procedures
- Falls
- Patient or family dissatisfaction with care
- Refusal of treatment or refusal to sign consent for treatment

Nursing is involved in all areas, but the medical staff may be primarily responsible in cases involving refusal of treatment or consent to treatment.

Medical records and incidence reports serve to document organizational, nurse, and physician accountability. For every reported occurrence, however, many more are unreported. If records are faulty, inadequate, or omitted, the organization is more likely to be sued and more likely to lose. **Incident reports** are used to analyze the severity, frequency, and causes of occurrences within the five risk categories. Such analysis serves as a basis for intervention.

## Incident Reports

Accurate and comprehensive reporting on both the patient's chart and in the incident report is essential to protect the organization and caregivers from litigation. Incident reporting is often the nurse's responsibility. Reluctance to report incidents is usually due to fear of the consequences. This fear can be alleviated by:

- Holding staff education programs that emphasize objective reporting
- Omitting inflammatory words and judgmental statements
- Having a clear understanding that the purposes of the incident reporting process are documentation and follow-up
- Never using the report, under any circumstances, for disciplinary action.

Nursing colleagues and nurse managers should not berate another employee for an incident, and never in front of other staff members, patients, or patients' family members. Peer review analysis, however, is a valuable tool to evaluate incidents (Hitchings et al., 2008).

A **reportable incident** should include any unexpected or unplanned occurrence that affects or could potentially affect a patient, family member, or staff. The report is only as effective as the form on which it is reported, so attention should be paid to the adequacy of the form as well as to the data required.

Reporting incidents involves the following steps:

1. *Discovery.* Nurses, physicians, patients, families, or any employee or volunteer may report actual or potential risk.

2. *Notification.* The risk manager receives the completed incident form within 24 hours after the incident. A telephone call may be made earlier to hasten follow-up in the event of a major incident.

3. *Investigation.* The risk manager or representative investigates the incident immediately.

4. *Consultation.* The risk manager consults with the referring physician, risk management committee member, or both to obtain additional information and guidance.

5. *Action.* The risk manager should clarify any misinformation to the patient or family, explaining exactly what happened. The patient should be referred to the appropriate source for help and, if needed, be assured that care for any necessary service will be provided free of charge.

6. *Recording.* The risk manager should be sure that all records, including incident reports, follow-up, and actions taken, if any, are filed in a central depository.

## Examples of Risk

The following are some examples of actual events in the various risk categories.

### Medication Errors

A reportable incident occurs when a medication or fluid is omitted, the wrong medication or fluid is administered, or a medication is given to the wrong patient, at the wrong time, in the wrong dosage, or by the wrong route. Here are some examples.

> *Patient A.* Weight was transcribed incorrectly from emergency room sheet. Medication dose was calculated on incorrect weight; therefore, patient was given double the dose

required. Error discovered after first dose and corrected. Second dose omitted per physician's order.

*Patient B.* Tegretol dosage written in Medex as "Tegretol 100 mg chewable tab—50 mg po BID." Tegretol 100 mg given po at 1400. Meds checked at 1430 and error noted. 50 mg Tegretol should have been given two times per day to total 100mg in 24 hours. Doctor notified. Second dose held.

*Patient C.* During rounds at 3:30 P.M. found .9% sodium chloride at 75 mLs per hour hanging. Order was written for D5W to run at 75 mLs per hour. Fluids last checked at 2:00 P.M. Changed to correct fluid. Doctor notified.

## Diagnostic Procedure

Any incident occurring before, during, or after such procedures as blood sample stick, biopsy, X-ray examination, lumbar puncture, or other invasive procedure is categorized as a diagnostic procedure incident.

*Patient A.* When I checked the IV site, I saw that it was red and swollen. For this reason, I discontinued the IV. When removing the tape, I noted a small area of skin breakdown where the tape had been. There was also a small knot on the medial aspect of the left antecubital above the IV insertion site. Doctor notified. Wound dressed.

*Patient B.* Patient found on the floor after lumbar puncture. Right side rail down. Examined by a physician, BP 120/80, T 98.6, P 72, R 18. No injury noted on exam. Patient returned to bed, side rail placed up. Will continue to monitor patient condition.

## Medical–Legal Incident

If a patient or family refuses treatment as ordered and prescribed or refuses to sign consent forms, the situation is categorized as a medical-legal incident.

*Patient A.* After a visit from a member of the clergy, patient indicated he was no longer in need of medical attention and asked to be discharged. Physician called. Doctor explained potential side effects if treatment were discontinued to patient. Patient continued to ask for discharge. Doctor explained "against medical advice" (AMA) form. Patient signed AMA form and left at 1300 without medications.

*Patient B.* Patient refused to sign consent for bone marrow biopsy. States side effects not understood. Doctor reviewed reasons for test and side effects three different times. Doctor informed the patient that without consent he could not perform the test. Offered to call in another physician for second opinion. Patient agreed. After doctor left, patient signed consent form.

## Patient or Family Dissatisfaction with Care

When a patient or family indicates general dissatisfaction with care and the situation cannot be or has not been resolved, then an incident report is filed.

*Patient A.* Mother complained that she had found child saturated with urine every morning (she arrived around 0800). Explained to mother that diapers and linen are changed at 0600 when 0600 feedings and meds are given. Patient's back, buttocks, and perineal areas are free of skin breakdown. Parents continue to be distressed. Discussed with primary nurse.

*Patient B.* Mr. Smith appeared very angry. Greeted me at the door complaining that his wife had not been treated properly in our emergency room the night before. Wanted to speak to someone from administration. Was unable to reach the administrator on call. Suggested Mr. Smith call administrator in the morning. Mr. Smith thanked me for my time and assured me that he would call the administrator the next day.

## Root Cause Analysis

**Root cause analysis** is a method to work backwards through an event to examine every action that led to the error or event that occurred; it is a complicated process. A simplified method to conduct an event analysis follows:

- Patient—what patient factors contributed to the event?
- Personnel—what personnel actions contributed to the event?
- Policies—are there policies for this type of event?
- Procedures—are there standard procedures for this type of event?
- Place—did the workplace environment contribute to the event?
- Politics—did institutional or outside politics play a role in the event? (Weiss, 2009)

Complaints have emerged, however, that the method uses too many resources for too few improvements (Wu, Lipshutz, & Pronovost, 2008). The authors posit that most organizations try to drill down to a single cause, ignoring system failures. Furthermore, they insist that corrective action is seldom taken due to lack of resources, professional disagreements, and absence of management support. They recommend improving system-wide dysfunctions and examining the broader health care environment to find improvements needed across hospitals.

## Role of the Nurse Manager

The nurse manager plays a key role in the success of any risk management program. Nurse managers can reduce risk by helping their staff view health and illness from the patient's perspective. Usually, the staff's understanding of quality differs from the patient's expectations and perceptions. By understanding the meaning of the course of illness to the patient and the family, the nurse will manage risk better because that understanding can enable the nurse to individualize patient care. This individualized attention produces respect and, in turn, reduces risk.

A patient incident or a patient's or family's expression of dissatisfaction regarding care indicates not only some slippage in quality of care but also potential liability. A distraught, dissatisfied, complaining patient is a high risk; a satisfied patient or family is a low risk. A risk management or liability control program should therefore emphasize a personal approach. Many claims are filed because of a breakdown in communication between the health care provider and the patient. In many instances, after an incident or bad outcome, a quick visit or call from an organization's representative to the patient or family can soothe tempers and clarify misinformation.

In the examples given, prompt attention and care by the nurse manager protected the patients involved and may have averted a potential liability claim. Once an incident has occurred, the important factors in successful risk management are:

- Recognition of the incident
- Quick follow-up and action
- Personal contact
- Immediate restitution (where appropriate)

The concerns of most patients' and their families' concerns can and should be handled at the unit level. When that first line of communication breaks down, however, the nurse manager needs a resource—usually the risk manager or nursing service administrator.

### Handling Complaints

Handling a patient's or family member's complaints stemming from an incident can be very difficult. These confrontations are often highly emotional; the patient or family member must be calmed down, yet have their concerns satisfied. Sometimes just an opportunity to release the anger or emotion is all that is needed.

The first step is to listen to the person to hear concerns and to help defuse the situation. Arguing or interrupting only increases the person's anger or emotion. After the patient or family member has had his or her say, the nurse manager can then attempt to solve the problem by asking what is expected in the form of a solution. The nurse manager should ensure that immediate patient care and safety needs are met, collect all facts relevant to the incident, and if possible, comply with the patient or family member's suggested resolution.

Sometimes, a simple apology from a staff member or moving a patient to a different room on the unit can resolve a difficult situation. If the patient and/or family member's requested resolution exceeds the nurse manager's authority, the nurse manager should seek the assistance of a nurse administrator or hospital legal counsel. Offering vague solutions (e.g., "everything will be taken care of") may only lead to more problems later on if expectations as to solution and timing differ.

All incidents must be properly documented. Information on the incident form should be detailed and include all the factors relating to the incident, as demonstrated in the previous examples. The documentation in the chart, however, should be only a statement of the facts and of the patient's physical response; no reference to the incident report should be made, nor should words such as *error* or *inappropriate* be used.

When a patient receives 100 mg of Demerol instead of 50 mg as ordered, the proper documentation in the chart is, "100 mg of Demerol administered. Physician notified." The remainder of the documentation should include any reaction the patient has to the dosage, such as "Patient's vital signs unchanged." If there is an adverse reaction, a follow-up note should be written in the chart, giving an update of the patient's status. A note related to the patient's reaction should be written as frequently as the status changes and should continue until the patient returns to his or her previous status.

The chart must never be used as a tool for disciplinary comments, action, or expressions of anger. Notes such as, "Incident would never have occurred if Doctor X had written the correct order in the first place" or "This carelessness is inexcusable" or "Paged the doctor eight times, as usual, no reply" are wholly inappropriate and serve no meaningful purpose. Carelessness and incorrect orders do indeed cause errors and incidents, but the place to address and resolve these issues is in the risk management committee or in the nurse manager's office, not on the patient chart.

Handling a complaint without punishing a staff member is a delicate situation. The manager must determine what happened in order to prevent another occurrence, but using an incident report for discipline might result in fewer or erroneous incident reports in the future. Learn how one manager handled a situation of this kind in Case Study 6-1.

### A Caring Attitude

With employees, the nurse manager sets the tone that contributes to a safe and low-risk environment. One of the most important ways to reduce risk is to instill a sense of confidence in both patients and families by emphasizing and recognizing that they will receive personalized attention and that their needs will be attended to with competence. This confidence is created environmentally and professionally.

Examples of environmental factors include cleanliness, attention to patients' privacy, promptly responding to patients' and family members' requests, an orderly looking unit, and engaging in minimal social conversations in front of patients. One example of portraying professional confidence is to provide patients and families with the name of the person in charge. A sincere visit by that person is reassuring. In addition, a thorough orientation creates independence for the patient and confidence in an efficient unit.

The nurse manager needs to foster the attitude that any mistake that does occur is perceived as an opportunity to improve a system or a process rather than to punish an individual. If the nurse manager has developed a patient-focused atmosphere in which patients believe their best interests are a priority, the potential for risk will be reduced.

### Creating a Blame-Free Environment

The health care environment is known to be a blame culture that "is a major source of medical errors and poor quality of patient care" (Khatri, Brown, & Hicks, 2009, p. 320). Such a culture inhibits reporting of inadequate practice, underreporting of adverse events, and inattention to possible safety problems.

## CASE STUDY 6-1

### RISK MANAGEMENT

Yasmine Dubois is the nurse manager for the cardiac catheterization lab and special procedures unit in a suburban hospital. The hospital has an excellent reputation for its cardiac care program, including the use of cutting-edge technology. The cath lab utilizes a specialized computer application that records the case for the nursing staff, requiring little handwritten documentation at the end of a procedure.

Last month, a 56-year-old woman was brought from the ER to the cath lab at approximately 1900 for placement of a stent in her left anterior descending coronary artery. During the procedure, the heart wall was perforated. The patient coded and was taken in critical condition to the OR, where she died during surgery.

Two days following the incident, the patient's husband requested a review of his wife's medical records. During his review, he pointed out to the medical records clerk that the documentation from the cath lab stated that his wife ". . . tolerated the procedure well and was taken in satisfactory condition to the recovery area." The documentation was signed, dated, and timed by Elizabeth Clark, RN. The medical records director notified the hospital's risk manager of the error. The risk manager investigated the incident and determined that Elizabeth Clark's charting was in error.

Following her meeting with the risk manager, Yasmine met with Elizabeth to discuss the incident. She showed Elizabeth a copy of the cath lab report. Elizabeth asked Yasmine if she could have the chart from medical records so she could correct her mistake. Yasmine informed Elizabeth that she couldn't correct her charting at this point in time. But, she could, however, write an addendum to the chart, with today's date and time, to clarify the documentation. Yasmine also told Elizabeth that the addendum would be reviewed by the risk manager and the hospital's attorney prior to inclusion in the chart.

To ensure compliance with the hospital's documentation standards and to determine if Elizabeth or any other cath lab nurse had committed any similar charting errors, Yasmine requested charts for all patients in the past 12 months who had been sent to surgery from the cath lab due to complications during a procedure. She conducted a retrospective audit and determined that this had been an isolated incident.

A **just culture**, in contrast, allows for reporting of errors without fear of undue retribution (Gorzeman, 2008). Khatri, Brown, & Hicks (2009) suggest that transitioning to a just culture does more than improve reporting mechanisms or initiate training programs. A just culture provides an environment in which employees can question policies and practices, express concerns, and admit mistakes without fear of retribution. A just culture requires organizational commitment, managerial involvement, employee empowerment, an accountability system, and a reporting system (Gorzeman, 2008).

Accountability for errors, however, must be maintained (Gorzeman, 2008). Errors can be categorized as:

- Human errors, such as unintentional behaviors that may cause an adverse consequence
- At-risk behaviors, such as unsafe habits, negligence, carelessness
- Reckless behaviors, such as conscious disregard for standards

A just culture is prepared to handle incidents involving human error. At-risk or reckless behaviors, however, are not tolerated.

Managing and improving quality requires ongoing attention to system-wide processes and individual actions. The nurse manager is in a key position to identify problems and encourage a culture of safety and quality.

## What You Know Now

- Total quality management is a philosophy committed to excellence throughout the organization.
- Continuous quality improvement is a process to improve quality and performance.
- Six Sigma is another quality management program that uses measures, has goals, and is a management system.
- Lean Six Sigma provides tools to improve flow and eliminate waste.
- DMAIC is a Six Sigma process improvement method to define, measure, analyze, improve, and control performance.
- A culture of safety and quality permeates efforts at the national level.
- Cost may increase or decrease with quality initiatives.
- Evidence-based practice, electronic medical records, and dashboards can be used to improve and monitor quality.
- Reducing medication errors is a priority for health care organizations and policy makers.
- A risk management program focuses on reducing accidents and injuries and intervening if either occurs.
- A caring attitude and prompt attention to complaints help to reduce risk.
- A just culture is more likely to encourage reporting of adverse events, including near misses, as well as point out unsafe practices.

## Tools for Managing and Improving Quality

1. Remember: Quality management is a system. When something goes wrong, it is usually due to a flaw in the system.
2. Become familiar with standards and outcome measures and use them to guide and improve your practice.
3. Strive for perfection, but be prepared to tolerate failure in order to encourage innovation.
4. Be sure that performance appraisals and incident reports are not used for discipline but rather are the bases for improvements to the system and/or development of individuals.
5. Remind yourself and your colleagues that a caring attitude is the best prevention of problems.

Following an incident:

1. Meet with the risk manager and hospital attorney to review documentation and determine which staff will be interviewed regarding the incident.
2. Provide any requested information to administration in a timely manner.
3. Audit documentation and processes to determine if an incident is part of a pattern or an isolated incident.
4. Provide the results of any audits or discussions with staff to appropriate administrators.
5. Educate staff as appropriate.
6. Determine if disciplinary action is required.
7. Follow up with risk management, nursing administration, and human resources as appropriate.
8. Continue to cooperate with the hospital attorney if the incident results in litigation.

## Questions to Challenge You

1. Imagine that an organization is debating among several quality management programs. What would you recommend? Why?
2. Do you know what standards and outcome measures are used in your clinical setting? How are data handled? Are they shared with employees?
3. What comparable groups, both internal and external, are used for benchmarking performance in your organization?
4. Universities also use benchmarking. What institutions does your college or university use to benchmark its performance? Find out.
5. Have you, a family member, or a friend ever had a serious problem in a health care organization that resulted in injury? What was the outcome? Is this how you would have handled it? What will you do in the future in a similar situation?
6. Have you or anyone you know ever made a mistake in a clinical setting? What happened? Would you assess the organization as a blame-free environment?

**Pearson Nursing Student Resources**

Find additional review materials at
**www.nursing.pearsonhighered.com**

Prepare for success with additional NCLEX®-style practice
questions, interactive assignments and activities, Web links,
animations and videos, and more!

# References

Anderson, E. F., Frith, K. H., &
Caspers, B. (2011). Linking
economics and quality:
Developing an evidence-
based nurse staffing tool.
*Nursing Administration
Quarterly, 35*(1), 53–60.

Brown, C. E., Wickline, M. A.,
Ecoff, L., & Glaser, D.
(2008). Nursing practice,
knowledge, attitudes and
perceived barriers to
evidence-based practice
at an academic medical
center. *Journal of Advanced
Nursing, 64*(4), 371–381.

Cebul, R. D. (2008). Using
electronic medical records
to measure and improve
performance. *Transactions
of the American Clinical
and Climatological Asso-
ciation, 119*, 65–76.

Chan, K. S., Fowles, J. B., &
Weiner, J. P. (2010).
Electronic medical records
and the reliability and
validity of quality mea-
sures: A review of the literature. *Medical Care
Research and Review,
67*(5), 503–527.

Chassin, M. R., Loeb, J. M.,
Schmaltz, S. P., & Wachter,
R. M. (2010). Accountability measures: Using mea-
surement to promote quality
improvement. *The New
England Journal of Medi-
cine, 363*(7), 683–688.

Davis, K. K., Capozzoli,
J., & Parks, J. (2009).
Implementing peer review:
Guidelines for managers
and staff. *Nursing Administration Quarterly, 33*(3),
251–257.

DMAIC tools: Six sigma
training tools. (2011).
Retrieved October 21,
2011 from http://www.
dmaictools.com

Federico, F. (2010). An overview
of error-reduction options.
*Nursing Management,
41*(9), 14–16.

Frith, K. H., Anderson, F., &
Sewell, J. P. (2010).
Assessing and selecting
data for a nursing services
dashboard. *Journal of
Nursing Administration,
40*(1), 10–16.

Frith, K. H., Tseng, R., &
Anderson, F. (2008). The
effect of nurse staffing on
patient outcomes in acute
care hospitals. *2008 Mini
Grant Proceedings.*
Huntsville, AL: University
of Alabama in Huntsville,
1–10.

Fujita, L. Y., Harris, M., Johnson,
K. G., Irvine, N. P., &
Latimer, R. W. (2009).
Nursing peer review:
Integrating a model in a
shared governance environ-
ment. *Journal of Nursing
Administration, 39*(12),
524–530.

Gorzeman, J. (2008). Balancing
just culture with regula-
tory standards. *Nursing
Administration Quarterly,
32*(4), 308–311.

Hader, R. (2010). The evident
that isn't . . . interpreting
research. *Nursing Management, 41*(9), 23–26.

Heath, C. & Heath, D. (2010).
*Switch: How to change
things when change is
hard.* New York: Crown.

Hedges, C. (2006). Research,
evidence-based practice,
and quality improvement.
*AACN Advanced Critical
Care, 17*(4), 457–458.

Hitchings, K. S., Davies-Hathen,
N., Capuano, T. A., &
Morgan, G. (2008). Peer
case review sharpens event
analysis. *Journal of
Nursing Care Quality,
23*(4), 296–304.

Hyun, W., Gakken, S., Douglas,
K., & Stone, P. (2008).
Evidence-based staffing:
Potential roles for informat-
ics. *Nursing Economics,
26*(3), 151.

Institute for Healthcare
Improvement (IHI) (2011).
*Current IHI strategic
initiatives.* Retrieved
May 26, 2011 from http://
www.ihi.org/IHI/Programs/
StrategicInitiatives/

Institute for Healthcare
Improvement (IHI) (2009).
*IHI Collaborative: Trans-
forming care at the bedside.*
Retrieved May 9, 2011
from http://www.ihi.org/
IHI/Programs/Collaboratives/

TransformingCareatthe Bedside.htm

Institute of Medicine. (1999). *To err is human: Building a safer health system.* Washington, DC: National Academy Press.

Institute of Medicine. (2003). *Health professions education: A bridge to quality.* Washington, DC: National Academy Press.

Joint Commission. (2011). *Hospital national patient safety goals.* Retrieved May 26, 2011 from http://www.jointcommission.org/assets/1/6/2011_NPSG_Hospital_3_17_11.pdf

Kazley, A. S., & Ozcan, Y. A. (2008). Do hospitals with electronic medical records (EMRs) provide higher quality care? *Medical Care Research and Review, 65*(4), 496–513.

Khatri, N., Brown, G. D., & Hicks, L. L. (2009). From a blame culture to a just culture in health care. *Health Care Management Review, 34*(4), 312–322.

National Quality Forum (NQF) (2011). *About NQF.* Retrieved May 26, 2011 from http://www.quality-forum.org/About_NQF/About_NQF.aspx

Needleman, J. (2008). Is what's good for the patient good for the hospital? *Policy, Politics, and Nursing Practice, 9*(2), 80–87.

Niemeijer, G. C., Trip, A., Ahaus, K. T. B., Does, R. J. M. M., & Wendt, K. W. (2010). Quality in trauma care: Improving the discharge procedure of patients by means of Lean Six Sigma. *Journal of Trauma Injury, Infection, and Critical Care, 69*(3), 614–619.

Reeves, K. (2207). New evidence report on nurse staffing and quality of patient care. *MEDSURG Nursing, 16*(2), 73–74.

Swearingen, S. (2009). A journey to leadership: Designing a nursing leadership development program. *Journal of Continuing Education in Nursing, 40*(3), 107–112.

Unruh, L., Agrawal, M., & Hassmiller, S. (2011). The business case for transforming care at the bedside among the "TCAB 10" and lessons learned. *Nursing Administration Quarterly, 35*(2), 97–109.

Westbrook, J. I., Woods, A., Rob, M. I., Dunsmuir, W. T., & Day, R. O. (2010). Association of interruptions with an increased risk and severity of medication administration errors. *Archives of Internal Medicine, 170*(8), 683–692.

Weiss, A. P. (2009). Quality improvement in healthcare: The six Ps of root-cause analysis. (Letter to the editor). *American Journal of Psychiatry, 166*(3), 372.

Wu, A. W., Lipshutz, A. K., & Pronovost, P. J. (2008). Effectiveness and efficiency of root cause analysis in medicine. *Journal of the American Medical Association, 299*(6), 685–687.

Yamamoto, J. J., Malatestinic, B., Lehman, A., & Juneja, R. (2010). Facilitating process changes in meal delivery and radiological testing to improve inpatient insulin timing using Six Sigma method. *Quality Management in Health Care, 19*(3), 189–200.

**Power Defined**

**Power and Leadership**

**Power: How Managers and Leaders Get Things Done**

**Using Power**

   IMAGE AS POWER

   USING POWER APPROPRIATELY

**Shared Visioning as a Power Tool**

**Power, Politics, and Policy**

   NURSING'S POLITICAL HISTORY

   USING POLITICAL SKILLS TO INFLUENCE POLICIES

   INFLUENCING PUBLIC POLICIES

**Using Power and Politics for Nursing's Future**

## Learning Outcomes

*After completing this chapter, you will be able to:*

1. Define power.
2. Describe how power is used.
3. Discuss how image is a source of power.
4. Explain how to use shared visioning as a power tool.

5. Discuss how politics influence policy.
6. Describe how nurses can use politics to influence policies.

## Key Terms

Coercive power
Connection power
Expert power
Information power
Legitimate power
Personal power

Policy
Politics
Position power
Power
Power plays
Punishment

Referent power
Reward power
Shared visioning
Stakeholders
Vision

# Power Defined

**Power** is the potential ability to influence others (Hersey, 2011). Power is involved in every human encounter, whether you recognize it or not. Power can be symmetrical when two parties have equal and reciprocal power, or it may be asymmetrical with one person or group having more control than another (Mason, Leavitt, & Chaffee, 2011). Power can be exclusive to one party or may be shared among many people or groups. To acquire power, maintain it effectively, and use it skillfully, nurses must be aware of the sources and types of power that they will use to influence and transform patient care.

# Power and Leadership

Real power—principle-centered power—is based on honor, respect, loyalty, and commitment. Principle-centered power is a model congruent with nursing's values. It is based on respect, honor, loyalty, and commitment. Originally conceived by Stephen Covey (1991), the model is increasingly used by leaders in many fields (Ikeda, 2009). Power sharing evolves naturally when power is centered on one's values and principles. In fact, the notion that power is something to be shared seems to contradict the usual belief that power is something to be amassed, protected, and used for one's own purposes.

Leadership power comes from the ability to sustain proactive influence, because followers trust and respect the leader to do the right thing for the right reason. As leaders in health care, nurses must understand and select behaviors that activate principle-centered leadership:

- Get to know people. Understanding what other people want is not always simple.
- Be open. Keep others informed. Trust, honor, and respect spread just as equally as fear, suspicion, and deceit.
- Know your values and visions. The power to define your goals is the power to choose.
- Sharpen your interpersonal competence. Actively listen to others and learn to express your ideas well.
- Use your power to enable others. Be attentive to the dynamics of power and pay attention to ground rules, such as encouraging dissenting voices and respecting disagreement.
- Enlarge your sphere of influence and connectedness. Power sometimes grows out of someone else's need.

# Power: How Managers and Leaders Get Things Done

Classically, managers relied on authority to rouse employees to perform tasks and accomplish goals. In contemporary health care organizations, managers use persuasion, enticement, and inspiration to mobilize the energy and talent of a work group and to overcome resistance to change.

A leader's use of power alters attitudes and behavior by addressing individual needs and motivations. There are seven generally accepted types of interpersonal power used in organizations to influence others (Hersey, 2011):

1. **Reward power** is based on the inducements the manager can offer group members in exchange for cooperation and contributions that advance the manager's objectives. The degree of compliance depends on how much the follower values the expected benefits. For example, a nurse manager may grant paid educational leave as a way of rewarding a staff nurse who agreed to work overtime. Reward power often is used in relation to a manager's formal job responsibilities.

2. **Coercive power** is based on the penalties a manager might impose on an individual or a group. Motivation to comply is based on fear of **punishment** (coercive power) or withholding of rewards. For example, the nurse manager might make undesirable job assignments, mete out

a formal reprimand, or recommend termination for a nurse who engages in disruptive behavior. Coercion is used in relation to a manager's perceived authority to determine employment status.

3. **Legitimate power** stems from the manager's right to make a request because of the authority associated with job and rank in an organizational hierarchy. Followers comply because they accept a manager's prerogative to impose requirements, sanctions, and rewards in keeping with the organization's mission and aims. For instance, staff nurses will comply with a nurse manager's directive to take time off without pay when the workload has dropped below projected levels because they know that the manager is charged with maintaining unit expenses within budget limitations.

4. **Expert power** is based on possession of unique skills, knowledge, and competence. Nurse managers, by virtue of experience and advanced education, are often the best qualified to determine what to do in a given situation. Employees are motivated to comply because they respect the manager's expertise. Expert power relates to the development of personal abilities through education and experience. Newly graduated nurses might ask the nurse manager for advice in learning clinical procedures or how to resolve conflicts with coworkers or other health professionals.

5. **Referent power** is based on admiration and respect for an individual. Followers comply because they like and identify with the manager. Referent power relates to the manager's likeability and success. For example, a new graduate might ask the advice of a more experienced and admired nurse about career planning.

6. **Information power** is based on access to valued data. Followers comply because they want the information for their own needs. Information power depends on a manager's organizational position, connections, and communication skills. For example, the nurse manager is frequently privy to information about pending organizational changes that affect employees' work situations. A nurse manager may exercise information power by sharing significant information at staff meetings, thereby improving attendance.

7. **Connection power** is based on an individual's formal and informal links to influential or prestigious persons within and outside an area or organization. Followers comply because they want to be linked to influential individuals. Connection power also relates to the status and visibility of the individual as well. If, for example, a nurse manager is a neighbor of an organization's board member, followers may believe that connection will protect or advance their work situation.

Managers have both personal and position power. **Position power** is determined by the job description, assigned responsibilities, recognition, advancement, authority, the ability to withhold money, and decision making. Legitimate, coercive, and reward power are positional because they relate to the "right" to influence others based on rank or role. The extent to which managers mete out rewards and punishment is usually dictated by organizational policy. Information and legitimate power are directly related to the manager's role in the organizational structure.

Expert, referent, information, and connection power are based, for the most part, on personal traits. **Personal power** refers to one's credibility, reputation, expertise, experience, control of resources or information, and ability to build trust. The extent to which one may exercise expert, referent, information, and connection power relates to personal skills and positive interpersonal relationships as well as employees' needs and motivations. Box 7-1 illustrates how nurses can learn to use power in organizations.

## Using Power

Despite an increase in pride and self-esteem that comes with using power and influence, some nurses still consider power unattractive. Power grabbing, which has been the traditionally accepted means of relating to power for one's own self-interests and use, is how nurses

## BOX 7-1    Guidelines for the Use of Power in Organizations

### Guidelines for Using Legitimate Authority

- Make polite, clear requests.
- Explain the reasons for a request.
- Don't exceed your scope of authority.
- Verify authority if necessary.
- Follow proper channels.
- Follow-up to verify compliance.
- Insist on compliance if appropriate.

### Guidelines for Using Reward Power

- Offer the type of rewards that people desire.
- Offer rewards that are fair and ethical.
- Don't promise more than you can deliver.
- Explain the criteria for giving rewards and keep it simple.
- Provide rewards as promised if requirements are met.
- Use rewards symbolically (not in a manipulative way).

### Guidelines for Using Coercive Power

- Explain rules and requirements and ensure that people understand the serious consequences of violations.
- Respond to infractions promptly and consistently without showing any favoritism to particular individuals.
- Investigate to get the facts before using reprimands or punishment and avoid jumping to conclusions or making hasty accusations.
- Except for the most serious infractions, provide sufficient oral and written warnings before resorting to punishment.

- Administer warnings and reprimands in private and avoid making rash threats.
- Stay calm and avoid the appearance of hostility or personal rejection.
- Express a sincere desire to help the person comply with role expectations and thereby avoid punishment.
- Invite the person to suggest ways to correct the problem and seek agreement on a concrete plan.
- Maintain credibility by administering punishment if noncompliance continues after threats and warnings have been made.

### Guidelines for Using Expert Power

- Explain the reasons for a request or proposal and why it is important.
- Provide evidence that a proposal will be successful.
- Don't make rash, careless, or inconsistent statements.
- Don't exaggerate or misrepresent the facts.
- Listen seriously to the person's concerns and suggestions.
- Act confidently and decisively in a crisis.

### Ways to Acquire and Maintain Referent Power

- Show acceptance and positive regard.
- Act supportive and helpful.
- Use sincere forms of ingratiation.
- Defend and back up people when appropriate.
- Do unsolicited favors.
- Make self-sacrifices to show concern.
- Keep promises.

Adapted from Yukl, G. (2007). *Leadership in organizations* (6th ed.) (pp. 150–156). Upper Saddle River, NJ: Prentice Hall. Reprinted by permission.

often think of power. Rather, nurses tend to be more comfortable with power sharing and empowerment: power "with" rather than power "over" others.

### Image as Power

A major source of power for nurses is an image of power. Even if one does not have actual power from other sources, the perception by others that one is powerful bestows a degree of power. The same is true for the profession as a whole. If the public sees the profession of nursing as powerful, the profession's ability to achieve its goals and agendas is enhanced.

Images emerge from interactions and communications with others. If nurses present themselves as caring and compassionate experts in health care through their interactions and communications with the public, then a strong, favorable image develops for both the individual nurse and the profession. Nurses, as the ambassadors of care, must understand the importance and benefits of positive therapeutic communications and image. Developing a positive image of power is important for both the individual and the profession.

Individual nurses can promote an image of power by a variety of means, such as:

1. Appropriately introducing yourself by saying your name, making eye contact, and shaking hands can immediately establish you as a powerful person. If nurses introduce themselves by first name to the physician, Dr. Smith, they have immediately set forth an unequal power relationship unless the physician also uses his or her first name. Although women are not socialized to initiate handshakes, it is a power strategy in male-dominated circles, including health care organizations. In Western cultures, eye contact conveys a sense of confidence and connection to the individual to whom one is speaking. These seemingly minor behaviors can have a major impact on how competent and powerful the nurse is perceived.

2. Attire can symbolize power and success (Sullivan, 2013). Although nurses may believe that they are limited in choice of attire by uniform codes, it is in fact the presentation of the uniform that can hold the key to power. For example, a nurse manager needs a powerful image both with unit staff and with administrators and other professionals who are setting organizational policy. An astute nurse manager might wear a suit rather than a uniform to work on the day of a high-level interdisciplinary committee meeting. Certainly, attention to details of grooming and uniform selection can enhance the power of the staff nurse as well.

3. Conveying a positive and energetic attitude sends the message that you are a "doer" and someone to be sought out for involvement in important issues. Chronic complaining conveys a sense of powerlessness, whereas solving problems and being optimistic promote a "can do" attitude that suggests power and instills confidence in others.

4. Pay attention to how you speak and how you act when you speak. Nonverbal signs and signals say more about you than words. Stand erect and move energetically. Speak with an even pace and enunciate words clearly. Make sure your words are reflected in your body language. Keep your facial expression consistent with your message.

5. Use facts and figures when you need to demonstrate your point. Policy changes usually evolve from data presented in a compelling story. Positioning yourself as a powerful player requires the ability to collect and analyze data. Technology facilitates data retrieval. For example, Chapter 6 lists various quality initiatives that yield useful data, including benchmarks and dashboards. Remember that power is a matter of perception; therefore, you must use whatever data are available to support your judgment.

6. Knowing when to be at the right place at the right time is crucial to gain access to key personnel in the organization. This means being invited to events, meetings, and parties not necessarily intended for nurses. It means demanding to sit at the policy table when decisions affecting staffing and patient care are made. Influence is more effective when it is based on personal relationships and when people see others in person: "If I don't see you, I can't ask you for needed information, analysis, and alternative recommendations." Become visible. Be available. Offer assistance. You can be invaluable in providing policy makers with information, interpreting data, and teaching them about the nursing side of health care.

7. In dealing with people outside of nursing, it is important to develop powerful partnerships. Learn how to share both credit and blame. When working on collaborative projects, use "we" instead of "they," and be clear about what is needed. If something isn't working well, say so. Never accept another's opinion as fact. Facts can be easily manipulated to fit one's personal agenda. Learn how to probe and obtain additional information. Don't assume you have all the information. Beware of unsolicited commentary. Don't be fearful of giving strong criticism, but always put criticisms in context. Before giving any criticism, give a compliment, if appropriate. Also, make sure your partners are ready to hear all sides of the issue. It's never superfluous to ask, "Do you want to talk about such and such right now?" Once an issue is decided—really decided—don't raise it again.

8. Make it a point to get to know the people who matter in your sphere of influence. Become a part of the power network so that when people are discussing issues or seeking people for important appointments of leadership, your name comes to mind. Be sure to deal with senior people. The more contact you have with the "power brokers," the more support you can generate in the future should the need arise. The more power you use, the more you get.

9. Know who holds the power. Identify the key power brokers. Develop a strategy for gaining access to power brokers through joining alliances and coalitions. Learn how to question others and how to become part of the organizational infrastructure. There is an art to determining when, what, and how much information is exchanged and communicated at any one time and to determining who does so. Powerful people have a keen sense of timing. Be sure to position yourself to be at the right place at the right time. Any strategy will involve a good deal of energy and effort. Direct influence and efforts toward issues of highest priority or when greatest benefits are likely to result.

10. Use power appropriately to promote consensus in organizational goals, develop common means to achieve these goals, and enhance a common culture to bind organizational members together. As the health care providers closest to the patient, nurses best understand patients' needs and wants. In the hospital, nurses are present on the first patient contact and thereafter for 24 hours a day, 7 days a week. In the clinic, the nurse may be the person the patient sees first and most frequently. By capitalizing on the special relationship that they have with patients, nurses can use marketing principles to enhance their position and image as professional caregivers.

Nursing as a profession must market its professional expertise and ability to achieve the objectives of health care organizations. From a marketing perspective, nursing's goal is to ensure that identified markets (e.g., patients, physicians, other health professionals, community members) have a clear understanding of what nursing is, what it does, and what it is going to do. In doing so, nursing is seen as a profession that gives expert care with a scientific knowledge base.

Nursing care often is seen as an indicator of an organization's overall quality. Regardless of the setting, quality nursing care is something that is desired and valued. Through understanding patients' needs and preferences for programs that promote wellness and maintain and restore health, nurses become the organization's competitive edge to enhancing revenues. Marketing an image of expertise linked with quality and cost can position nursing powerfully and competitively in the health care marketplace.

## Using Power Appropriately

Using power not only affects what happens at the time, but also has a lasting effect on your relationships. Therefore, it is best to use the least amount of power necessary to accomplish your goals. Also, use power appropriate to the situation (Sullivan, 2013). Table 7-1 lists rules for using power.

Improper use of power can destroy a manager's effectiveness. Power can be overused or underused. Overusing power occurs when you use excessive power relative to the situation. If you fail to use power when it is needed, you are underusing your power. In addition to the immediate loss of influence, you may lose credibility for the future.

Power plays are another way that power is used inappropriately. **Power plays** are attempts by others to diminish or demolish their opponents. Typical power plays include:

"Let's be fair."

"Can you prove that?"

"It's either this or that; which is it? Take your pick."

"But you said . . . and now you say. . . ."

| TABLE 7-1 | Rules for Using Power |
|---|---|

1. Use the least amount of power you can to be effective in your interactions with others.
2. Use power appropriate to the situation.
3. Learn when not to use power.
4. Focus on the problem, not the person.
5. Make polite requests, never arrogant demands.
6. Use coercion only when other methods don't work.
7. Keep informed to retain your credibility when using your expert power.
8. Understand you may owe a return favor when you use your connection power.

From Sullivan, E. J. (2013). *Becoming influential: A guide for nurses* (2nd ed.). Upper Saddle River, NJ: Prentice Hall. Reprinted by permission.

Such statements engender feelings of insecurity, incompetence, confusion, embarrassment, and anger. You do not need to respond directly in these situations but, rather, you can simply restate your initial point in a firm manner. Keep your expression neutral, ignore accusations, and restate your position, if appropriate. If you refuse to respond to these thinly veiled attacks, your opponent is unable to intimidate and manipulate you.

Nursing must perceive power for what it really is—the ability to mobilize and focus energy and resources. What better position can nurses be in but to assume power to face new problems and responsibilities in reshaping nursing practice to adapt to environmental changes? Power is the means, not the end, to seek new ways for doing things in this uncertain and unsettling time in health care.

## Shared Visioning as a Power Tool

Shared visioning is a powerful tool to influence the organization's future. **Shared visioning** is an interactive process in which both leaders and followers commit to the organization's goals (Kantabutra, 2009; Pearce, Conger, & Locke, 2008). A **vision** is a mental model of a possible future (Kantabutra, 2008). It should inspire and challenge both leaders and followers to accomplish the organization's goals set forth in the vision.

Top-down management is an out-of-date concept (Pearce, Conger, & Locke, 2008). Today's leaders recognize that their power must be shared and that integrated leadership styles—bottom-up and lateral—are essential for success. Consensus about the organization's future can motivate leaders and employees alike to envision their preferred future and do their best to achieve it. In addition, a shared vision makes implementing the necessary, and often difficult, changes easier.

Kantabutra (2009) posits that the leader is not a passive participant in the visioning process. The leader should be an active group member, leading the group toward the desired vision in a participative fashion. The leader helps guide the group toward consensus.

Furthermore, innovation is necessary for organizations to effect positive change (McKeown, 2008). Innovation requires employee buy-in to flourish (Melnyk & Davidson, 2009). Shared visioning is a strategy that encourages innovation.

## Power, Politics, and Policy

While power is the potential ability to influence others, **politics** is the art of influencing others to achieve a goal (Mason, Chaffee, & Leavitt, 2011).

Politics:

- Is an interpersonal endeavor—uses communication and persuasion
- Is a collective activity—requires the support and action of many people
- Calls for analysis and planning—requires an assessment of the issue and a plan to resolve it
- Involves image—hinges on the image people have of change makers

## Nursing's Political History

Nurses' political activities began with Florence Nightingale, continued with the emergence of nursing schools and women's suffrage, and improved with the establishment of nursing organizations and the feminist movement (Sullivan, 2013). Establishing the National Center for Nursing Research (later changed to the National Institute of Nursing Research) within the National Institutes of Health is an example of nurses' powerful political action.

*A Brief History of the National Institute of Nursing Research*

*After the Institute of Medicine report recommended a federal nursing research entity as part of the mainstream scientific community in the early 1980s, nursing leaders in the United States began promoting establishment of a nursing institute at the National Institutes of Health. This effort involved lobbying Congress, the Reagan administration, and the other institutes at NIH—a formidable task. A few members of Congress were interested in the potential that nursing science had for improving health, but the administration was not in favor of another institute at NIH, and the other institutes seemed puzzled as to why nursing would need its own institute to do research. Couldn't nurse researchers receive funding through existing institutes? Medicine did so without a separate institute.*

*Step by step, nursing leaders persuaded (harassed?) institute directors and Congress, insisting that nursing research would improve human response to illness and assist in maintaining and enhancing health. A bill was born. Concern about cost and increasing bureaucracy emerged and was overcome. The bill passed only to be vetoed by President Reagan. Then a funny thing happened. Nursing made an unprecedented move. The profession came together, united with one goal: to override President Reagan's veto (none had been successfully overridden before).*

*One by one, across the country, nurses called their senators and congressional representatives urging support for a nursing institute, explaining that nurses were represented only among a few funded researchers at other institutes who did not understand the impact of nursing interventions on health and recovery. A modest investment, they explained, would yield exponentially greater results. Thanks to a few persuasive members of Congress, a compromise was negotiated and the National Center for Nursing Research was established in 1985. Through a statutory revision in 1993, the Center became an Institute.*

Similarly, Georgia nurses successfully changed that state's practice act to include prescriptive authority for advanced practice nurses, overcoming fierce opposition from the medical association (Beall, 2007). Working in concert with each other and with consumers and the media, they generated a letter-writing campaign that countered every obstacle the medical association tried. Georgia became the last state to grant prescribing privileges to nurse practitioners.

**Policy**, on the other hand, is the decision that determines action. Policies result from political action.

## Using Political Skills to Influence Policies

Political skill, per se, is not included in nursing education (nor is it tested on state board exams), yet it is a vital skill for nurses to acquire. To improve your political skill:

- Learn self-promotion—report your accomplishments appropriately.
- Be honest and tell the truth—say what you mean and mean what you say.
- Use compliments—recognize others' accomplishments.

| **TABLE 7-2** Steps in Political Action |
| --- |
| 1. Determine what you want. |
| 2. Learn about the players and what they want. |
| 3. Gather supporters and form coalitions. |
| 4. Be prepared to answer opponents. |
| 5. Explain how what you want can help them. |

From Sullivan, E. J. (2013). *Becoming influential: A guide for nurses* (2nd ed.). Upper Saddle River, NJ: Prentice Hall. Reprinted by permission.

- Discourage gossip—silence is the best response.
- Learn and use quid pro quo—do and ask for favors.
- Remember: appearance matters—attend to grooming and attire.
- Use good manners—be courteous. (Green & Chaney, 2006)

Health care involves multiple special-interest groups all competing for their share of a limited pool of resources. The delivery of nursing services occurs at many levels in health care organizations. The effectiveness of care delivery is linked to the application of power, politics, and marketing. Nurses belong to a complex organization that is continually confronted with limited resources and is in competition for those resources.

How politically savvy are you? Ask yourself the following questions:

- Do you get credit for your ideas?
- Do you know how to deal with a difficult colleague?
- Do you have a mentor?
- Are you "in the loop"?
- Can you manage and influence others' perceptions of you and your work?
- Are you able to convert enemies to friends?
- Do your ideas get a fair hearing?
- Do you know when and how to present them? (Reardon, 2011)

To take action, first decide what you want to accomplish. Is it realistic? Will you have supporters? Who will be the detractors? The steps in political action are shown in Table 7-2.

Try to find out what other people involved, called **stakeholders**, want. Maybe you could piggyback on their ideas. Members of Congress do this all the time by adding amendments to proposed bills in an attempt to satisfy their opponents.

Start telling your supporters about your idea and see if they will join with you in a coalition. This is not necessarily a formal group but allows you to know who you can count on in the discussions.

Find out exactly what objections your opponents have. Try to figure out a way to alter your plan accordingly or help your opponents understand how your proposal might help them. Political action is never easy, but the most politically astute people accomplish goals far more often than those who don't even try.

A case study that exemplifies a nurse using organizational politics is shown in Case Study 7-1.

## Influencing Public Policies

What happens in the workplace both depends on and influences what is happening in the larger community, professional organizations, and government. Developing influence in each of these three groups takes time and a long-range plan of action. Although the nurse's first priority should be to establish influence in the workplace, the nurse can gradually increase connections and influence with other groups and, later on, make these other groups a priority.

## CASE STUDY 7-1

### USING ORGANIZATIONAL POLITICS FOR PERSONAL ADVANTAGE

Juanita Pascheco has been nurse manager of medical and surgical ICUs in a large, urban, for-profit hospital for the past seven years. Two years ago, Juanita completed her master's degree in nursing administration. Her thesis research centered on the acceptance of standardized and computerized documentation methods for critical care units. Juanita is well respected in her current role and is a member of several key committees addressing the need for a replacement health information system (HIS) for the hospital. She reports directly to the director of critical care services.

Although Juanita enjoys her work as nurse manager, she believes she is ready to assume additional responsibilities at the director level. Through her work on the hospital's HIS selection team and as the nursing representative to the physician's technology committee, Juanita identifies the need for a clinical informatics director role. One of Juanita's responsibilities on the HIS selection team is to identify talent from clinical areas who could support the HIS implementation. Juanita has also agreed to chair several working committees that will assist in determining required clinical functionality for the HIS.

During her tenure at the hospital, Juanita has cultivated solid working relationships with several key decision makers within the organization. The human resources director, Ken Harding, has worked with Juanita on several large projects over the past two years, including implementation of multidisciplinary teams in the ICUs. Juanita schedules a lunch with Ken to discuss growth opportunities in the information technology department, the process for creating new roles, and in particular, who will determine the need for and approval of new information technology positions. Using this knowledge and her experience on the HIS selection team and the physicians' technology committee, Juanita develops a proposal for the clinical informatics director position.

As the HIS selection team draws closer to selecting a final vendor for the computerized health information system and an implementation timeline is established by the information technology department, Juanita approaches her supervisor, Sherrie Wright, with her proposal. Juanita also provides Sherrie with an overview of the clinical support that will be necessary for successful implementation of the HIS product. Since the critical care units are targeted for the initial phase of implementation, Sherrie is aware that Juanita's high interest in technology and her clinical expertise in the ICU would be invaluable for successful implementation. As a strong manager, Juanita can build acceptance of this change among the nurses, physicians, and other members of the health care team.

Sherrie agrees to take Juanita's proposal to the chief nursing officer for formal consideration.

### Manager's Checklist

The nurse manager is responsible for:

- Knowing and understanding the formal lines of authority within the organization.
- Identifying key decision makers and understanding their priorities and how those priorities affect any new initiatives.
- Recognizing the importance of timing when initiating change.
- Being ready to take advantage of new opportunities
- Building strong and credible working relationships with decision makers.
- Being willing to take on new and challenging tasks that may lead to more responsibility.

---

In order to influence public policies, nurses need to know how to work with the public officials who enact those policies. Table 7-3 lists guidelines for working with public officials.

First, be respectful. Public officials have many constituents and demands on their support. Build relationships with officials. Don't just contact them when you have a request. Keep in touch at other times.

### Communicating with Elected Officials

Nurses often wish to contact elected officials to support or oppose legislation. You can call, e-mail, tweet, or write to public officials. (Links to state legislators and contact information for federal government officials are listed in the Web resources for this chapter.)

Here's how to contact state or federal elected officials. Call the official's staff and ask to speak to the person who handles the issue that concerns you. Tell the aide that you support or oppose a certain bill and state the reasons why. Name the bill by number.

| TABLE 7-3 | How to Work with Public Officials |
|---|---|
| 1. Be respectful. | 5. Understand the issue. |
| 2. Build relationships. | 6. Be a constructive opponent. |
| 3. Keep in touch. | 7. Be realistic. |
| 4. Arrive informed. | 8. Be helpful. |

From Sullivan, E. J. (2013). *Becoming influential: A guide for nurses* (2nd ed.). Upper Saddle River, NJ: Prentice Hall. Reprinted by permission.

E-mail or write directly to the official. Identify the bill in question, state your position on the bill, and explain why you support or oppose it. Keep your comments brief, and address only one issue per correspondence. Hand-written letters get more attention than form letters distributed by organizations.

Use this format to address members of the U.S. Senate:

> The Honorable (full name of senator)
> __(Rm.#)__(name of) Senate Office Building
> United States Senate
> Washington, DC 20510

Dear Senator:

To contact the member of the U.S. Congress, use a similar format.

> The Honorable (full name)
> __(Rm.#)__(name of) House Office Building
> United States House of Representatives
> Washington, DC 20515

Dear Representative:

### Meeting with Elected Officials

To meet in person with an elected official, make an appointment, arrive on time, and come prepared. Understand the pros and cons of the issue you are bringing to the person's attention. Be a constructive opponent. Argue for your position and be prepared with additional information and alternative suggestions. Still, be realistic. What you want may not be possible, or it may not be likely at the present time. Always be helpful. Show how your issue benefits the official's constituents and, thus, the representative.

The American Association of Critical-Care Nurses suggests pointers for working with public officials (AACN, 2010). In addition, the American Nurses Association (ANA) has legislative and government information for nurses (ANA, 2011). (See links to these organizations in the Web resources for this chapter.)

## Using Power and Politics for Nursing's Future

Kelly (2007) suggests that apathy prevents nurses from using their political skills. Becoming active in professional associations, learning the legislative issues that affect nursing, gaining political skills, and being willing to advocate for nursing's causes are necessary for the profession to flex its considerable political muscles. All nurses can participate to some extent in these activities.

Nurses can have a tremendous impact on health care policy. The best impact is often made with a bit of luck and timing, but never without knowledge of the whole system. This includes knowledge of the policy agenda, the policy makers, and the politics that are involved. Once you gain this knowledge, you are ready to move forward with a political base to promote nursing.

To convert your policy ideas into political realities, consider the following power points:

- *Use persuasion over coercion.* Persuasion is the ability to share reasons and rationale when making a strong case for your position while maintaining a genuine respect for another's perspective.
- *Use patience over impatience.* Despite the inconveniences and failings caused by health care restructuring, impatience in the nursing community can be detrimental. Patience, along with a long-term perspective on the health care system, is needed.
- *Be open-minded rather than closed-minded.* Acquiring accurate information is essential if you want to influence others effectively.
- *Use compassion over confrontation.* In times of change, errors and mistakes are easy to pinpoint. It takes genuine care and concern to change course and make corrections.
- *Use integrity over dishonesty.* Honest discourse must be matched with kind thoughts and actions. Control, manipulations, and malice must be pushed aside for change to occur.

By using their political skills, nurses can improve patient care in individual institutions, help organizations survive and thrive, and influence public officials.

## What You Know Now

- Power is the potential ability to influence others.
- Power can be positional or personal.
- Types of power include reward, coercive, legitimate, expert, referent, information, and connection.
- Image is a source of power.
- Power can be overused, underused, or used inappropriately. To be effective, the power used must be appropriate to the situation.
- Shared visioning is an interactive process in which both leaders and followers commit to the organization's goals.
- Politics is the art of influencing others to achieve a goal.
- Policy is the decision that determines action. Policies result from political action.
- Nurses can use political action to influence policies in the organization and to influence public policies.

## Tools for Using Power and Politics

1. Learn the formal lines of authority within your organization.
2. Identify key decision makers and build strong and credible relationships with them.
3. Identify decision makers' priorities and how those affect any new initiatives.
4. Learn the rules for using power and put them into practice.
5. Offer solutions to problems and take advantage of new opportunities.
6. Exhibit a willingness to take on new and challenging tasks that may lead to more responsibility.
7. Pay attention to people who are influential and adopt their strategies if appropriate.
8. Learn strategies for working with public officials.

## Questions to Challenge You

1. Consider a person you believe to have power. What are the bases of that person's power?
2. Evaluate how the person you named uses his or her power. Is it positive or negative?
3. Have you observed people using power inappropriately? Describe what they did and what happened as a result.

4. Assess your own power using the seven types of power discussed in the chapter. Name three ways you could increase your power.
5. How politically savvy are you? Did you discover areas to challenge you?
6. Have you been involved in developing policies in your organization or have you worked with public officials? Explain.

## Pearson Nursing Student Resources

Find additional review materials at
**www.nursing.pearsonhighered.com**

Prepare for success with additional NCLEX®-style practice questions, interactive assignments and activities, Web links, animations and videos, and more!

## Web Resources

American Association of Critical-Care Nurses: www.aacn.org
American Nurses Association: www.nursingworld.org
United States House of Representatives: www.house.gov
United States Senate: www.senate.gov
National Conference of State Legislatures: www.ncsl.org

## References

American Association of Critical Care Nurses. (2010). *Advocacy 101: Golden rules for those who work with public officials*. Retrieved October 22, 2010 from http://www.aacn.org/wd/practice/content/publicpolicy/goldenrules.pcms?pid=1&mid=2874&menu=Community

American Nurses Association. (2011). RN activist kit. Retrieved June 3, 2011 from www.nursingworld.org/gova

Beall, F. (2007). Overview and summary: Power to influence patient care: Who holds the keys? *Online Journal of Issues in Nursing, 12*(1). Retrieved October 22, 2010 from http://www.nursingworld.org/MainMenuCategories/ANAMarketplace/ANAPeriodicals/OJIN/TableofContents/Volume122007/No1Jan07/tpc32ntr16088.aspx

Covey, S. R. (1991). *Principle-centered leadership*. New York: Simon & Schuster.

Green, C. G., & Chaney, L. H. (2006). The game of office politics. *Supervision, 67*(8), 3–6.

Hersey, P. H. (2011). *Management of organizational behavior* (10th ed.). Upper Saddle River, NJ: Prentice Hall.

Ikeda, J. (2009). Principle centered power. Retrieved April 12, 2011 from http://www.leadwithhonor.com/blog/2009/03/26/principle-centered-power/

Kantabutra, S. (2008). What do we know about vision? *Journal of Applied Business Research, 24*(2), 323–342.

Kantabutra, S. (2009). Toward a behavioral theory of vision in organizational settings. *Leadership & Organizational Development Journal, 30*(4), 319–337.

Kelly, K. (2007). From apathy to political activism. *American Nurse Today, 2*(8), 55–56.

Mason, D. J., Leavitt, J. K., & Chaffee, M. W. (2011). *Policy and politics in nursing and health care* (6th ed.). Philadelphia: W. B. Saunders.

McKeown, M. (2008). *The truth about innovation*. Great Britain: Pearson Education Limited.

Melnyk, B. M., & Davidson, S. (2009). Creating a culture of innovation in nursing education through shared vision, leadership, interdisciplinary partnerships, and positive deviance. *Nursing Administration Quarterly, 33*(4), 288–295.

Pearce, C. L., Conger, J. A., & Locke, E. A. (2008). Shared leadership theory. *The Leadership Quarterly, 19*(3), 622–628.

Sullivan, E. J. (2013). *Becoming influential: A guide for nurses* (2nd ed.). Upper Saddle River, NJ: Prentice Hall Health.

# Thinking Critically, Making Decisions, Solving Problems

## Learning Outcomes

*After completing this chapter, you will be able to:*

1. Discuss how to use the critical-thinking process.
2. Describe ways to foster creativity.
3. Develop a plan to improve your decision-making and problem-solving skills.
4. Compare and contrast individual and collective decision-making processes in various situations.
5. Recognize stumbling blocks to making decisions and solving problems.
6. Foster innovation in your work and that of others.

## Key Terms

Adaptive decisions
Artificial intelligence
Brainstorming
Creativity
Critical thinking
Decision making
Democratic leadership
Descriptive rationality model
Experimentation

Expert systems
Groupthink
Innovation
Innovative decisions
Objective probability
Political decision-making model
Probability
Probability analysis

Problem solving
Rational decision-making model
Routine decisions
Satisficing
Subjective probability
Trial-and-error method

Nurse managers are expected to use knowledge from various disciplines to solve problems with patients, staff, and the organization as well as problems in their own personal and professional lives. They must make decisions in dynamic situations, such as:

- After a position vacates should we refill it, given the tighter economy?
- Is the present policy requiring 12-hour shifts adequate for both patients and nurses?
- Which is the best staffing pattern to prevent turnover and ensure quality patient care?
- What is the best time to have staff meetings and council meetings in order to involve the night shift too?

This chapter explains and differentiates critical thinking, decision making, and problem solving and describes processes and techniques for using each.

## Critical Thinking

**Critical thinking** is the process of examining underlying assumptions, interpreting and evaluating arguments, imagining and exploring alternatives, and developing a reflective criticism for the purpose of reaching a conclusion that can be justified. Critical thinking is not the same as criticism, though it does call for inquiring attitudes, knowledge about evidence and analysis, and skills to combine them.

Critical-thinking skills can be used to resolve problems rationally. Identifying, analyzing, and questioning the evidence and implications of each problem stimulate and illuminate critical thought processes. Critical thinking is also an essential component of decision making. However, compared to problem solving and decision making, which involve seeking a single solution, critical thinking is a higher-level cognitive process that includes creativity, problem solving, and decision making (Figure 8-1).

### Critical Thinking in Nursing

The need for critical thinking in nursing has long been accepted. Zori, Nosek, and Musil (2010) used the California Critical Thinking Disposition Inventory to measure critical thinking in nurses. The researchers found that the nurses supervised by managers with higher critical thinking skills perceived their work environment to be more positive than those whose managers scored lower on critical-thinking skills.

Case scenarios and discussion of clinical experiences taught newly licensed nurses critical thinking and improved their retention rate in one facility (Ashcraft, 2010). Bittner and Gravlin (2009) studied nurses' critical-thinking skills when delegating to assistive personnel. They found that the nurse's lack of critical thinking more often resulted in missed or omitted routine care.

**Figure 8-1** ●
Critical-thinking model.

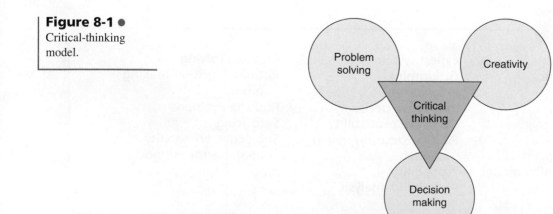

The Carnegie Foundation's call for reform in nursing education argues, however, that nursing should move beyond critical thinking toward clinical reasoning and diverse thinking (Benner et al., 2009).

## Using Critical Thinking

The critical-thinking process seems abstract unless it can be related to practical experiences. One way to develop this process is to consider a series of questions when examining a specific problem or making a decision, such as:

1. *What are the underlying assumptions?*  Underlying assumptions are unquestioned beliefs that influence an individual's reasoning. They are perceptions that may or may not be grounded in reality. For example, some people believe the AIDS epidemic is punishment for homosexual behavior. This attitude toward people with AIDS could alter one's approach to care for an AIDS patient.

2. *How is evidence interpreted?*  What is the context? Interpretation of information also can be value laden. Is the evidence presented completely and clearly? Can the facts be substantiated? Are the people presenting the evidence using emotional or biased information? Are there any errors in reasoning?

3. *How are the arguments to be evaluated?*  Is there objective evidence to support the arguments? Have all value preferences been determined? Is there a good chance that the arguments will be accepted? Are there enough people to support decisions? Health care organizations were able to change to smoke-free environments once societal values favored nonsmokers, and public policies reflected those values.

4. *What are the possible alternative perspectives?*  Using different basic assumptions and paradigms can help the critical thinker develop several different views of an issue. Compare how a nurse manager who assumes that more RNs equal better care will deal with a budget cut with a manager who is committed to adding assistive personnel instead. What evidence supports the alternatives? What solutions do staff members, patients, physicians, and others propose? What would be the ideal alternative?

Critical-thinking skills are used throughout the nursing process (see Table 8-1). Nurses can build on the knowledge base they began acquiring in school to make the critical-thinking process a conscious one in daily activities. Learning to be a critical thinker requires a commitment over time, but the skills can be learned. The characteristics of an expert critical thinker are shown in Box 8-1.

## Creativity

Creativity is an essential part of the critical-thinking process. **Creativity** is the ability to develop and implement new and better solutions. Creativity demands a certain amount of exposure to outside contacts, receptiveness to new and seemingly strange ideas, a certain amount of freedom, and some permissive management.

Most nurses, however, are employed in bureaucratic settings that do not foster creativity. Control is exercised over staff, and rigid adherence to formal channels of communication jeopardizes innovation. In addition, there is little room for failure, and when failures do occur they are not well tolerated. When staff are afraid of the consequences of failure, their creativity is inhibited and innovation does not take place. (See later section on innovation.)

Maintaining a certain level of creativity is one way to keep an organization alive. New employees, who are not encumbered with details of accepted practices often can make suggestions based on their prior experiences or insights before they get set in their ways or have their innovative ideas "turned off." The advantages offered by new employees should be explored because all staff gain from such use of valuable human resources.

**TABLE 8-1    Critical Thinking Through the Nursing Process**

| The Nursing Process | Critical-Thinking Skills |
|---|---|
| Assessment | Observing |
| | Distinguishing relevant from irrelevant data |
| | Distinguishing important from unimportant data |
| | Validating data |
| | Organizing data |
| | Categorizing data |
| Diagnosis | Finding patterns and relationships |
| | Making inferences |
| | Stating the problem |
| | Suspending judgment |
| Planning | Generalizing |
| | Transferring knowledge from one situation to another |
| | Hypothesizing |
| Implementation | Applying knowledge |
| | Testing hypotheses |
| Evaluation | Deciding whether hypotheses are correct |
| | Making criterion-based evaluations |

From Wilkinson, J. (1992). *Nursing process in action: A critical thinking approach*. Redwood City, CA: Addison-Wesley Nursing, p. 29.

---

**BOX 8-1    Characteristics of an Expert Critical Thinker**

- Outcome-directed
- Open to new ideas
- Flexible
- Willing to change
- Innovative
- Creative
- Analytical
- Communicator
- Assertive

- Persistent
- Caring
- Energetic
- Risk taker
- Knowledgeable
- Resourceful
- Observant
- Intuitive
- "Out of the box" thinker

From Ignatavicius, D.D. (2001). Six critical thinking skills for at-the-bedside success. *Nursing Management, 32*(1), 37–39.

The climate must promote the survival of potentially useful ideas. The nurse manager can foster a climate of support by giving new ideas a fair and adequate hearing, and thereby reduce the tendency to discourage the creative process in individuals and within groups. The challenge for nurse managers is to know when, for whom, and to what extent control is appropriate. If creativity does have a priority in the health care setting, then the reward system should be geared to and commensurate with that priority.

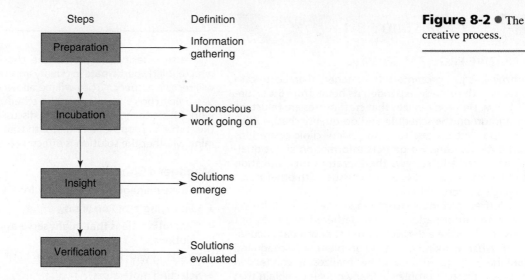

**Figure 8-2** ● The creative process.

Creativity has four stages: preparation, incubation, insight, and verification. Even people who think they are not naturally creative can learn this process (Figure 8-2).

1. *Preparation.* A carefully designed planning program is essential. First, acquire information necessary to understand the situation. Individuals can do this on their own, or groups can work together.

   The process follows this sequence:

   • Pick a specific task
   • Gather relevant facts
   • Challenge every detail
   • Develop preferred solutions
   • Implement improvements

2. *Incubation.* After all the information available has been gathered, allow as much time as possible to elapse before deciding on solutions.

3. *Insight.* Often solutions emerge after a period of reflection that would not have occurred to anyone without this time lapse.

4. *Verification.* Once a solution has been implemented, evaluate it for effectiveness. You may need to restart the process or go back to another step and create a different solution.

   Case Study 8-1 describes how one nurse manager used creativity to solve a problem.

## Decision Making

Considering all the practice individuals get in making decisions, it would seem they might become very good at it. However, the number of decisions a person makes does not correspond to the person's skill at making them. The assumption is that decision making comes naturally, like breathing. It does not.

The decision-making process described in this chapter provides nurses with a system for making decisions that is applicable to any decision. It is a useful procedure for making practical choices. A decision not to solve a problem is also a decision.

Although *decision making* and *problem solving* appear similar, they are not synonymous. **Decision making** may or may not involve a problem, but it always involves selecting one of several alternatives, each of which may be appropriate under certain circumstances. **Problem solving**, on the other hand, involves diagnosing a problem and solving it, which may or may not entail deciding on one correct

## CASE STUDY 8-1

### CREATIVE PROBLEM SOLVING

Jeffrey was just promoted to manager of an acute care clinic, which recently expanded its hours from 6 A.M. until 10 P.M. He soon realizes that staff nurses are reluctant to sign up on the schedule and do quality chart audits, an important process used to review clinic operations and patients' care. He gathers information about quality improvement, reviews the literature on motivation and incentives, and discusses the issue with other nurse managers (preparation).

Jeffrey continues to manage the clinic, thinking about the information he has gathered but does not consciously make a decision or reject new ideas (incubation). When working on a new problem, self-scheduling for the change in hours, he realizes a connection between the two problems. Many nurses complain that by the time they receive the schedule the day shifts are filled.

Jeffrey decides to review the chart audits. Nurses who regularly participate in quality improvement projects will receive a "perk." They will be allowed, on a rotating basis, first choice at selecting the schedule they want to work (this is the insight stage). He discusses the plan with the staff and proposes a two-month trial period to determine whether the solution is effective (verification).

### Manager's Checklist

The nurse manager is responsible for:

- Identifying problem areas
- Generating ideas that might serve as possible solutions
- Checking with others for advice
- Selecting motivators
- Implementing a solution
- Evaluating the results

---

solution. Most of the time, decision making is a subset of problem solving. However, some decisions are not of a problem-solving nature, such as decisions about scheduling, equipment, or in-services.

### Types of Decisions

The types of problems nurses and nurse managers encounter and the decisions they must make vary widely and determine the problem-solving or decision-making methods they should use. Relatively well defined, common problems can usually be solved with **routine decisions**, often using established rules, policies, and procedures. For instance, when a nurse makes a medication error, the manager's actions are guided by policy and the report form. Routine decisions are more often made by first-level managers than by top administrators.

**Adaptive decisions** are necessary when both problems and alternative solutions are somewhat unusual and only partially understood. Often they are modifications of other well-known problems and solutions. Managers must make **innovative decisions** when problems are unusual and unclear and when creative, novel solutions are necessary.

### Decision-Making Conditions

The conditions surrounding decision making can vary and change dramatically. Consider the total system. Whatever solutions are created will succeed only if they are compatible with other parts of the system. Decisions are made under conditions of certainty, risk, or uncertainty.

#### Decision Making Under Certainty

When you know the alternatives and the conditions surrounding each alternative, a state of certainty is said to exist. Suppose a nurse manager on a unit with acutely ill patients wants to decrease the number of venipunctures a patient experiences when an IV is started, as well as reduce costs resulting from failed venipunctures. Three alternatives exist:

- Establish an IV team on all shifts to minimize IV attempts and reduce costs
- Establish a reciprocal relationship with the anesthesia department to start IVs when nurses experience difficulty
- Set a standard of two insertion attempts per nurse per patient, although this does not substantially lower equipment costs

The manager knows the alternatives (IV team, anesthesia department, standards) and the conditions associated with each option (reduced costs, assistance with starting IVs, minimum attempts and some cost reduction). A condition of strong certainty is said to exist and the decision can be made with full knowledge of what the payoff probably will be.

### Decision Making Under Uncertainty and Risk

Seldom do decision makers know everything there is to know about a subject or situation. If everything was known, the decision would be obvious for all to realize.

Most critical decision making in organizations is done under conditions of *uncertainty* and *risk*. The individual or group making the decision does not know all the alternatives, attendant risks, or possible consequences of each option. Uncertainty and risk are inevitable because of the complex and dynamic nature of health care organizations.

Here is an example: If the weather forecaster predicts a 40 percent chance of snow, the nurse manager is operating in a situation of risk when trying to decide how to staff the unit for the next 24 hours.

In a risk situation, availability of each alternative, potential successes, and costs are all associated with probability estimates. **Probability** is the likelihood, expressed as a percentage, that an event will or will not occur. If something is certain to happen, its probability is 100 percent. If it is certain not to happen, its probability is 0 percent. If there is a 50–50 chance, its probability is 50 percent.

Here is another example: Suppose a nurse manager decides to use agency nurses to staff a unit during heavy vacation periods. Two agencies look attractive, and the manager must decide between them. Agency A has had modest growth over the past 10 years and offers the manager a three-month contract, freezing wages during that time. In addition, the unit will have first choice of available nurses. Agency B is much more dynamic and charges more but explains that the reason they have had a high rate of growth is that their nurses are the best and the highest paid in the area. The nurse manager can choose Agency A, which will provide a safe, constant supply of nursing personnel, or B, which promises better care but at a higher cost.

The key element in decision making under conditions of risk is to determine the probabilities of each alternative as accurately as possible. The nurse manager can use a **probability analysis**, whereby expected risk is calculated or estimated. Using the probability analysis shown in Table 8-2, it appears as though Agency A offers the best outcome. However, if the second agency had a 90 percent chance of filling shifts and a 50 percent chance of fixing costs, a completely different situation would exist.

The nurse manager might decide that the potential for increased costs was a small trade-off for having more highly qualified nurses and the best probability of having the unit fully staffed during vacation periods. **Objective probability** is the likelihood that an event will or will not occur based on facts and reliable information. **Subjective probability** is

| TABLE 8-2 | Probability Analysis |
| --- | --- |
| **Probability Analysis** | |
| Agency A | 60% Filling shifts<br>100% Fixed wages |
| Agency B | 50% Filling shifts<br>70% Fixed wage |

the likelihood that an event will or will not occur based on a manager's personal judgment and beliefs.

> *Janeen, a nurse manager of a specialized cardiac intensive care unit, faces the task of recruiting scarce and highly skilled nurses to care for coronary artery bypass graft patients. The obvious alternative is to offer a salary and benefits package that rivals that of all other institutions in the area. However, this means Janeen will have costly specialized nursing personnel in her budget who are not easily absorbed by other units in the organization. The probability that coronary artery bypass graft procedures will become obsolete in the future is unknown. In addition, other factors (e.g., increased competition, government regulations regarding reimbursement) may contribute to conditions of uncertainty.*

### The Decision-Making Process

The **rational decision-making model** is a series of steps that managers take in an effort to make logical, well-grounded rational choices that maximize the achievement of objectives. First identify all possible outcomes, examine the probability of each alternative, and then take the action that yields the highest probability of achieving the most desirable outcome. Not all steps are used in every decision nor are they always used in the same order. The rational decision-making model is thought of as the ideal but often cannot be fully used.

Individuals seldom make major decisions at a single point in time and often are unable to recall when a decision was finally reached. Some major decisions are the result of many small actions or incremental choices the person makes without regarding larger issues. In addition, decision processes are likely to be characterized more by confusion, disorder, and emotionality than by rationality. For these reasons, it is best to develop appropriate technical skills and the capacity to find a good balance between lengthy processes and quick, decisive action.

The **descriptive rationality model**, developed by Simon in 1955 and supported by research in the 1990s (Simon, 1993), emphasizes the limitations of the rationality of the decision maker and the situation. It recognizes three ways in which decision makers depart from the rational decision-making model:

- The decision maker's search for possible objectives or alternative solutions is limited because of time, energy, and money
- People frequently lack adequate information about problems and cannot control the conditions under which they operate
- Individuals often use a satisficing strategy

**Satisficing** is not a misspelled word; it is a decision-making strategy whereby the individual chooses an alternative that is not ideal but either is good enough (suffices) under existing circumstances to meet minimum standards of acceptance or is the first acceptable alternative. Many problems in nursing are ineffectively solved with satisficing strategies.

> *Elena, a nurse manager in charge of a busy neurosurgical floor with high turnover rates and high patient acuity levels, uses a satisficing alternative when hiring replacement staff. She hires all nurse applicants in order of application until no positions are open. A better approach would be for Elena to replace staff only with nurse applicants who possess the skills and experiences required to care for neurosurgical patients, regardless of the number of applicants or desire for immediate action. Elena also should develop a plan to promote job satisfaction, the lack of which is the real reason for the vacancies.*

Individuals who solve problems using satisficing may lack specific training in problem solving and decision making. They may view their units or areas of responsibility as drastically simplified models of the real world and be content with this simplification because it allows them to make decisions with relatively simple rules of thumb or from force of habit.

The **political decision-making model** describes the process in terms of the particular interests and objectives of powerful stakeholders, such as hospital boards, medical staffs, corporate officers, and regulatory bodies. Power is the ability to influence or control how problems and objectives are defined, what alternative solutions are considered and selected, what information flows, and, ultimately, what decisions are made (see Chapter 7).

The decision-making process begins when a gap exists between what is actually happening and what should be happening, and it ends with action that will narrow or close this gap. The simplest way to learn decision-making skills is to integrate a model into one's thinking by breaking the components down into individual steps. The seven steps of the decision-making process (Box 8-2) are as applicable to personal problems as they are to nursing management problems. Each step is elaborated by pertinent questions clarifying the statements, and they should be followed in the order in which they are presented.

## Decision-Making Techniques

Decision-making techniques vary according to the nature of the problem or topic, the decision maker, the context or situation, and the decision-making method or process. For routine decisions, choices that are tried and true can be made for well-defined, known situations or problems. Well-designed policies, rules, and standard operating procedures can produce satisfactory results with a minimum of time. **Artificial intelligence**, including programmed computer systems such as **expert systems** that can store, retrieve, and manipulate data, can diagnose problems and make limited decisions.

For adaptive decisions involving moderately ambiguous problems and modification of known and well-defined alternative solutions, there are a variety of techniques. Many types of decision grids or tables can be used to compare outcomes of alternative solutions. Decisions about units or services can be facilitated, with analyses comparing output, revenue, and costs over time or under different conditions. Analyzing the costs and revenues of a proposed new service is an example.

Regardless of the decision-making model or strategy chosen, data collection and analysis are essential. In many health care organizations, quality teams are using a variety of tools to gather, organize, and analyze data about their work such as decision grids, flow

| BOX 8-2 | Steps in Decision Making |
| --- | --- |
| 1. Identify the purpose: | Why is a decision necessary? What needs to be determined? State the issue in the broadest possible terms. |
| 2. Set the criteria: | What needs to be achieved, preserved, and avoided by whatever decision is made? The answers to these questions are the standards by which solutions will be evaluated. |
| 3. Weigh the criteria: | Rank each criterion on a scale of values from 1 (totally unimportant) to 10 (extremely important). |
| 4. Seek alternatives: | List all possible courses of action. Is one alternative more significant than another? Does one alternative have weaknesses in some areas? Can these be overcome? Can two alternatives or features of many alternatives be combined? |
| 5. Test alternatives: | First, using the same methodology as in step 3, rank each alternative on a scale of 1 to 10. Second, multiply the weight of each criterion by the rating of each alternative. Third, add the scores and compare the results. |
| 6. Troubleshoot: | What could go wrong? How can you plan? Can the choice be improved? |
| 7. Evaluate the action: | Is the solution being implemented? Is it effective? Is it costly? |

**Figure 8-3** ●

Brainstorming session of a nursing quality focus team.

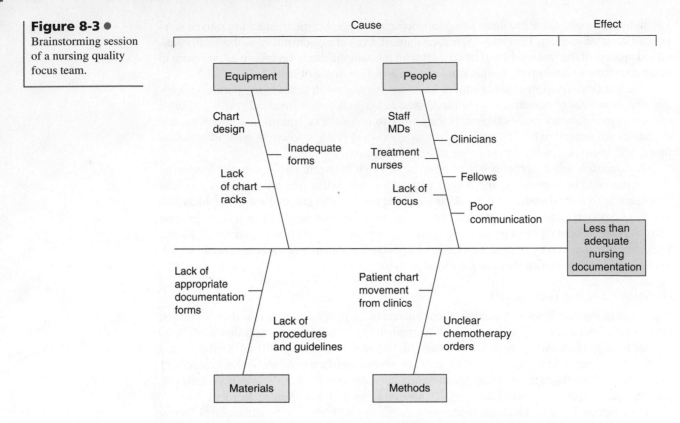

charts, or cause-and-effect diagrams. Figure 8-3 illustrates a cause-and-effect diagram that a team of nurses created to help them improve the documentation process for their ambulatory oncology unit.

Another example of a decision tool is the Dynamic Network Analysis Decision Support (DyNADS) project at the University of Arizona College of Nursing (see http://www.dynads.nursing. arizona.edu). This simulation product enables the manager to predict the consequences of decisions on patient safety and quality outcomes. The tool simulates virtual nursing units, identifies potential errors, and predicts the likely result. Using the tool, the manager can discover if an innovation or a combination of innovations is likely to be successful (Effkenet al., 2010). DyNADS is a decision support tool that improves predictability in today's complex environment.

### Group Decision Making

The widespread use of participative management, quality improvement teams, and shared governance in health care organizations requires every nurse manager to determine when group, rather than individual, decisions are desirable and how to use groups effectively. A number of studies have shown that professional people do not function well in a micromanaged environment. As an alternative, group problem solving of substantial issues casts the manager in the role of facilitator and consultant. Compared to individual decision making, groups can provide more input, often produce better decisions, and generate more commitment. One group decision-making technique is brainstorming.

In **brainstorming**, group members meet together and generate many diverse ideas about the nature, cause, definition, or solution to a problem without consideration of their relative value. The focus team whose work is shown in Figure 8-3 used brainstorming.

With brainstorming, a premium is placed on generating lots of ideas as quickly as possible and on coming up with unusual ideas. Most importantly, members do not critique ideas as they are proposed. Evaluation takes place after all the ideas have been generated. Members are encouraged to improve on each other's ideas. These sessions are enjoyable but are often unsuccessful because members inevitably begin to critique ideas, and as a result, meetings shift to the ordinary interacting group format. Criticisms of this approach are the high cost factor, the time consumed, and the superficiality of many solutions.

# Problem Solving

People use problem solving when they perceive a gap between an existing state (what is going on) and a desired state (what should be going on). How one perceives the situation influences how the problem is identified or solved. Therefore, perceptions need to be clarified before problem solving can occur.

## Problem-Solving Methods

A variety of methods can be used to solve problems. People with little management experience tend to use the **trial-and-error method**, applying one solution after another until the problem is solved or appears to be improving. These managers often cite lack of experience and of time and resources to search for alternative solutions.

> *In a step-down unit with an increasing incidence of medication errors, Max, the nurse manager, uses various strategies to decrease errors, such as asking nurses to use calculators, having the charge nurse check medications, and posting dosage and medication charts in the unit. After a few months, by which time none of the methods has worked, it occurs to Max that perhaps making nurses responsible for their actions would be more effective. Max develops a point system for medication errors: When nurses accumulate a certain amount of points, they are required to take a medication test; repeated failure of the test may eventually lead to termination. Max's solution is effective and a low level of medication errors is restored.*

As the above example shows, a trial-and-error process can be time-consuming and may even be detrimental. Although some learning can occur during the process, the nurse manager risks being perceived as a poor problem solver who has wasted time and money on ineffective solutions.

**Experimentation**, another type of problem solving, is more rigorous than trial and error. Pilot projects or limited trials are examples of experimentation. Experimentation involves testing a theory (hypothesis) or hunch to enhance knowledge, understanding, or prediction. A project or study is carried out in either a controlled setting (e.g., in a laboratory) or an uncontrolled setting (e.g., in a natural setting such as an outpatient clinic). Data are collected and analyzed and results interpreted to determine whether the solution tried has been effective.

> *Lin, a nurse manager of a pediatric floor, has received many complaints from mothers of children who think the nurses are short-tempered. Lin has a hunch that 12-hour shifts, which have been recently implemented on her floor, are contributing to the problem; she believes that nurses who must interact frequently with families would perform better on eight-hour shifts. She can test her theory by setting up a small study comparing the two staffing patterns with patient satisfaction.*

Experimentation may be creative and effective or uninspired and ineffective, depending on how it is used. As a major method of problem solving, experimentation may be inefficient because of the amount of time and control involved. However, a well-designed experiment can be persuasive in situations in which an idea or activity, such as a new staffing system or care procedure, can be tried in one of two similar groups and results objectively compared.

Still other problem-solving techniques rely on *past experience* and *intuition*. Everyone has various and countless experiences. Individuals build a repertoire of these experiences and base future actions on what they considered successful solutions in the past. If a particular course of action consistently resulted in positive outcomes, the person will try it again when similar circumstances occur. In some instances, an individual's past experience can determine how much risk he or she will take in present circumstances.

The nature and frequency of the experience also contribute significantly to the effectiveness of this problem-solving method. How much the person has learned from these experiences, positive or negative, can affect the current viewpoint and can result in either subjective, narrow judgments or wise ones. This is especially true in human relations problems. Intuition relies heavily on past experience and trial and error. The extent to which past experience is related to intuition is difficult to determine, but nurses' wisdom, sensitivity, and intuition are known to be valuable in solving problems.

Some problems are self-solving: if permitted to run a natural course, they are solved by those personally involved. This is not to say that a uniform laissez-faire management style solves all problems. The nurse manager must not ignore managerial responsibilities, but often difficult situations become more manageable when participants are given time, resources, and support to discover their own solutions.

This typically happens, for example, when a newly graduated nurse joins a unit where most of the staff are associate degree RNs who resent the new nurse's level of education as well as the nurse's lack of experience. If the nurse manager intervenes, a problem that the staff might have worked out on their own becomes an ongoing source of conflict. The important skill required here is knowing when to act and when not to act. (See Chapter 12 for a discussion of conflict.)

## The Problem-Solving Process

Many nursing problems require immediate action. Nurses don't have time for formalized processes of research and analysis specified by the scientific method. Therefore, learning an organized method for problem solving is invaluable. One practical method for problem solving is to follow this seven-step process, which is also outlined in Box 8-3.

1. *Define the problem.* The definition of a problem should be a descriptive statement of the state of affairs, not a judgment or conclusion. If one begins the statement of a problem with a judgment, the solution may be equally judgmental, and critical descriptive elements could be overlooked.

   Suppose a nurse manager reluctantly implements a self-scheduling process and finds that each time the schedule is posted, evenings and some weekend shifts are not adequately covered. The manager might identify the problem as the immaturity of the staff and their inability to function under **democratic leadership**. The causes may be lack of interest in group decision making, minimal concern over providing adequate patient coverage, or, perhaps more correctly, a few nurses' lack of understanding of the process.

   If the nurse manager defines the above problem as immaturity and reverts to making out the schedules without further fact-finding, a minor problem could develop into a major upheaval.

---

**BOX 8-3**    Steps in Problem Solving

1. Define the problem.
2. Gather information.
3. Analyze the information.
4. Develop solutions.
5. Make a decision.
6. Implement the decision.
7. Evaluate the solution.

Premature interpretation can alter one's ability to deal with facts objectively. For example, are there other explanations for the apparent behavior that do not entail negative assumptions about the maturity of the staff?

Accurate assessment of the scope of the problem also determines whether the manager needs to seek a lasting solution or just a stopgap measure. Is this just a situational problem requiring only intervention with a simple explanation, or is it more complex, involving the leadership style of the manager? The manager must define and classify problems in order to take action.

To define a problem, ask:

- Do I have the authority to do anything about this myself?
- Do I have all the information? The time?
- Who else has important information and can contribute?
- What benefits could be expected? A list of potential benefits provides the basis for comparison and choice of solutions. The list also serves as a means for evaluating the solution.

2. *Gather information.* Problem solving begins with collecting facts. This information gathering initiates a search for additional facts that provides clues to the scope and solution of the problem. This step encourages people to report facts accurately. Everyone involved can contribute. Although this may not always provide objective information, it reduces misinformation and allows everyone an opportunity to tell what he or she thinks is wrong with a situation.

Experience is another source of information—one's own experience as well as the experience of other nurse managers and staff. The people involved usually have ideas about what should be done. Some data will be useless, some inaccurate, but some will be useful to develop innovative ideas worth pursuing.

3. *Analyze the information.* Analyze the information only when all of it has been sorted into some orderly arrangement as follows:

- Categorize information in order of reliability.
- List information from most important to least important.
- Set information into a time sequence. What happened first? Next? What came before what? What were the concurrent circumstances?
- Examine information in terms of cause and effect. Is A causing B, or vice versa?
- Classify information into categories: *human factors,* such as personality, maturity, education, age, relationships among people, and problems outside the organization; *technical factors,* such as nursing skills or the type of unit; *temporal factors,* such as length of service, overtime, type of shift, and double shifts; and *policy factors,* such as organizational procedures or rules applying to the problem, legal issues, and ethical concerns.
- Consider how long the situation has been going on.

Because no amount of information is ever complete or comprehensive enough, critical-thinking skills, discussed earlier, help the manager examine the assumptions, evidence, and potential value conflicts.

4. *Develop solutions.* As an individual or a group analyzes information, numerous possible solutions will suggest themselves. Do not consider only simple solutions, because that may stifle creative thinking and cause over concentration on detail. Developing alternative solutions makes it possible to combine the best parts of several solutions into a superior one. Also, alternatives are valuable in case the first-order solutions prove impossible to implement.

When exploring a variety of solutions, maintain an uncritical attitude toward the way the problem has been handled in the past. Some problems have had a long-standing history by the time they reach you, and attempts may have been made to resolve them over a period of time. "We tried this before and it didn't work" is often said and may apply—or more likely, may not apply—in a changed situation. Past experience may not always supply an answer, but it can aid the critical-thinking process and help prepare for future problem solving.

5. *Make a decision.* After reviewing the list of potential solutions, select the one that is most applicable, feasible, satisfactory, and has the fewest undesirable consequences. Some solutions have to be put into effect quickly; matters of discipline or compromises in patient safety, for example, need immediate intervention. You must have legitimate authority to act in an emergency and know the penalties to be imposed for various infractions.

   If the problem is a technical one and its solution brings about a change in the method of doing work (or using new equipment), expect resistance. Changes that threaten individuals' personal security or status are especially difficult. In those cases, the change process must be initiated before solutions are implemented. If the solution involves change, the manager should fully involve those who will be affected by it, if possible, or at least inform them of the process. (See Chapter 5 for discussion of the change process.)

6. *Implement the decision.* Implement the decision after selecting the best course of action. If unforeseen new problems emerge after implementation, evaluate these impediments. Be careful, however, not to abandon a workable solution just because a few people object; a minority always will. If the previous steps in the problem-solving process have been followed, the solution has been carefully thought out, and potential problems have been addressed, implementation should move forward.

7. *Evaluate the solution.* After the solution has been implemented, review the plan and compare the actual results and benefits to those of the idealized solution. People tend to fall back into old patterns of habit, only giving lip service to change. Is the solution being implemented? If so, are the results better or worse than expected? If they are better, what changes have contributed to its success? How can we ensure that the solution continues to be used and to work? Such a periodic checkup gives you valuable insight and experience to use in other situations and keeps the problem-solving process on course.

See Case Study 8-2 to learn how one nurse manager used critical thinking to solve a problem.

## Group Problem Solving

Traditionally, managers solved most problems in isolation. This practice, however, is outdated. Both the complexity of problems and the staff's desire for meaningful involvement create the impetus for using group approaches to problem solving. Today consensus-based problem solving, inherent in shared governance, is the norm.

### Advantages of Group Problem Solving

Groups collectively possess greater knowledge and information than any single member and may access more strategies to solve a problem. Under the right circumstances and with appropriate leadership, groups can deal with more complex problems than a single individual, especially if there is no one right or wrong solution to the problem. Individuals tend to rely on a small number of familiar strategies; a group is more likely to try several approaches.

Group members may have a greater variety of training and experiences and approach problems from more diverse points of view. Together, a group may generate more complete, accurate, and less biased information than one person. Groups may deal more effectively with problems that cross organizational boundaries or involve change that requires support from other units or

## CASE STUDY 8-2

### CRITICAL THINKING AND PROBLEM SOLVING

Latonia Wilson is nurse manager for a busy 20-bed telemetry unit. In addition to providing postsurgical care for cardiac patients, nurses also prepare patients for cardiac catheterization lab procedures. Latonia's staff includes eight new graduate nurses, almost half of her nursing staff. The new nurses have attended most of the required nursing orientation for the hospital.

Three times in one month, telemetry unit patients who had orders for heparin drips were administered heparin flush instead. Premixed IV bags for heparin drips as well as heparin flush for indwelling arterial catheters are stocked on the IV solutions cart in the medication room. While no adverse patient outcomes had been reported, procedures have been delayed.

Geena Donati is a graduate nurse on the telemetry unit. Recently, she took a bag of heparin drip from the IV cart and started to attach it to the IV tubing. She noticed that the label stated heparin flush instead of heparin. Upon returning to the med room, she checked the heparin drip bin and found heparin flush bags mixed in with the heparin drip. The pharmacy technician came into the med room and began stocking the IV cart. Geena noticed that the pharmacy technician put extra heparin drip bags in the heparin flush bin. She questioned the pharmacy technician and he told Geena that since the unit used a lot of heparin

solution, he had started bringing extra to decrease his trips to the unit.

Geena met with Latonia later during her shift. She told her manager about the extra heparin bags being mixed into the wrong bins. Latonia asked Geena if she would be interested in working with two other RNs on the unit to develop new procedures to decrease heparin medication errors. Geena and the task force worked with the pharmacy department to change the label color for heparin drip and heparin flush solutions, physically separated the bins on the IV cart onto different shelves, and provided a short educational segment at the monthly staff meeting. Since the new procedures were developed, no further heparin errors have occurred on the telemetry unit.

### Manager's Checklist

The nurse manager is responsible for:

- Tracking and identifying recurring negative performance issues on the unit
- Analyzing adverse outcomes to determine what factors contributed to the outcome
- Empowering staff to improve work processes on the unit
- Understanding the organizational structure and helping staff work with other departments within the organization

departments. Participative problem solving has additional advantages: it increases the likelihood of acceptance and understanding of the decision, and it enhances cooperation in implementation.

### Disadvantages of Group Problem Solving

Group problem solving also has disadvantages: it takes time and resources and may involve conflict. Group problem solving also can lead to the emergence of benign tyranny within the group. Members who are less informed or less confident may allow stronger members to control group discussion and problem solving. A disparity in participation may contribute to a power struggle between the nurse manager and a few assertive group members.

Also managers may resist using groups to make decisions. They may fear that they may not agree with the decision the group makes or that they will not be needed if all decisions are made by the group. Neither is the case. Some decisions are rightfully the managers' (e.g., handling the budget), others are staff decisions (e.g., peer review, self-scheduling), and some are shared (e.g., joint hiring decisions). Figure 8-4 illustrates this.

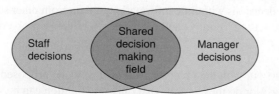

**Figure 8-4** ●
Shared decision making goal. From Shiparski, L. (2005). Engaging in shared decision making: Leveraging staff and management expertise. *Nurse Leader, 3*(1), 40.

Group problem solving also can be affected by **groupthink**. Groupthink is a negative phenomenon that occurs in highly cohesive groups that become isolated. Through prolonged close association, group members come to think alike and have similar prejudices and blind spots, such as stereotypical views of outsiders. They exhibit a strong tendency to seek concurrence, which interferes with critical thinking about important decisions. In addition, the leadership of such groups suppresses open, free-wheeling discussion and controls what ideas will be discussed and how much dissent will be tolerated. Groupthink seriously impairs critical thinking and can result in erroneous and damaging decisions.

Also groups tend to make riskier decisions than individuals. Groups are more likely to support unusual or unpopular positions (e.g., public demonstrations). Groups tend to be less conservative than individual decision makers and frequently display more courage and support for unusual or creative solutions to problems.

Individuals who lack information about alternatives may make a safe choice, but after group discussion they acquire additional information and become more comfortable with a less secure alternative. The group setting also allows for the diffusion of responsibility. If something goes wrong, others also can be assigned the blame or risk. In addition, leaders may be greater risk takers than individuals, and group members may attach a social value to risk taking because they identify it with leadership.

## Stumbling Blocks

The leader's personality traits, inexperience, lack of adaptability, and preconceived ideas may be obstacles to decision making and problem solving.

### Personality

The leader's personality can and often does affect how and why certain decisions are made. Managers are often selected because of their expert clinical, not managerial, skills. Inexperienced in management, they may resort to various unproductive actions. On the one hand, a nurse manager who is insecure may base decisions primarily on approval seeking. When a truly difficult situation arises, the manager, rather than face rejection from the staff, makes a decision that will placate people rather than one that will achieve the larger goals of the unit and organization.

On the other hand, a nurse manager who demonstrates an authoritative type of personality might make unreasonable demands on the staff, fail to reward staff for long hours because he or she has a "workaholic" attitude, or give the staff little control over unit decisions. Similarly, an inexperienced manager may cause a unit to flounder because the manager is not inclined to act on new ideas or solutions to problems. Optimism, humor, and a positive approach are crucial to energizing staff and promoting creativity.

### Rigidity

Rigidity, an inflexible management style, is another obstacle to problem solving. It may result from ineffective trial-and-error solutions, fear of risk taking, or inherent personality traits. Avoid ineffective trial-and-error problem solving by gathering sufficient information and determining a means for early correction of wrong or inadequate decisions. Also, to minimize risk in problem solving, understand alternative risks and expectations.

The person who uses a rigid style in problem solving easily develops tunnel vision—the tendency to look at new things in old ways and from established frames of reference. It then becomes difficult to see things from another perspective, and problem solving becomes a process whereby one person makes all of the decisions with little information or data from other sources. In today's rapidly changing health care setting, rigidity can be a barrier to effective problem solving.

### Preconceived Ideas

Effective leaders do not start out with the preconceived idea that one proposed course of action is right and all others wrong. Nor do they assume that only one opinion can be voiced and others will be silent. They start out with a commitment to find out why others disagree. If the staff, other professionals, or patients see a different reality or even a different problem, leaders need to integrate this information into developing additional problem-solving alternatives.

## Innovation

**Innovation** is a strategy to bridge the gap between an existing state and a desired state (Porter-O'Grady & Malloch, 2010). Organized nursing has recognized the importance of innovation to solve health care's many problems (Lachman, Glasgow, & Donnelly, 2009). The American Academy of Nursing's campaign "Raise the Voice" highlights "edge runners," those nurses who create innovative solutions for the health care system (see www.aannet.org).

To stimulate innovation, several techniques include:

- Simulations—uses actors representing standardized patients or high-tech mannequins
- Case studies—encourages participants to use critical thinking to analyze actual patient situations
- Problem-based learning—incorporates additional information into the case study over time
- Debate—helps participants examine an issue from more than one viewpoint (Lachman, Glasgow, & Donnelly, 2009)

One university has even developed a post-master's certificate program in innovation (Dreher, 2008). Using a case-study model, Drexel University's College of Nursing offers an online program in innovation and entrepreneurship (see www.Drexel.edu) designed to foster creative thinking to solve internal and external problems (Lachman, Glasgow, & Donnelly, 2009).

Critical thinking, creativity, and innovative thinking, along with the appropriate tools and techniques, will enable nurses and their managers to make decisions and solve problems in the least time and with the best outcomes.

## What You Know Now

- Critical thinking requires examining underlying assumptions about current evidence, interpreting information, and evaluating the arguments presented to reach a new and exciting conclusion.
- The creative process involves preparation, incubation, insight, and verification, which can be learned by individuals and groups.
- Problem-solving and decision-making processes use critical-thinking skills.
- The decision-making process may employ several models: rational, descriptive rationality, satisficing, and political.
- Decision-making techniques vary according to the problem and the degree of risk and uncertainty in the situation.
- Methods of problem solving include trial and error, intuition, experimentation, past experience, tradition, and recognizing that some problems are self-solving.
- The problem-solving process involves defining the problem, gathering information, analyzing information, developing solutions, making a decision, implementing the decision, and evaluating the solution.
- Group problem solving can be positive, providing more information and knowledge than an individual. It can also be negative if it generates disruptive conflict or groupthink.
- Stumbling blocks to making decisions and solving problems include the leader's personality, rigidity, or preconceived ideas.
- Innovation helps bridge the gap between the existing state and the desired state.

## Tools for Making Decisions and Solving Problems

1. Identify problem areas.
2. Ask questions, interpret data, and consider alternatives to make decisions and solve problems.
3. Evaluate the level of certainty, uncertainty, and risk, and consider appropriate alternatives.

4. Identify opportunities to use groups appropriately to make decisions and solve problems.
5. Follow the problem-solving process described in the chapter.
6. Challenge yourself to look for creative and innovation solutions.

## Questions to Challenge You

1. Identify someone you believe has critical-thinking skills. What critical thinking attributes does this person possess?
2. Describe a situation when you made an important decision. What content in the chapter applied to that situation? What was the outcome?
3. Have you been involved in group decision making at school or at work? What techniques were used? Were they effective?
4. A number of ways that problem solving might fail were discussed in the chapter. Name three more.
5. Have you ever proposed a creative or innovative idea at work or school? Describe the idea and explain what happened.

## Web Resources

DyNADS project: http://www.dynads.nursing.arizona.edu
Post-Master's Certificate Program in Innovation and Intra/Entrepreneurship: http://www.drexel.edu/gradnursing/msn/post-MastersCertOnline/innovationEntrepreneurship/
American Academy of Nursing Edge Runners: http://www.aannet.org/edgerunners
American Academy of Nursing Raise the Voice: http://www.aannet.org/raisethevoice

**Pearson Nursing Student Resources**
Find additional review materials at
**www.nursing.pearsonhighered.com**
Prepare for success with additional NCLEX®-style practice questions, interactive assignments and activities, Web links, animations and videos, and more!

## References

Ashcraft, T. (2010). Solving the critical thinking puzzle. *Nursing Management, 41*(1), 8–10.

Benner, P., Sutphen, M., Leonard, V., & Day, L. (2009). *Educating Nurses: A call for radical transformation.* San Francisco: Jossey-Bass.

Bittner, N. P., & Gravlin, G. (2009). Critical thinking, delegation, and missed care in nursing practice. *Journal of Nursing Administration, 39*(3), 142–146.

Dreher, H. M. (2008). Innovation in nursing education:

Preparing for the future of nursing. *Holistic Nursing Practice, 22*(2), 77–80.

Effken, J. A., Verrn, J. A., Logue, M. D., & Hsu, Y. C. (2010). Nurse managers' decisions. *Journal of Nursing Administration, 40*(4), 188–195.

Lachman, V. D., Smith Glasgow, M. E., & Donnelly, G. F. (2009). Teaching innovation. *Nursing Administration Quarterly, 33*(3), 205–211.

Porter-O'Grady, T. & Malloch, K. (2010). *Innovation leadership:*

*Creating the landscape of healthcare.* Sudbury, MA: Jones & Bartlett.

Simon, H. A. (1993). Decision making: Rational, non-rational, and irrational. *Education Administration Quarterly, 29*(3), 392–411.

Zori, S., Nosek, L. J., & Musil, C. M. (2010). Critical thinking of nurse managers related to staff RNs' perceptions of the practice environment. *Journal of Nursing Scholarship, 42*(3), 305–313.

# Communicating Effectively

**Communication**

MODES OF COMMUNICATION

DISTORTED COMMUNICATION

DIRECTIONS OF COMMUNICATION

EFFECTIVE LISTENING

**Effects of Differences in Communication**

GENDER DIFFERENCES IN COMMUNICATION

GENERATIONAL AND CULTURAL DIFFERENCES IN COMMUNICATION

DIFFERENCES IN ORGANIZATIONAL CULTURE

**The Role of Communication in Leadership**

EMPLOYEES

ADMINISTRATORS

COWORKERS

MEDICAL STAFF

OTHER HEALTH CARE PERSONNEL

PATIENTS AND FAMILIES

**Collaborative Communication**

**Enhancing Your Communication Skills**

## Learning Outcomes

*After completing this chapter, you will be able to:*

1. Identify the factors that influence communication.
2. Discuss how communication can be distorted and misunderstood.
3. Choose which communication mode to use depending on the message and the relationship.
4. Explain how communication strategies vary according to the situation and those involved.
5. Improve your collaborative communication skills.
6. Develop a plan to enhance your communication skills.

## Key Terms

| | | |
|---|---|---|
| Communication | Intersender conflict | Negative assertion |
| Diagonal communication | Intrasender conflict | Negative inquiry |
| Downward communication | Lateral communication | Upward communication |
| Fogging | Metacommunications | |

# Communication

**Communication** is a complex, ongoing, dynamic process in which the participants simultaneously create shared meaning in an interaction. The goal of communication is to approach, as closely as possible, a common understanding of the message sent and the one received. At times, this can be difficult because both participants are influenced by past conditioning; the present situation; each person's purpose in the current communication; and each person's attitudes toward self, the topic, and each other. It is important that participants construct messages as clearly as possible, listen carefully, monitor each other's response, and provide feedback.

## Modes of Communication

Messages may be oral (face-to-face, one-on-one, or in groups; by telephone, text, voice mail or posted on a social media site; or written (handwritten or typed) and sent by mail, e-mail, or fax. The purpose of the message determines the best mode to use. In general, the more important or delicate the issue, the more intimate the mode should be. Any difficult issue should be communicated face-to-face, such as terminating an individual's employment. Conflict or confrontation also is usually best handled in person so that the individual's response, especially nonverbal signals (discussed later), can be seen and answered appropriately.

What mode to use depends on the level of intimacy required based on the person, your relationship, and the message. The levels of intimacy, in descending order, are:

- in person
- by phone
- voice mail
- text
- e-mail
- postal mail
- posting on social media sites, including blogs

Meeting someone face-to-face is the most intimate contact. The individual can see your face, see your body movements, and hear your words simultaneously. The telephone is slightly less intimate than in-person communication. Tone of voice, for instance, can be conveyed, and phone conversations can be two-way. Voice mail is the next level of communication. Voice mail is useful to convey information that is not necessarily sensitive and may or may not require a reply. The time and place of an upcoming meeting, for example, can be communicated by voice mail, which has the added advantage of avoiding "phone tag."

E-mail is useful for information similar to that conveyed by voice mail and, like some voice mail systems, can be broadcast to large groups at once. The dates and times for a blood drive are a good example of a broadcast message. Conveying complicated information that may require thought before the receiver replies is another value of using e-mail. Texting is similar to e-mail, although briefer. Posting on social media sites or blogs is the least personal communication (Kaplan & Haenlein, 2010).

The level of formality of the communication also affects the mode used. Applying for a position requires a written format even if the letter is e-mailed rather than mailed. The relationship between the sender and receiver also affects the mode. If a staff nurse, for example, wants to nominate a coworker for an award given by the hospital board of directors, a written letter or e-mail is required. Memos are less formal than written messages and can be e-mailed, faxed, or mailed. Social media postings are public and impersonal (Raso, 2010; Trossman, 2010).

## Distorted Communication

Oral messages are accompanied by a number of nonverbal messages known as **metacommunications**. These behaviors include head or facial agreement or disagreement; eye contact; tone, volume, and inflection of the voice; gestures of the shoulders, arms, hands, or fingers; body posture and position; dress and appearance; timing; and environment.

Nonverbal communication is more powerful than the words one speaks and can distort the meaning of the spoken words. When a verbal message is incongruent with the nonverbal message, the recipient has difficulty interpreting the intended meaning; this results in **intrasender conflict**. For example, a manager who states, "Come talk to me anytime," but keeps on typing at the keyboard while you talk, sends a conflicting message to the staff. **Intersender conflict** occurs when a person receives two conflicting messages from differing sources. For example, the risk manager may encourage a nurse to report medication errors, but the nurse manager follows up with discipline over the error. The nurse is caught between conflicting messages from the two managers.

Other common causes of distorted communication are:

- Using inadequate reasoning
- Using strong, judgmental words
- Speaking too fast or too slowly
- Using unfamiliar words
- Spending too much time on details

Distortion also occurs when the recipient is busy or distracted, bases understanding on previous unsatisfactory experience with the sender, or has a biased perception of the meaning of the message or the messenger. Consider the example of distortion of written communication provided in Box 9-1.

## BOX 9-1    Distortion in Written Communication

There is ample opportunity for distortion in the complicated process of sending, receiving, and responding to messages, as demonstrated by the following correspondence between a plumber and an official of the National Bureau of Standards (Donaldson & Scannell, 1979).

Bureau of Standards
Washington, D.C.
Gentlemen:
    I have been in the plumbing business for over 11 years and have found that hydrochloric acid works real fine for cleaning drains. Could you tell me if it's harmless?

Sincerely,
Tom Brown, Plumber

Mr. Tom Brown, Plumber
Yourtown, U.S.A.
Dear Mr. Brown:
    The efficacy of hydrochloric acid is indisputable, but the chlorine residue is incompatible with metallic permanence!

Sincerely,
Bureau of Standards

Bureau of Standards
Washington, D.C.
Gentlemen:
    I have your letter of last week and am mightily glad you agree with me on the use of hydrochloric acid.

Sincerely,
Tom Brown, Plumber

Mr. Tom Brown, Plumber
Yourtown, U.S.A.
Dear Mr. Brown:
    We wish to inform you we have your letter of last week and advise that we cannot assume responsibility for the production of toxic and noxious residues with hydrochloric acid and further suggest you use an alternate procedure.

Sincerely,
Bureau of Standards

Bureau of Standards
Washington, D.C.
Gentlemen:
    I have your most recent letter and am happy to find you still agree with me.

Sincerely,
Tom Brown, Plumber

Mr. Tom Brown, Plumber
Yourtown, U.S.A.
Dear Mr. Brown:
    Don't use hydrochloric acid, it eats the hell out of pipes!

Sincerely,
Bureau of Standards

For communication among more than two people, the chance of distortion increases proportionally.

E-mail is particularly fraught with opportunities for misunderstanding. From the greeting (e.g., dear, hi, hello, or no salutation) to the sign-off (e.g., warm regards, best wishes, best, or no sign-off), the sender conveys more than the choice of words. A speedy reply is expected and encourages a response, sometimes without adequate thought. Finally, the possibility of sending the message to the wrong person, especially the dreaded "reply to all," is another chance for your message to be misinterpreted. Texting shares many of the same dangers as e-mail and has added pressure for a faster response.

## Directions of Communication

Formal or informal communication may be downward, upward, lateral, or diagonal. **Downward communication** (manager to staff) is often directive. The staff is told what needs to be done or given information to facilitate the job to be done. **Upward communication** occurs from staff to management or from lower management to middle or upper management. Upward communication often involves reporting pertinent information to facilitate problem solving and decision making. **Lateral communication** occurs between individuals or departments at the same hierarchical level (e.g., nurse managers, department heads). **Diagonal communication** involves individuals or departments at different hierarchical levels (e.g., staff nurse to chief of the medical staff). Both lateral and diagonal communication involve information sharing, discussion, and negotiation.

An informal channel commonly seen in organizations is the grapevine (e.g., rumors and gossip). Grapevine communication is usually rapid, haphazard, and prone to distortion. It can also be useful. Sometimes the only way to learn about a pending change is through the grapevine. One problem with grapevine communication, however, is that no one is accountable for any misinformation that is relayed. Keep in mind, too, that information gathered this way is a slightly altered version of the truth, changing as the message passes from person to person.

## Effective Listening

Most nurses believe they are good listeners. Observing and listening to patients are skills nurses learn early in their careers and use every day. Being a good listener, however, involves more than just hearing words and watching body language (Sullivan, 2013). Maintaining eye contact is misleading; it may or may not signal that a person is listening. Barriers to effective listening include preconceived beliefs, lack of self-confidence, flagging energy, defensiveness, and habit (Donaldson, 2007).

### Preconceived Beliefs

The longer your relationship with someone is, the more apt you are to think you know what the person says or means and, thus, the more likely you are to not listen. This holds true in personal as well as professional relationships and applies to groups of people (known as stereotyping). Not expecting others to have anything worthwhile to say also is an example of preconceptions about them.

### Lack of Self-Confidence

Listening is difficult if you are nervous, and weak self-confidence frequently is the cause. People tend to talk too much or think about what they're planning to say next to pay attention to the person speaking. Often their mind is racing and they may not be listening even when they're talking themselves.

### Flagging Energy

Listening takes energy and sometimes we simply don't have enough energy to listen carefully. Too many people speaking at once, having too much to do, being worried, or being too tired can all interfere with our ability to listen.

Defensiveness

Survival required that we learned to hear danger approaching, but today humans have translated defense mechanisms into a way to avoid hearing bad news. Then, we think, we don't have to deal with it. The opposite is true, however. Only when we can hear and consider information can we handle it.

Habit

Over time, many people develop the habit of thinking ahead during conversations. Thinking ahead is valuable in most aspects of life, but it's deadly when you need to be listening. Like all behaviors that have become habits, changing this one is not easy. Reminding yourself to refocus on the speaker can help.

# Effects of Differences in Communication

## Gender Differences in Communication

Men and women communicate differently (Feldhahn, 2009; Tannen, 2001). They have become socialized through communication patterns that reflect their societal roles. Men tend to talk more, longer, and faster, whereas women are more descriptive, attentive, and perceptive. Women tend to use tag questions (e.g., "I can take off this weekend, can't I?") and tend to self-disclose more than men. Women tend to ask more questions and solicit more input than their male counterparts. Table 9-1 lists differences in the ways that men and women communicate.

Helgeson and Johnson (2010) suggest ways that women can improve their communication at work. Neither men nor women should raise their voices no matter what the provocation. Nor should one omit important details or assume everyone knows what you mean. Not allowing questions or objections also should be avoided, and never walk away and talk at the same time (Donaldson, 2007).

Using gender-neutral language in communication helps bridge the gap between the way men and women communicate. Men and women can improve their ability to communicate with each other by following the recommendations for gender-neutral communication found in Table 9-2.

## Generational and Cultural Differences in Communication

Generational differences, discussed in Chapter 1, affect communication styles, patterns, and expectations. Traditionals tend to be more formal, following the chain of command without question. Baby boomers question more. They enjoy the process of group problem solving

| TABLE 9-1    Gender Differences in Communication | |
| --- | --- |
| Men tend to | Women tend to |
| Interrupt more frequently | Wait to be noticed |
| Talk more, longer, louder, and faster | Use qualifiers (prefacing and tagging) |
| Disagree more | Use questions in place of statements |
| Focus on the issue more than the person | Relate personal experiences |
| Boast about accomplishments | Promote consensus |
| Use banter to avoid a one-down position | Withdraw from conflict |

From Sullivan, E. J. (2013). *Becoming influential: A guide for nurses.* (2nd ed.). Upper Saddle River, NJ: Prentice Hall, p. 57. Reprinted by permission.

**TABLE 9-2    Recommendations for Gender-Neutral Communication**

| Men may need to | Women may need to |
|---|---|
| Listen to objections and suggestions | State your message clearly and concisely |
| Listen without feeling responsible | Solve problems without personalizing them |
| Suspend judgment until information is in | Say what you want without hinting |
| Explain your reasons | Eliminate unsure words ("sort of") and nonwords ("truly") |
| Not yell | Not cry |

From Sullivan, E. J. (2013). *Becoming influential: A guide for nurses*. (2nd ed.). Upper Saddle River, NJ: Prentice Hall, p. 58. Reprinted by permission.

and decision making. Independent Generation X members are just the opposite and want decisions made without unnecessary discussion. Collegial millennials (Generation Y) expect immediate feedback to their messages. E-mail, text, or voice mail is the best way to connect with them. Mutual respect and understanding of the unique differences between and among groups will help to minimize conflict and maximize satisfaction for both managers and staff (Hahn, 2009).

Cultural attitudes, beliefs, and behaviors also affect communication (Robertson-Malt, Herrin-Griffith, & Davies, 2010). Such elements as body movement, gestures, tone, and spatial orientation are culturally defined. A great deal of misunderstanding results from a lack of understanding of each other's cultural expectations. For example, people of Asian descent take great care in exchanges with supervisors so that there is no conflict or "loss of face" for either person.

Understanding the cultural heritage of employees and learning to interpret cultural messages is essential to communicate effectively with staff from diverse backgrounds. Personal and professional cultural enrichment training is recommended. This includes reading the literature and history of the culture; participating in open, honest, respectful communication; and exploring the meaning of behavior. It is important to recognize, however, that subcultures exist within all cultures; therefore, what applies to one individual will not be true for everyone else in that culture.

### Differences in Organizational Culture

As discussed in Chapter 2, the customs, norms, and expectations within an organization are powerful forces that shape behavior. Focusing on relevant issues regarding the organizational culture can identify failures in communication. Poor communication is a frequent source of job dissatisfaction as well as a powerful determinant of an organization's effectiveness. Just as violation of other norms within the organization results in repercussions, so does violation of communication rules.

To discover what rules affect communication in your organization, ask yourself:

- Who has access to what information? Is information withheld? Is it shared widely?
- What modes of communication are used for which messages? Are they used appropriately?
- How clear are the messages? Or are they often distorted?
- Does everyone receive the same information?
- Do you receive too much information? Not enough?
- How effective is the message?

# The Role of Communication in Leadership

Although communication is inherent in the manager's role, the manager's ability to communicate often determines his or her success as a leader. Leaders who engage in frank, open, two-way communication and whose nonverbal communication reinforces the verbal communication are seen as informative. Communication is enhanced when the manager listens carefully and is sensitive to others. The major underlying factor, however, is an ongoing relationship between the manager and employees.

Successful leaders are able to persuade others and enlist their support. The most effective means of persuasion is the leader's personal characteristics. Competence, emotional control, assertiveness, consideration, and respect promote trustworthiness and credibility. A participative leader is seen as a careful listener who is open, frank, trustworthy, and informative.

## Employees

Depending on the organization's policies, the nurse manager's responsibilities may include selecting, interviewing, evaluating, counseling, and disciplining employees; handling their complaints; and settling conflicts. The principles of effective communication are especially pertinent in these activities because good communication is the adhesive that builds and maintains an effective work group.

Giving direction is not, in itself, communication. If the manager receives an appropriate response from the subordinate, however, communication has occurred. To give directions and achieve the desired results, develop a message strategy. The techniques that follow can help improve effective responses from others.

- *Know the context of the instruction.*   Be certain you know exactly what you want done, by whom, within what time frame, and what steps should be followed to do it. Be clear in your own mind what information a person needs to carry out your instruction, what the outcome will be if the instruction is carried out, and how that outcome can or will be evaluated. When you have thought through these questions, you are ready to give the proper instruction.
- *Get positive attention.*   Avoid factors that interfere with effective listening. Informing the person that the instructions will be given is one simple way to try to get positive attention. Highlighting the background, giving a justification, or indicating the importance of the instructions also may be appropriate.
- *Give clear, concise instructions.*   Use an inoffensive and nondefensive style and tone of voice. Be precise, and give all the information receivers need to carry out your expectations. Follow a step-by-step procedure if several actions are needed.
- *Verify through feedback.*   Make sure the receiver has understood your specific request for action. Ask for a repeat of the instructions.
- *Provide follow-up communication.*   Understanding does not guarantee performance. Follow up to discover if your instruction is clear and if the person has any questions.

The nurse manager is responsible both for the quality of the work life of individual employees and for the quality of patient care in the entire unit. To carry out this job, acknowledge the needs of individual employees, especially if the needs of one conflict with needs of the unit, speak directly with those involved, and state clearly and accurately the rationale for the decisions made.

## Administrators

The manager's interaction with higher administration is comparable to the interaction between the manager and an employee, except that the manager is now the subordinate. Higher administration is responsible for the consequences of decisions made for a larger area, such as all of nursing service or the entire organization. The principles used in communicating with subordinates are equally appropriate. Managers should be organized and prepared to state their needs clearly, explain the rationale for requests, suggest benefits for the larger organization, and use appropriate channels. Listen objectively to your supervisor's response and be willing to consider reasons for possible conflict with needs of other areas.

Working effectively with an administrator is important because this person directly influences personal success in a career and within the organization. Managing a supervisor, or managing upward, is a crucial skill for nurses. To manage upward, remember that the relationship requires participation from both parties. Managing upward is successful when power and influence move in both directions. Rules for managing your supervisor are found in Box 9-2.

One aspect of managing upward is to understand the supervisor's position from her or his frame of reference. This will make it easier to propose solutions and ideas that the supervisor will accept. Understand that a supervisor is a person with even more responsibility and pressure. Learn about the supervisor from a personal perspective: What pressures, both personal and professional, does the supervisor face? How does the supervisor respond to stress? What previous experiences are liable to affect today's issues? This assessment will allow you to identify ways to help your supervisor with his or her job and for your supervisor to help you with yours.

### Influencing Your Supervisor

Nurses need to approach their supervisor to exert their influence on a variety of issues and problems. Support for the purchase of capital equipment, for changes in staffing, or for a new policy or procedure all require communicating with a supervisor. Your rationale, choice of form or format, and possible objections all are important factors to consider as you prepare to make such a request. Timing is critical; choose an opportunity when the supervisor has time and appears receptive. Also, consider the impact of your ideas on other events occurring at that time.

Should ideas be presented in spoken or written form? Usually some combination is used. Even if you have a brief meeting about a relatively small request, it is a good idea to follow up with an e-mail, detailing your ideas and the plans to which you both agreed. Sometimes the procedure works in reverse. If you provide the supervisor with a written proposal prior to a meeting, both of you will be familiar with the idea at the start. In the latter case, careful preparation of the written material is essential.

What can be done if, in spite of careful preparation, your supervisor says no? First, make sure you have understood the objections and associated feelings. **Negative inquiry** (e.g., "I don't understand") is a helpful technique to use. Do not interrupt or become defensive or distraught; remain diplomatic. **Fogging**, agreeing with part of what was said, or **negative assertion**, accepting some blame, are two additional techniques that you can use.

The next step is confrontation. Keep your voice low and measured; use "I" language; and avoid absolutes, why questions, put-downs, inflammatory statements, and threatening gestures. Finally, if you feel you have lost and compromise is unlikely, table the issue by saying, "Could

---

**BOX 9-2    Rules for Managing Your Boss**

- Give immediate positive feedback for good things that the supervisor does; positive feedback is a welcome change.
- Never let your supervisor be surprised; keep her or him informed.
- Always tell the truth.
- Find ways to compensate for weaknesses of your supervisor. Fill in weak areas tactfully. Volunteer to do something the supervisor dislikes doing.

- Be your own publicist. Don't brag, but keep your supervisor informed of what you achieve.
- Keep aware of your supervisor's achievements and acknowledge them.
- If your supervisor asks you to do something, do it well and ahead of the deadline if possible. If appropriate, add some of your own suggestions.
- Establish a positive relationship with the supervisor's assistant.

we continue discussing this at another time?" Then, think through your supervisor's reasoning and evaluate it.

Afterward ask yourself: "What new information did I get from the supervisor?" "What are ways I can renegotiate?" "What do I need to know or do to overcome objections?" Once you can answer these questions, approach your supervisor again with the new information. This behavior shows that the proposal is a high priority, and the new information may cause him or her to reevaluate.

Managers often succeed in influencing supervisors through persistence and repetition, especially if supporting data and documentation are supplied. If the issue is important enough, you may want to take it to a higher authority. If so, tell your supervisor you would like an administrator at a higher level to hear the proposal. Keep an open mind, listen, and try to meet objections with suggestions of how to solve problems. Be prepared to compromise, which is better than no movement at all, or to be turned down.

### Taking a Problem to Your Supervisor

No one wants to hear about a problem, and your boss is no different. Nonetheless, work involves problems, and the manager's job is to solve them. Go to your supervisor with a goal to problem solve together. Have some ideas about solving the problem in hand if you can but do not be so wedded to them that you are unable to listen to your supervisor's ideas. Keep an open mind. Use the following steps to take a problem to your supervisor:

- Find an appropriate time to discuss a problem, scheduling an appointment if necessary.
- State the problem succinctly and explain why it is interfering with work.
- Listen to your supervisor's response and provide more information if needed.
- If you agree on a solution, offer to do your part to solve it. If you cannot discover an agreeable solution, schedule a follow-up meeting or decide to gather more information.
- Schedule a follow-up appointment.

By solving the problem together and, if necessary, by taking active steps together, you and your supervisor are more likely to accept the decision and be committed to it. Setting a specific follow-up date can prevent a solution from being delayed or forgotten.

### If All Else Fails

Sometimes no matter what you do, working with your supervisor seems nearly impossible. Some managers foster a negative work environment, and employees become dissatisfied, angry, and depressed. High absenteeism and turnover result. As a manager you are charged with supporting your supervisor. If working with that person is too difficult for you to manage your work satisfactorily, you may have to transfer elsewhere or leave.

## Coworkers

Interactions with coworkers are inevitable. Relationships can vary from comfortable and easy to challenging and complex. Coworkers often share similar concerns. Camaraderie may be present; coworkers can exchange ideas and address problems creatively. They can provide support, and the strengths of one can be developed in the other.

Conversely, there may also be competition or conflicts (e.g., battles over territory, personality clashes, differences of opinion) affected by history, the organization's mores, or generational or cultural differences. Even when there are conflicts, coworkers should interact on a professional level. Chapter 12 suggests ways to handle conflict.

## Medical Staff

Communication with the medical staff may be difficult for the nurse manager because the relationship of physicians and nurses has been that of superior and subordinate (Kripalani et al., 2007). Complicating physician–nurse relationships is the employee status of the medical staff.

They may not be employees of the organization but still have considerable power because of their ability to attract patients to the organization, and, finally, the medical staff is in itself diverse, consisting of physicians who are organizational employees, residents, physicians in private practice, and consulting physicians.

One program designed to help physicians improve their communication skills is LegacyMd (see http://legacymd.com/). Using improvisational techniques, participants practice interacting in scenes depicting workplace examples, receive feedback, and replay the scene with enhanced skills.

(See the next section on collaborative communication for how to interact more effectively with physicians.)

### Other Health Care Personnel

The nurse manager has the overwhelming task of coordinating the activities of a number of personnel with varied levels and types of preparation and different kinds of tasks. The patient may receive regular care from a registered nurse, unlicensed assistive personnel, a respiratory therapist, a physical therapist, and a dietitian, among others. The nurse manager may supervise all of them. Regardless, the manager needs considerable skill to communicate effectively with diverse personnel, recognize their commonalities, and deal with their differences.

### Patients and Families

Nurse managers deal with many difficult issues. Patient or family complaints about the delivery of care (e.g., complaints about a staff member, violations of policy) are one example. When dealing with patient or family complaints, keep the following principles in mind:

- *The patient and family are the principal customers of the organization.* Treat patients and families with respect; keep communication open and honest. Dissatisfied customers fail to continue to use a service and also inform their friends and families about their negative experiences. Handle complaints or concerns tactfully and expeditiously. Many times lawsuits can be avoided if the patient or family feels that someone has taken the time to listen to their complaints. (See the section on risk management in Chapter 6.)
- *Most individuals are unfamiliar with medical jargon.* Use words that are appropriate to the recipient's level of understanding. However, take care not to be condescending or intimidating. It is just as important to assess the person's knowledge base and level of understanding as it is to know his or her vital signs or liver status.
- *Maintain privacy and identify a neutral location for dealing with difficult interactions.*
- *Make special efforts to find interpreters if a patient or family does not speak English.* Have readily available a list of individuals who are able to communicate in a variety of languages. The list also should include individuals experienced in sign language and Braille. Another resource is AT&T's language line service (800-752-6096), which provides interpreters for over 140 languages 24 hours a day.
- *Recognize cultural differences in communicating with patients and their families.* People in some cultures do not ask questions for fear of imposing on others (Huber, 2009). Some cultures prefer interpreters from their own culture; others do not. Cultural education for the staff can help identify some of these differences and teach them appropriate, culturally sensitive responses (Raingruber et al., 2010).

## Collaborative Communication

Collaboration is central to patient safety, according to a study by Vitalsmarts™ (Maxfield et al., 2005). The researchers found seven areas where health care workers found it difficult to speak up, including seeing colleagues make mistakes, perform incompetently, disrespect others, break rules, fail to support colleagues, exhibit poor teamwork, or micromanage inappropriately.

| **TABLE 9-3    Improving Communication** |
| --- |

1. Consider your relationship to the receiver.
2. Craft your message, including your goal and how to answer responses.
3. Decide on the medium based on your relationship, the content, and the setting.
4. Check your timing.
5. Deliver your message.
6. Attend to verbal or written responses.
7. Reply appropriately.
8. Conclude when both parties' messages have been understood.
9. Evaluate communication process.

Propp and colleagues (2010) found that two processes were critical to ensuring collaboration with physicians and other members of the health care team. These were ensuring quality decisions and promoting team synergy (see Table 9-3). Developing a collaborative practice model, nurses can build their credibility with physicians and enhance the workplace environment.

Another study found that communication and role understanding crucial to collaborative practice (Suter et al., 2009). Appreciation of one another's roles was key to improving communication and positive patient outcomes. Focusing educational objectives on communication and understanding others' roles, rather than more diffuse skills, such as respect, is more likely to lead to better practices, the researchers assert.

To support greater collaboration between nurses and physicians and to improve the product of nursing service—patient care—keep these principles in mind:

- Respect physicians as persons, and expect them to respect you.
- Consider yourself and your staff equal partners with physicians in health care.
- Build your staff's clinical competence and credibility. Ensure that your staff has the clinical preparation necessary to meet required standards of care.
- Actively listen and respond to physician complaints as customer complaints. Create a problem-solving structure. Stop blaming physicians exclusively for communication problems.
- Use every opportunity to increase your staff's contact with physicians and to include your staff in meetings that include physicians. Remember that limited interactions contribute to poor communication.
- Establish a collaborative practice committee on your unit whose membership is composed equally of nurses and physicians. Identify problems, develop mutually satisfactory solutions, and learn more about each other. Emphasize similarities and the need for quality care. Begin with those physicians who have a positive attitude toward collaboration.
- Serve as a role model to your staff in nurse–physician communication.
- Support your staff in participating in collaborative efforts by words and by your actions.

If you are confronted with power plays or intimidation, what is the best way to respond? Intimidation can be counteracted by increasing self-confidence and personal feelings of power. Four ways that generate power are:

1. With words:
   - Use the other person's name frequently.
   - Use strong statements.
   - Avoid discounters, such as "I'm sorry, but . . . ?"
   - Avoid clichés, such as "hit the nail on the head," "goes without saying," "easier said than done."
   - Avoid fillers (such as "ah," "uh," and "um").

2. Through delivery:
   - Be enthusiastic.
   - Speak clearly and forcefully.
   - Make one point at a time.
   - Do not tolerate interruptions.

3. By listening:
   - Listen for facts.
   - Pay attention to emotions.
   - Listen for what is not being said (e.g., body language, mixed messages, hidden messages).

4. Through body posture and body language:
   - Sit next to your antagonist; turn 30 degrees toward the person when you address him or her.
   - Lean forward.
   - Expand your personal space.
   - Use gestures.
   - Stand when you talk.
   - Smile when you are pleased, not in order to please.
   - Maintain eye contact, but do not stare.

One nurse manager handled a problem with a physician as shown in Case Study 9-1. Additional techniques to counteract intimidation and threat are included in Chapters 12, 21, and 22.

## CASE STUDY 9-1

### COMMUNICATION

Josie Randolph is nurse manager of a perioperative unit, including responsibility for the preoperative testing unit, 18 OR suites, pre-op holding, and sterile processing. The OR department supports the hospital's Level I trauma service as well as all other surgical services.

Dr. Jonas Welborne is a plastic surgeon with a history of aggressive behavior. He has several cases on today's OR schedule. While he is in his first surgery, a trauma case is brought to the OR. Susan Richardson, the OR charge nurse, decides to bump Dr. Welborne's second case out of OR #3 to make room for the trauma case. When Dr. Welborne has finished his first case, he is informed of the delay in his second case. Dr. Welborne storms into the OR scheduling office and begins yelling at Susan. The situation quickly escalates to the point where Dr. Welborne uses obscenities and throws several charts on the floor. Loretta Donnelly, an OR tech, runs to Josie's office and asks her to come immediately to the OR scheduling office.

Susan and Dr. Welborne continue to yell at one another, in full view of patients in the pre-op area. Josie immediately steps between Dr. Welborne and Susan and firmly asks both of them to lower their voices. She instructs Susan to wait in the staff lounge while she speaks with Dr. Welborne. Josie asks Dr. Welborne to step into her office so they can calmly discuss the situation. Dr. Welborne is still visibly agitated but agrees to discuss the problem.

After hearing his side of the story, Josie apologizes for the inconvenience, but reminds him of the OR policies. Emergent cases take precedence over elective cases, and no other elective cases were on the schedule at that time. She asks Dr. Welborne if there are alternatives to scheduling his cases that would minimize delays or bumps. As they talk, Dr. Welborne becomes calmer.

Josie informs Dr. Welborne that his earlier behavior is unacceptable. Within a few minutes, he apologizes to Josie and asks to speak with Susan. He also apologizes to Susan. Josie and Susan discuss the incident and ways Susan can help diffuse similar situations in the future. As with Dr. Welborne, Josie indicates that Susan's behavior was unprofessional and, as the OR charge nurse, she is always expected to act as a nursing professional and role model.

### Manager's Checklist

The nurse manager is responsible for:

- Mediating conflict in a timely manner
- Knowing organizational policies and procedures that support staff decisions
- Allowing open and complete discussion of the problem
- Actively listening to both participants
- Using assertive communication to facilitate problem solving

# Enhancing Your Communication Skills

Communication skills can be learned. Suggestions to improve your communication skills are shown in Table 9-3.

To communicate effectively, first consider your relationship to the receiver (e.g., boss or patient). Then craft your message. Be clear about your goal in your mind so that you can communicate it appropriately. Then think about what the other person is liable to say and consider how you might respond.

Next decide on the medium. Is this message best conveyed in person, by phone, e-mail, or text? Should you leave a message if the person isn't available? Note the personal intimacy content earlier in the chapter for guidance.

Timing plays a critical role in successful communication. Catch your boss in the midst of planning for a budget shortfall and you are less apt to get a receptive hearing.

Be prepared when you deliver your message. The best-crafted message, delivered by the appropriate medium can misfire by a sender who fails to listen carefully, avoids responding out of fear of consequences, or undermines the message with qualifiers, such as "I don't know if you're interested."

(For more information on communicating effectively, see Sullivan, E. J. (2013). *Becoming influential: A guide for nurses* (2nd ed.). Upper Saddle River, NJ: Prentice Hall.

## What You Know Now

- Communication is a complex, ongoing, dynamic process.
- How to deliver a message depends on the purpose, the content, and the relationship.
- Messages can be distorted or misconstrued.
- Gender, generation, cultural background, and the organizational culture influence communication and its outcome.
- Expert communication skills are essential for a leader to be successful.
- Communication strategies vary according to the situation and the roles of people involved.
- Collaborative communication is challenging, and specific skills can help.
- Nurses can enhance their communication skills with effort and practice.

## Tools for Communicating Effectively

1. Identify and use the appropriate method (in person, phone, voice mail, text, e-mail, letter) for your communications.
2. Evaluate your communication skills in various situations. Think of ways to improve.
3. Practice using the skills described in specific situations, such as with your coworkers, the medical staff, and with patients and their families.
4. Become sensitive to others' responses, both verbal and nonverbal, and craft your messages appropriately.
5. Gather feedback and continue to assess the effectiveness of your communications.
6. Strive to improve your communication skills.

## Questions to Challenge You

1. Consider a recent interaction you witnessed.
   Did the sender express the message clearly?
   Use the appropriate medium?
   Listen and respond to questions and comments?
   What was the outcome?
2. Now think about a recent interaction where you were the sender using the above criteria. If you could replay the interaction, what would you do differently?
3. How well does communication function in your workplace, school, or clinical site?
4. To improve your communication, practice the skills described in the chapter by role playing or recording yourself (Sullivan, 2013).

**Pearson Nursing Student Resources**

Find additional review materials at
**www.nursing.pearsonhighered.com**

Prepare for success with additional NCLEX®-style practice questions, interactive assignments and activities, Web links, animations and videos, and more!

## Web Resources

LegacyMD: http://legacymd.com
Silence Kills: The Seven Crucial Conversations in HealthCare:
   http://silenttreatmentstudy.com/Silent%20Treatment%20Executive%20Summary.pdf

## References

Donaldson, M. C. (2007). *Negotiating for dummies* (2nd ed.). New York: Wiley Publishing.

Feldhahn, S. (2009). *The male factor: The unwritten rules, misperceptions, and secret beliefs of men in the workplace.* New York: Crown Business.

Hahn, J. (2009). Effectively manage a multigenerational staff. *Nursing Management, 40*(9), 8–10.

Helgesen, S., & Johnson, J. (2010). *The female vision: Women's real power at work.* San Francisco: Berrett-Koehler Publications.

Huber, L. M. (2009). Making community health care culturally correct. *American Nurse Today, 4*(5), 13–15.

Kaplan, A. M., & Haenlein, M. (2010). Users of the world, unite! The challenges and opportunities of social media. *Business Horizons, 53*(1), 59–68.

Kripalani, S., LeFevre, F., Phillips, C., Williams, M., Basaviah, P., & Baker, D. (2007). Deficits in communication and information transfer between hospital-based and primary care physicians. *Journal of American Medical Association, 297*(8), 831–841.

Maxfield, D., Grenny, J., Lavandero, R., & Groah, L. (2005). The silent treatment: Why safety tools and checklists aren't enough to save lives. Retrieved April 11, 2011 from http://www.silencekills.com/UPDL/SilenceKillsExecSummary.pdf

Propp, K. M., Apker, J., Zabava Ford, W. S., Wallace, N., Servenski, M., & Hofmeister, N. (2010). Meeting the complex needs of the health care team: Identification of nurse-team communication practices perceived to enhance patient outcomes. *Qualitative Health Research, 20*(1), 15–28.

Raingruber, B., Teleten, O., Curry, H., Vang-Yang, B., Kuzmenko, L., Marquez, V., & Hill, J. (2010). Improving nurse-patient communication and quality of care: The transcultural, linguistic care team. *Journal of Nursing Administration, 40*(6), 258–260.

Raso, R. (2010). Social media for nurse managers: What does it all mean? *Nursing Management, 41*(8), 23–25.

Robertson-Malt, S., Herrin-Griffith, D. M., & Davies, J. (2010). Designing a patient care model with relevance to the cultural setting. *Journal of Nursing Administration, 40*(6), 277–282.

Sullivan, E. J. (2013). *Becoming influential: A guide for nurses* (2nd ed.). Upper Saddle River, NJ: Prentice Hall.

Suter, E., Arndt, J., Arthur, N., Parboosingh, J., Taylor, E., & Deutschlander, S. (2009). Role understanding and effective communication as core competencies for collaborative practice. *Journal of Interprofessional Care, 23*(1), 41–51.

Tannen, D. (2001). *Talking from 9 to 5: How women's and men's conversational styles affect who gets heard, who gets credit, and what gets done at work.* New York: Harper.

Trossman, S. (2010). Sharing too much? Nurses nationwide need more information on social networking pitfalls. *American Nurse Today, 5*(11), 38–39.

# Delegating Successfully

**Delegation**

**Benefits of Delegation**

BENEFITS TO THE NURSE

BENEFITS TO THE DELEGATE

BENEFITS TO THE MANAGER

BENEFITS TO THE ORGANIZATION

**The Five Rights of Delegation**

**The Delegation Process**

**Accepting Delegation**

**Ineffective Delegation**

ORGANIZATIONAL CULTURE

LACK OF RESOURCES

AN INSECURE DELEGATOR

AN UNWILLING DELEGATE

UNDERDELEGATION

REVERSE DELEGATION

OVERDELEGATION

## Learning Outcomes

*After completing this chapter, you will be able to:*

1. Describe how delegation involves responsibility, accountability, and authority.
2. Describe how effective delegation benefits the delegator, the delegate, the unit, and the organization.
3. Discuss how to be an effective delegator.
4. Identify obstacles that can impede effective delegation.
5. Explain how liability affects delegation.

## Key Terms

Accountability
Assignment
Authority

Delegation
Overdelegation
Responsibility

Reverse delegation
Underdelegation

# Delegation

**Delegation** is the process by which responsibility and authority for performing a task (function, activity, or decision) is transferred to another individual who accepts that authority and responsibility. Although the delegator remains accountable for the task, the delegate is also accountable to the delegator for the responsibilities assumed. Delegation can help others to develop or enhance their skills, promote teamwork, and improve productivity.

It is easy to say delegate, but delegation is a difficult leadership skill for nurses to learn and one that may not be taught in undergraduate education. Given the confusion over what tasks assistive personnel can perform and what are those that are the unique purview of RNs, nurses and nurse managers may be reluctant to delegate. Never before, however, has delegation been as critical a skill for nurses and nurse managers to perfect as it is today, with the emphasis on doing more with less.

The benefits of delegating appropriately are many. (See the next section.) In fact, a leader who models delegation promotes collaboration between nurses and support personnel (Orr, 2010) as well as a positive workplace environment (Standing & Anthony, 2008).

Responsibility, accountability, and authority are concepts related to delegation. Although *responsibility* and *accountability* are often used synonymously, the two words represent different concepts that go hand in hand. **Responsibility** denotes an obligation to accomplish a task, whereas **accountability** is accepting ownership for the results or lack thereof. Responsibility can be transferred, but accountability is shared.

You can delegate only those tasks for which you are responsible. If you have no direct responsibility for the task, then you can't delegate that task. For instance, if a manager is responsible for filling holes in the staffing schedule, the manager can delegate this responsibility to another individual. However, if staffing is the responsibility of a central coordinator, the manager can make suggestions or otherwise assist the staffing coordinator, but cannot delegate the task.

Likewise, if an orderly who is responsible for setting up traction is detained and a nurse asks a physical therapist on the unit to assist with traction, this is not delegation, because setting up traction is not the responsibility of the nurse. However, if the orderly (the person responsible for the task) had asked the physical therapist to help, this could be an act of delegation if the other principles of delegation are met.

Along with responsibility, you must transfer authority. **Authority** is the right to act. Therefore, by transferring authority, the delegator is empowering the delegate to accomplish the task. Too often this principle of delegation is neglected. Nurses retain authority, crippling the delegate's abilities to accomplish the task, setting the individual up for failure, and minimizing efficiency and productivity.

Delegation is often confused with work assignment. Delegation involves transfer of responsibility and authority. In **assignment** no transfer of authority occurs. Instead, assignments are a bureaucratic function that reflect job descriptions and patient or organizational needs. Effective delegation benefits the delegator, the delegate, the manager, and the organization.

# Benefits of Delegation

### Benefits to the Nurse

Nurses also benefit from delegation. If the nurse is able to delegate some tasks to UAPs, more time can be devoted to those tasks that cannot be delegated, especially complex patient care. Thus, patient care is enhanced, the nurse's job satisfaction increases, and retention is improved.

*Nancy, RN, has three central line dressing changes to complete as well as two patients to transfer to another unit before the end of shift in one hour. Nancy delegates the transfer duties to Shelley, LPN, and completes the central line dressing changes.*

### Benefits to the Delegate

The delegate also benefits from delegation. The delegate gains new skills and abilities that can facilitate upward mobility. In addition, delegation can bring trust and support, and thereby build self-esteem and confidence. Subsequently, job satisfaction and motivation are enhanced as individuals feel stimulated by new challenges. Morale improves; a sense of pride and belonging develops as well as greater awareness of responsibility. Individuals feel more appreciated and learn to appreciate the roles and responsibilities of others, increasing cooperation and enhancing teamwork.

### Benefits to the Manager

Delegation also yields benefits for the manager. First, if staff are using UAPs appropriately, the manager will have a better functioning unit. Also the manager may be able to delegate some tasks to staff members and devote more time to management tasks that cannot be delegated. With more time available, the manager can develop new skills and abilities, facilitating the opportunity for career advancement.

### Benefits to the Organization

As teamwork improves, the organization benefits by achieving its goals more efficiently. Overtime and absences decrease. Subsequently, productivity increases, and the organization's financial position may improve. As delegation increases efficiency, the quality of care improves. As quality improves, patient satisfaction increases.

## The Five Rights of Delegation

Fear of liability often keeps nurses from delegating. State nurse practice acts determine the legal parameters for practice, professional associations set practice standards, and organizational policy and job descriptions define delegation appropriate to the specific work setting. Also guidelines from the National Council of State Boards of Nursing (NCSBN) can help.

The NCSBN identified the five rights of delegation shown in Table 10-1. In addition, each state board of nursing has its own rules regarding delegation.

- The right task specifies what can be safely delegated to a specific patient. These are commonly assigned tasks. Tasks that require nursing assessment or judgment should not be delegated (Austin, 2008).
- The right circumstances include an appropriate setting and available resources. Evaluate the patient's needs and the skills of personnel who could be assigned to meet those specific needs.
- The right person refers to both the delegator and the delegate. The delegator must have the authority and responsibility for the patient's care and for the task to be assigned. The delegate must be capable of performing the task and be available to assist. Give the right task to the right person for the right patient.

---

**TABLE 10-1    The Five Rights of Delegation**

- Right task
- Right circumstances
- Right person
- Right direction and communication
- Right supervision

National Council of State Boards of Nursing. (2007). The five rights of delegation. Retrieved June 28, 2011 at https://www.ncsbn.org/Joint_statement.pdf

**Figure 10-1** ●
Decision tree for delegation to nursing assistive personnel. Source: Adapted from National Council of State Boards of Nursing. (2006). Joint statement on delegation. Retrieved December 2007 from www.ncsbn.org/Joint_statement.pdf

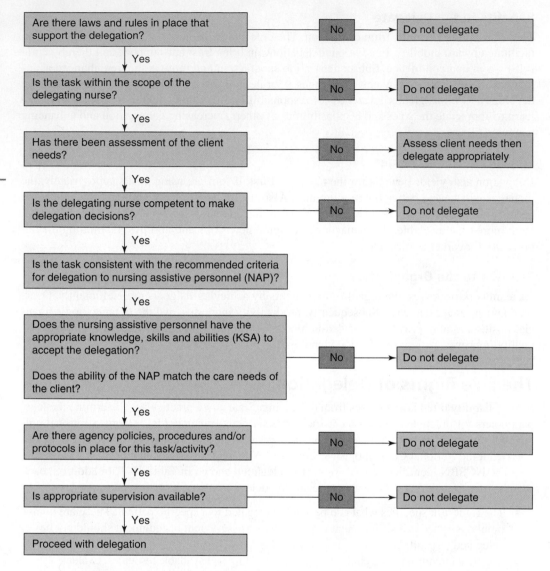

• The right direction and communication requires the delegator to give clear, concise description of the task as well as describe the objectives, the limits, and the expectations as a result. The delegate should be able to recognize that the patient is responding as expected.
• The right supervision includes monitoring the delegate, evaluating the person's performance, giving feedback as required, and intervening if necessary. The delegator remains responsible for the patient's care regardless of who performs it.

Also the National Council of State Boards of Nursing decision tree can help guide nurses' decisions about delegation. (See Figure 10-1.)

## The Delegation Process

The delegation process has five steps as shown in Table 10-2.

1. **Define the task.** Delegate only an aspect of your own work for which you have responsibility and authority. These include:
   • Routine tasks
   • Tasks for which you do not have time
   • Tasks that have moved down in priority

| **TABLE 10-2**   **Delegation Process** |
| --- |
| 1. Define the task. |
| 2. Decide on delegate. |
| 3. Determine the task. |
| 4. Reach agreement. |
| 5. Monitor performance and provide feedback. |

Define the aspects of the task. Ask yourself:

- Does the task involve technical skills or cognitive abilities?
- Are specific qualifications necessary?
- Is performance restricted by practice acts, standards, or job descriptions?
- How complex is the task?
- Is training or education required?
- Are the steps well defined, or are creativity and problem solving required?
- Would a change in circumstances affect who could perform the task?

While you are trying to define the complexity of the task and its components, it is important not to fall into the trap of thinking no one else is capable of performing this task. Often others can be prepared to perform a task through education and training. The time taken to prepare others can be recouped many times over. Also know well the task to be delegated.

An alternative would be to subdivide the task into component parts and delegate the components congruent with the available delegate's capabilities. For example, developing a budget is a managerial responsibility that cannot be delegated, but someone else could explore the types of tympanic thermometers on the market, their costs, advantages, and so on. A committee of staff nurses could evaluate the options and make a recommendation that you could include in the budget justification.

But how do you know what should not be delegated?

Before a task is delegated, determine what areas of authority and what resources you control to achieve the expected results. A unit manager who is responsible for maintaining adequate supplies needs budget authority. The authority to spend money on supplies, however, may be limited to a specific amount for specific supplies or may be allocated to supplies in general.

Certain tasks should never be delegated. Discipline should not be delegated, nor should a highly technical task. Also any situation that involves confidentiality or controversy should not be delegated to others.

2. *Decide on delegate.* Match the task to the individual. Analyze individuals' skill levels and abilities to evaluate their capability to perform the various tasks; also determine characteristics that might prevent them from accepting responsibility for the task. Conversely experience and individual characteristics, such as initiative, intelligence, and enthusiasm, can expand the individual's capabilities. A rule of thumb is to delegate to the lowest person in the hierarchy who has the requisite capabilities and who is allowed to do the task legally and by organizational policy.

Next determine availability. For example, Su Ling might be the best candidate, but she leaves for vacation tomorrow and won't be back before the project is due. Then ask who would be willing to assume responsibility. Delegation is an agreement that is entered into voluntarily.

3. *Determine the task.* The next step in delegation is to clearly define your expectations for the delegate. Also plan when to meet. Attempting to delegate in the middle of a crisis is not delegation; that is directing. Provide for enough time to describe the task and your expectations and to entertain questions. Also, meet in an environment as devoid of distractions as possible.

| **TABLE 10-3** | **Key Behaviors in Delegating Tasks** |
| --- | --- |

- Describe the task using "I" statements.
- Discuss the importance to the organization.
- Explain the expected outcome and timeline for completion.
- Identify any constraints for completing the task.
- Validate understanding of the task and your expectations.

Key behaviors in delegating tasks are shown in Table 10-3

a. Describe the task using "I" statements, such as "I would like . . ." and appropriate non-verbal behaviors—open body language, face-to-face positioning, and eye contact. The delegate needs to know what is expected, when the task should be completed, and where and how, if that is appropriate. The more experienced delegates may be able to define for themselves the where and how. Decide whether written reports are necessary or if brief oral reports are sufficient. If written reports are required, indicate whether tables, charts, or other graphics are necessary. Be specific about reporting times. Identify critical events or milestones that might be reached and brought to your attention. For patient care tasks, determine who has responsibility and authority to chart certain tasks. For example, UAPs can enter vital signs, but if they observe changes in patient status, the RN must investigate and chart the assessment.

b. Discuss the importance to the organization, you, the patient, and the delegate. Provide the delegate with an incentive for accepting both the responsibility and the authority to do the task.

c. Explain the expected outcome and the timeline for completion. Establish how closely the assignment will be supervised. Monitoring is important because you remain accountable for the task, but controls should never limit an individual's opportunity to grow.

d. Identify any constraints for completing the task or any conditions that could change. For example, you may ask an assistant to feed a patient for you as long as the patient is coherent and awake, but you might decide to feed the patient if he were confused.

e. Validate understanding of the task and your expectations by eliciting questions and providing feedback.

4. ***Reach agreement.*** Once you have outlined your expectations, you must be sure that the delegate agrees to accept responsibility and authority for the task. You need to be prepared to equip the delegate to complete the task successfully. This might mean providing additional information or resources or informing others about the arrangement as needed to empower the delegate. Before meeting with the individual, anticipate areas of negotiation, and identify what you are prepared and able to provide.

5. ***Monitor performance and provide feedback.*** Monitoring performance provides a mechanism for feedback and control that ensures that the delegated tasks are carried out as agreed. Give careful thought to monitoring efforts when objectives are established. When defining the task and expectations, clearly establish the where, when, and how. Remain accessible. Support builds confidence and reassures the delegate of your interest in the delegate and negates any concerns about dumping undesirable tasks.

Monitoring the delegate too closely, however, conveys distrust. Analyze performance with respect to the established goal. If problem areas are identified, privately investigate and explain the problem, provide an opportunity for feedback, and inform the individual how to correct the mistake in the future. Provide additional support as needed. Also, be sure to give the praise and recognition due, and don't be afraid to do so publicly.

# Accepting Delegation

Accepting delegation means that you accept full responsibility for the outcome and its benefits or liabilities. Just as the delegator has the option to delegate parts of a task, you also have the option to negotiate for those aspects of a task you feel you can accomplish. Recognize, however, that this may be an opportunity for growth. You may decide to capitalize on it, obtaining new skills or resources in the process.

When you accept delegation, you must understand what is being asked of you. First, acknowledge the delegator's confidence in you, but realistically examine whether you have the skills and abilities for the task and the time to do it. If you do not have the skills, you must inform the delegator. However, it does not mean you cannot accept the responsibility. See whether the person is willing to train or otherwise equip you to accomplish the task. If not, then you need to refuse the offer.

Once you agree on the role and responsibilities you are to assume, make sure you are clear on the time frame, feedback mechanisms, and other expectations. Don't assume anything. As a minimum, repeat to the delegator what you heard said; better yet, outline the task in writing.

Throughout the project, keep the delegator informed. Report any concerns you have as they come up. Foremost, complete the task as agreed. Successful completion can open more doors in the future.

If you are not qualified or do not have the time, do not be afraid to say no. Thank the delegator for the offer and clearly explain why you must decline at this time. Express your interest in working together in the future.

See how a school nurse handled delegation in Case Study 10-1.

## CASE STUDY 10-1

### DELEGATION

Lisa Ford is a school nurse for a suburban school district. She has responsibility for three school buildings, including a middle school, a high school, and a vocational rehabilitation workshop for mentally and physically handicapped secondary students. Her management responsibilities include providing health services for 1,000 students, 60 faculty members, and 25 staff members, as well as supervising two unlicensed school health aides and three special education health aides. The logistics of managing multiple school sites results in the delegation of many daily health room tasks, including medication administration, to the school-based health aides.

Nancy Andrews is an unlicensed health aide at the middle school. This is her first year as a health aide and she has a limited background in health care. The nurse practice act in the state allows for the delegation of medication administration in the school setting. Lisa is responsible for training Nancy to safely administer medication to students, documenting the training, evaluating Nancy's performance, and providing ongoing supervision. Part of Nancy's training will also include a discussion of those medication-related decisions that must be made by a registered nurse.

### Manager's Checklist

The nurse manger is responsible for:

- Understanding the state nurse practice act and its applicability to the school setting
- Implementing school district policies related to health services and medication administration
- Developing and implementing an appropriate training program
- Limiting opportunities for error and decreasing liability by ensuring that unlicensed health aides are appropriately trained to handle delegated tasks
- Maintaining documentation related to training and observing medication administration by unlicensed staff
- Auditing medication administration records to ensure accuracy and completeness
- Conducting several "drop in" visits during the school year to track competency of health aides
- If necessary, reporting any medication errors to administration and following up with focused training and closer supervision

# Ineffective Delegation

Ineffective delegation results in missed or omitted routine care, such as feeding, turning, ambulating, and toileting (Bittner & Gravlin, 2009; Gravlin & Bittner, 2010). Poor communication and interpersonal relationship between nurses and unlicensed assistive personnel (UAP) has been found to result in ineffective delegation (Standing & Anthony, 2008).

The RN/UAP unit is a microsystem in health care and when that unit is dysfunctional or functioning at less than optimal performance, the quality of care suffers. One reason for problems with delegation is the assignment of a single UAP to more than one RN. The UAP's workload may be more than one person can handle but each nurse may be unaware of the assistant's overload.

Another reason for ineffective delegation is that nurses define delegation differently (Standing & Anthony, 2008). Some nurses define delegation as explicit instructions to carry out a specific task. Others think that delegation is both specific and implicit in expected tasks, such as ambulating or toileting.

Potential barriers to effective delegation include organizational factors or the delegator's or delegate's beliefs or inexperience.

## Organizational Culture

The culture within the organization may restrict delegation. Hierarchies, management styles, and norms may all preclude delegation. Rigid chains of command and autocratic leadership styles do not facilitate delegation and rarely provide good role models. The norm is to do the work oneself because others are not capable or skilled. An atmosphere of distrust prevails as well as a poor tolerance for mistakes. A norm of crisis management or poorly defined job descriptions or chains of command also impede successful delegation.

## Lack of Resources

Another difficulty frequently encountered is a lack of resources. For example, there may be no one to whom you can delegate. Consider the sole registered nurse in a skilled nursing facility. If practice acts define a task as one that only a registered nurse can perform, there is no one else to whom that nurse can delegate that task.

Financial constraints also can interfere with delegation. For instance, someone from your department must attend the annual conference in your nursing specialty area. However, the organization will only pay the manager's travel and conference expenses, which precludes anyone else from attending.

Educational resources may be another limiting factor. Perhaps others could learn how to do a task if they could practice with the equipment, but the equipment or a trainer is not available.

Time can also be a limiting factor. For example, it is Friday, and the schedule needs to be posted on Monday. No one on your staff has experience developing schedules and you need to go out of town for a family emergency, so there is no one else to do the schedule.

## An Insecure Delegation

The majority of the barriers to delegation arise from the delegator. Reasons people give to fail to delegate include:

"I can do it better."

"I can do it faster."

"I'd rather do it myself."

"I don't have time to delegate."

Often underlying these statements are erroneous beliefs, fears, and inexperience in delegation. Certainly, the experienced person can do the task better and faster. Indeed, delegation takes time, but failing to delegate is a time waster. Time invested in developing staff today is later repaid many times over.

Common fears are:

- *Fear of competition or criticism.* What if someone else can do the job better or faster than I? Will I lose my job? Be demoted? What will others think? Will I lose respect and control? This fear is unfounded if the delegator has selected the right task and matched it with the right individual. In fact, the delegate's success in the task provides evidence of the delegator's leadership and decision-making abilities.
- *Fear of liability.* Some individuals are not risk takers and shy away from delegation for this reason. There are risks associated with delegation, but the delegator can minimize these risks by following the steps of delegation. A related concern is a fear of being blamed for the delegate's mistakes. If the delegator selected the task and delegate appropriately, then the responsibility for any mistakes made are solely those of the delegate; it is not necessary to take on guilt for another's mistakes.

   Review the five rights of delegation and the decision tree for the National Council of State Boards of Nursing as well as the state's nurse practice act and the organization's policies. RNs often fear blame from management if something goes wrong when a task has been delegated to an LPN or UAP, but those fears can be relieved if state law, organizational policies, and job descriptions are followed.
- *Fear of loss of control.* Will I be kept informed? Will the job be done right? How can I be sure? The more one is insecure and inexperienced in delegation, the more this fear is an issue. This is also a predominant concern in individuals who tend toward autocratic styles of leadership and perfectionism. The key to retaining control is to clearly identify the task and expectations and then to monitor progress and provide feedback.
- *Fear of overburdening others.* They already have so much to do; how can I suggest more? Everyone has work to do. Such a statement belittles the decisional capabilities of others. Recall that delegation is a voluntary, contractual agreement; acceptance of a delegated task indicates the availability and willingness of the delegate to perform the task. Often, the delegate welcomes the diversion and stimulation, and what the delegator perceives as a burden is actually a blessing. The onus is on the delegator to select the right person for the right reason.
- *Fear of decreased personal job satisfaction.* Because the type of tasks recommended to delegate are those that are familiar and routine, the delegator's job satisfaction should actually increase with the opportunity to explore new challenges and obtain other skills and abilities.

## An Unwilling Delegate

Inexperience and fear of failure can motivate a potential delegate to refuse to accept a delegated task. Much reassurance and support are needed. In addition, the delegate should be equipped to handle the task. If proper selection criteria are used and the steps of delegation followed, then the delegate should not fail. The delegator can boost the delegate's lack of confidence by building on simple tasks. The delegate needs to be reminded that everyone was inexperienced at one time. Another common concern is how mistakes will be handled. When describing the task, the delegator should provide clear guidelines for handling problems, guidelines that adhere to organizational policies.

Another barrier is the individual who avoids responsibility or is overdependent on others. Success breeds success; therefore, it is important to use an enticing incentive to engage the individual in a simple task that guarantees success.

When the steps of delegation are not followed or barriers remain unresolved, delegation is often ineffective. Inefficient delegation can result from unnecessary duplication, underdelegation, reverse delegation, and overdelegation.

## Underdelegation

**Underdelegation** occurs when

- The delegator fails to transfer full authority to the delegate;
- The delegator takes back responsibility for aspects of the task; or
- The delegator fails to equip and direct the delegate.

As a result, the delegate is unable to complete the task, and the delegator must resume responsibility for its completion.

> *Sharon, RN, is a school nurse with three separate buildings under her direction. UAPs, called health clerks, operate in the school health office when Sharon is at another building. Joye, a first-year health clerk, has had minimal medication administration instruction and experience. During the first week of school, Joye tries to "speed up" the medication administration process and sets out all of the noon medications in individual, unlabeled cups for the students. The cups are rearranged by students trying to find their meds and Joye cannot identify what meds belong to which students. Sharon is called back to the school to administer the correct medications, students are late to class, and Joye is frustrated that she couldn't handle the task.*

It may be that the RN fears liability or lacks confidence or experience in delegating and decides to do all the tasks rather than delegate to an assistant (Mitty et al., 2010). Conversely, the assistant may not be prepared for the tasks or may not believe the task is within the assistant's scope of practice. In addition, the assistant may not be able to complete all the tasks, especially if the person is assigned to several nurses.

## Reverse Delegation

In **reverse delegation**, someone with a lower rank delegates to someone with more authority.

> *Thomas is a nurse practitioner for the burn unit. He recently arrived on the unit to find several patients whose dressing changes have not been completed due to a code situation earlier in the morning. Dawn, LPN, asks Thomas to help the staff complete dressing changes before physician rounds begin.*

## Overdelegation

**Overdelegation** occurs when the delegator loses control over a situation by providing the delegate with too much authority or too much responsibility. This places the delegator in a risky position, increasing the potential for liability. In this instance, the nurse assumes that any task that doesn't involve nursing assessment or judgment should be assigned to assistive personnel.

> *Ellen, GN, is in her sixth week of orientation in the trauma ICU. Her mentor, Dolores, RN, notes that Mr. Anderson is scheduled for an MRI off the unit. Dolores delegates the task of escorting Mr. Anderson to the MRI unit to Ellen who is not ACLS certified. During the MRI, Mr. Anderson is accidentally extubated and suffers respiratory and cardiac arrest. A code is called in the MRI suite and ER nurses must respond since an ACLS certified nurse is not with the patient.*

Not delegating appropriately negatively affects other staff on the unit as well. Here are two examples:

> *Sally, RN, always says she "likes to do everything herself" for her patients. She doesn't like to ask aides for assistance. Her patients are usually happy, but Sally is extremely busy all day and doesn't ever have time to help a peer RN when asked or answer call lights to help the team. Sally's peers get frustrated because her lack of delegating*

*appropriate tasks to her nurse's aide partner makes the aide feel not valued, Sally feels too busy in her job, and her peers feel like they get no help from Sally when needed.*

*Bridgett, RN, feels that she has spent her time doing aide work while she was in nursing school. Now that she has taken NCLEX boards and is working as a nurse, she won't help patients to the bathroom or empty a bedpan, or change bed linens. She will call an aide to do these tasks even if she is in the room and has time to do the tasks herself. Bridgett's inappropriate delegation causes aides to be angry, peer RNs to be frustrated because the aides don't have time to help them because they are always doing Bridgett's work, and results in inconsistency in the practice between Bridgett and other nurses, which Bridget' patients' notice.*

Delegation is a skill that can be learned. Like other skills, successfully delegating requires practice. Sometimes it seems it might be easier to do it yourself. But it is not. Once you learn how to delegate, you will extend your ability to accomplish more by using others' help.

By delegating appropriately, managers can role model this behavior and teach their staff to do likewise. In addition, it is the best use of their time.

No one in health care today can afford not to delegate.

## What You Know Now

- Delegation is a contractual agreement in which authority and responsibility for a task is transferred by the person accountable for the task to another individual.
- Delegation benefits the delegator, delegate, the manager, the unit, and the organization.
  - The five rights of delegation are the right task, the right circumstances, the right person, the right direction, and the right supervision.
  - Delegation involves skill in identifying and determining the task and level of responsibility, deciding who has the requisite skills and abilities, describing expectations clearly, reaching mutual agreement, and monitoring performance and providing feedback.
  - Delegatable tasks are personal, routine tasks that the delegator can perform well; that do not involve discipline, highly technical tasks, or confidential information; and that are not controversial.
  - To accept delegation, agree on roles and responsibilities, the time frame for completion, feedback mechanisms, and expectations.
  - Ineffective delegation can occur with organizational constraints or the delegate's or delegator's lack of experience or beliefs.
  - Managers can role model appropriate delegation.
- Delegation is essential in health care today.

## Tools for Delegating Successfully

1. Delegate only tasks for which you have responsibility.
2. Transfer authority when you delegate responsibility.
3. Be sure you follow state regulations, job descriptions, and organizational policies when delegating.
4. Follow the delegation process and key behaviors for delegating described in the chapter.
5. Accept delegation when you are clear about the task, time frame, reporting, and other expectations.
6. Review the five rights of delegation and the NCSBN's decision tree to delegate appropriately.

## Questions to Challenge You

1. Review your state's nurse practice act. How is delegation defined? What tasks can and cannot be delegated? How is supervision defined? Are there any other guidelines for supervision? Are responsibilities regarding advanced practice delineated? How does the scope of practice differ between registered and licensed practical/vocational nurses? What is the scope of practice of other health care providers?
2. What are your organization's policies on delegation?

3. Describe a situation when you delegated a task to someone else. Did you follow the steps of delegation explained in the chapter? Was the outcome positive? If not, what went wrong?

4. Describe a situation when someone else delegated a task to you. Did your delegator explain what to do? Did you receive too much information? Not enough? Was supervision appropriate to the task and to your abilities? What was the outcome?

**Pearson Nursing Student Resources**

Find additional review materials at

**www.nursing.pearsonhighered.com**

Prepare for success with additional NCLEX®-style practice questions, interactive assignments and activities, Web links, animations and videos, and more!

## References

Austin, S. (2008). 7 legal tips for safe nursing practice. *Nursing 2008, 38*(3), 34–39.

Bittner, N. P., & Gravlin, G. (2009). Critical thinking, delegation, and missed care in nursing practice. *Journal of Nursing Administration, 39*(3), 142–146.

Gravlin, G., & Bittner, N. P. (2010). Nurses' and nursing assistants' reports of missed care and delegation. *Journal*

*of Nursing Administration, 40*(7/8), 329–335.

Mitty, E., Resnick, B., Bakerjian, D., Gardner, W., Rainbard, S., Mezey, M. (2010). Nursing delegation and medication administration in assisted living. *Nursing Administration Quarterly, 34*(2), 162–171.

National Council of State Boards of Nursing. (2007). The five rights of delegation. Retrieved June 28, 2011 at

https://www.ncsbn.org/Joint_statement.pdf

Orr, S. E. (2010). Characteristics of positive working relationships between nursing and support service employees. *Journal of Nursing Administration, 40*(3), 129–134.

Standing, T. S., & Anthony, M. K. (2008). Delegation: What it means to acute care nurses. *Applied Nursing Research, 21*(1), 8–14.

# Building and Managing Teams

## Learning Outcomes

*After completing this chapter, you will be able to:*

1. Describe how groups and teams function.
2. Differentiate between team building and managing teams.
3. Describe various methods of team building.
4. Discuss factors that influence team management.
5. Explain why the nurse manager's leadership skills are essential to team performance.
6. Discuss how to lead groups, task forces, and patient care conferences.

## Key Terms

Additive task
Adjourning
Clinical ladder
Cohesiveness
Committees or task
   forces
Competing groups
Conjunctive task
Disjunctive task
Divisible task
Formal committees
Formal groups

Forming
Group
Hidden agendas
Informal committees
Informal groups
Norming
Norms
Ordinary interacting
   groups
Performing
Pooled interdependence
Productivity

Real (command) groups
Reciprocal interdependence
Re-forming
Role
Sequential interdependence
Status
Status incongruence
Storming
Task forces
Task group
Team building
Teams

Most often, nursing occurs in a team environment. Work groups that share common objectives function in a harmonious, coordinated, purposeful manner as teams. The staff nurse is constantly involved in teamwork. The nurse/aide/unit secretary team works together every day on a nursing unit. With shared governance more often the norm and interprofessional team work common, the nurse may participate or lead a team broader in scale than one unit. For example, a nurse might lead the acute care practice council or be on a team to implement supplies at the bedside.

High-performance teams require expert leadership skills. In a health care delivery system integrated across settings, a team environment becomes increasingly essential. Nurse managers must skillfully orchestrate the activity and interactions of interprofessional teams as well as conventional nursing work groups. Understanding the nature of groups and how groups are transformed into teams is essential for the nurse to be effective.

## Groups and Teams

A **group** is an aggregate of individuals who interact and mutually influence each other. Both formal and informal groups exist in organizations. **Formal groups** are clusters of individuals designated temporarily or permanently by an organization to perform specified organizational tasks. Formal groups may be structured laterally, vertically, or diagonally. Task groups, teams, task forces, and committees may be structured in all of these ways, whereas command groups generally are structured vertically.

Group members include:

- Individuals from a single work group (e.g., nurses on one unit) or individuals at similar job levels from more than one work group (e.g., all professional staff)
- Individuals from different job levels (e.g., nurses and UAPs)
- Individuals from different work groups and different job levels in the organization (e.g., committee to review staff orientation classes)

Groups may be permanent or temporary. Command groups, teams, and committees usually are permanent, whereas task groups and task forces are often temporary.

**Informal groups** evolve naturally from social interactions. Groups are informal in the sense that they are not defined by an organizational structure. Examples of informal groups include individuals who regularly eat lunch together or who convene spontaneously to discuss a clinical dilemma.

**Real (command) groups** accomplish tasks in organizations and are recognized as a legitimate organizational entity. Its members are interdependent, share a set of norms, generally differentiate roles and duties among themselves, are organized to achieve ongoing organizational goals, and are collectively held responsible for measurable outcomes.

The group's manager has line authority in relation to group members individually and collectively. The group's assignments are usually routine and designed to fulfill the specific mission of the agency or organization. The regularly assigned staff who work together under the direction of a single manager constitute a command group.

A **task group** is composed of several persons who work together, with or without a designated leader, and are charged with accomplishing specific time-limited assignments. A group of nurses selected by their colleagues to plan an orientation program for new staff constitute a task group. Usually, several task groups exist within a service area and may include representatives from several disciplines (e.g., nurse, physician, dietitian, social worker).

Other special groups include **committees or task forces** formed to deal with specific issues involving several service areas. A committee responsible for monitoring and improving patient safety or a task force assigned to develop procedures to adhere to patient privacy regulations are examples of special work groups.

Health care organizations depend on numerous committees, which nurses participate in and often lead. Some of these committees are mandated by accrediting and regulatory bodies, such as committees for education, standards, disaster, and patient care evaluation. Others are established to meet a specific need (e.g., to formulate a new policy on substance abuse).

**Teams** are real groups in which individuals must work cooperatively with each other in order to achieve some overarching goal. Teams have command or line authority to perform tasks, and membership is based on the specific skills required to accomplish the tasks. Similar to groups described above, teams may include individuals from a single work group or individuals at similar job levels from more than one work group, individuals from different job levels, or individuals from different work groups and different job levels in the organization. They may have a short life span or exist indefinitely.

*Metropolitan Hospital has established a **clinical ladder** system for nursing staff. Each quarter, members of the clinical excellence committee meet to review applications from staff nurses who are seeking promotion to the next clinical ladder level. The committee is made up of staff nurses and nurse managers from each service line. Each applicant is responsible for completing a comprehensive application. The committee members evaluate each application and make recommendations to the vice president for patient care on those nurses who should be considered for promotion.*

Not all work groups, however, are teams. For example, groups of individuals who perform their tasks independently of each other are not teams. **Competing groups**, in which members compete with each other for resources to perform their tasks or compete for recognition, are also not teams.

A work group becomes a team when the individuals must apply group process skills to achieve specific results. They must exchange ideas, coordinate work activities, and develop an understanding of other team members' roles in order to perform effectively. Members appreciate the talents and contributions of each individual on the team and find ways to capitalize on them. Most work teams have a leader who maintains the integrity of the team's function and guides the team's activities, performance, and development. Teams may be self-directed, that is, led jointly by group members who decide together about work objectives and activities on an ongoing basis.

In a given service area, the entire staff might not function as a team, but a subgroup may. For example, case managers for the inpatient and ambulatory cystic fibrosis population in a children's medical center might be called a team. Individual members of an interdisciplinary team, such as this one, may report formally to different managers, but in delivering care to the cystic fibrosis population there is no designated individual in charge. In meetings, the team members discuss clients' problems and jointly decide on plans of action.

Many different types of groups and teams are used throughout organizations. Examples are ad hoc task groups, quality improvement teams, quality circles, self-directed work teams, shared governance councils, and focus groups.

*Nurse managers at a large university hospital are responsible for educating their staff about patient satisfaction. Patient satisfaction surveys are sent to randomly selected patients. Results are compiled, and each department receives a detailed report of the results. Staff members review the data at monthly staff meetings, using both positive and negative comments to guide their patient care activities. As needed, department standards and protocols are updated to reflect improved processes.*

Most groups are considered **ordinary interacting groups**. These groups usually have a designated formal leader, but they may be leaderless. Most work teams, task groups, and committees are ordinary interacting groups. Discussions usually begin with a statement of the problem by the group leader followed by an open, unstructured conversation. Normally, the final decision is made by consensus (without formal voting; members indicate concurrence with a group agreement that everyone can live with and support publicly). The decision may also be made by the leader or someone in authority, majority vote, an average of members' opinions, minority control, or an expert member. Interacting groups enhance the cohesiveness and *esprit de corps* among group members. Participants are able to build strong social ties and will be committed to the solution decided on by the group.

> *Infection control nurses have been tracking occurrences of MRSA infections among patients in their hospital system. In addition to implementing patient care protocols as recommended by federal and state infectious disease agencies, the nurses track compliance in high-risk units and tailor education programs to meet the needs of nursing and assistive staffs.*

Ordinary interacting groups, however, may be dominated by one or a few members. If the group is highly cohesive, its decision-making ability may be affected by groupthink (discussed in Chapter 8). Groupthink results in pressure for every member to conform, usually to the leader's beliefs, even to violating personal norms.

Sometimes groups spend excessive time dealing with socioemotional relationships, reducing the time spent on the problem and slowing consensus. Ordinary groups may reach compromise decisions that may not really satisfy any of the participants. Because of these problems, the functioning of ordinary groups is dependent on the leader's skills.

Each type of group presents unique opportunities and challenges. An important role of the nurse manager is to link service areas with groups at higher levels in the organization. This link facilitates problem solving, coordination, and communication throughout the organization. Leadership roles in work groups are important and may also be either formal or informal. For example, the nurse manager formally leads the unit or service area staff but may also informally lead a support group of nurse managers.

The leader's influence on group processes, formal or informal, and the ability of the group to work together as a team often determine whether the group accomplishes its goals. Nurse managers may effectively manage work groups and turn them into teams by understanding principles of group processes and applying them to group decision making, team building, and leading committees and task forces.

## Group and Team Processes

The modified version of Homans's (1950, 1961) social system conceptual scheme presented in Figure 11-1 provides a framework for understanding group inputs, processes, and outcomes. The schematic depicts the effects of organizational and individual background factors on group leadership, including dynamics (tasks, activities, interactions, attitudes) and processes (forming, storming, norming, performing, adjourning). Elements of the required group system and processes influence each other and the emergent group system and social structure.

This system determines the productivity of the group as well as members' quality of work life, such as job satisfaction, development, growth, and similarity in thinking. The framework distinguishes required factors that are imposed by the external system from factors that emerge from the internal dynamics of the group.

According to Homans's framework, the three essential elements of a group system are activities, interactions, and attitudes. Activities are the observable behaviors of group members. Interactions are the verbal or nonverbal exchanges of words or objects among two or more group members. Attitudes are the perceptions, feelings, and values held by individual group members, which may be both positive and negative. To understand and guide group functioning, a manager should analyze the activities, interactions, and attitudes of work group members.

Homans's framework indicates that background factors, the manager's leadership style, and the organizational system influence the normal development of the group. Groups, whether formal or informal, typically develop in these phases: form, storm, norm, perform, and adjourn or re-form. In the initial stage, **forming**, individuals assemble into a well-defined cluster. Group members are cautious in approaching each other as they come together as a group and begin to understand requirements of group membership. At this stage, the members often depend on a leader to define purpose, tasks, and roles.

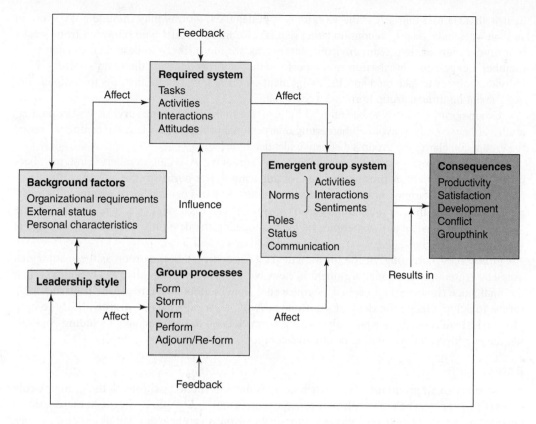

**Figure 11-1** ●
Conceptual scheme of a basic social system. *Source:* Adapted from Homans, G. (1950). *The human group.* New York: Harcourt Brace Jovanovich; and Homans, G. (1961). *Social behavior: Its elementary forms.* New York: Harcourt Brace. By permission of Transaction Publishers.

As the group begins to develop, **storming** occurs. Members wrestle with roles and relationships. Conflict, dissatisfaction, and competition arise on important issues related to procedures and behavior. During this stage, members often compete for power and status, and informal leadership emerges. During the storming stage, the leader helps the group to acknowledge the conflict and to resolve it in a win–win manner.

In the third stage, **norming**, the group defines its goals and rules of behavior. The group determines what are or are not acceptable behaviors and attitudes. The group structure, roles, and relationships become clearer. Cohesiveness develops. The leader explains standards of performance and behavior, defines the group's structure, and facilitates relationship building.

In the fourth stage, **performing**, members agree on basic purposes and activities and carry out the work. The group's energy becomes task-oriented. Cooperation improves, and emotional issues subside. Members communicate effectively and interact in a relaxed atmosphere of sharing. The leader provides feedback on the quality and quantity of work, praises achievement, critiques poor work and takes steps to improve it, and reinforces interpersonal relationships within the group.

The fifth stage is either **adjourning** (the group dissolves after achieving its objectives) or **re-forming**, when some major change takes place in the environment or in the composition or goals of the group that requires the group to refocus its activities and recycle through the four stages. When a group adjourns, the leader must prepare group members for dissolution and facilitate closure through celebration of success and leave-taking. If the group is to refocus its activities, the leader will explain the new direction and provide guidance in the process of re-forming.

## Norms

**Norms** are the informal rules of behavior shared and enforced by group members. Norms emerge whenever humans interact. Groups develop norms that members believe must be adhered to for fruitful, stable group functioning. Nursing groups often establish norms related to how members deal with absences that affect the workload of colleagues. Norms may include not calling in sick on weekends, readily accommodating requests for trading shifts, and returning from breaks in a timely manner. In a team environment, norms are more likely to be linked to each team member's expected contribution to the performance and products of the team's efforts. If an individual agrees to take on a specific assignment on the team's behalf and fails to complete the assignment on time, a group norm has been violated.

Group norms are likely to be enforced if they serve to facilitate group survival, ensure predictability of behavior, help avoid embarrassing interpersonal problems, express the central values of the group, and clarify the group's distinctive identity.

Groups go through several stages in enforcing norms with deviant members. First, members use rational argument or present reasons for adhering to the norms to the deviant individual. Second, if rational argument is not effective, members may use persuasive or manipulative techniques, reminding the deviant of the value of the group. The third stage is attack. Attacks may be verbal or even physical and sometimes include sabotaging the deviant's work. The final stage is ignoring the deviant.

It becomes increasingly difficult for a deviant to acquiesce to the group as these strategies escalate. Agreeing to rational argument is easy, but agreeing after an attack is difficult. When the final stage (ignoring) is reached, acquiescence may be impossible because group members refuse to acknowledge the deviant's surrender. A nurse manager has a responsibility to help groups deal with members who violate group norms related to performance, including counseling the employee and preventing destructive conflict.

### Roles

Norms apply to all group members, whereas roles are specific to positions in the group. A **role** is a set of expected behaviors that fit together into a unified whole and are characteristic of persons in a given context. Roles commonly seen in groups can be classified as either task roles or socioemotional (nurturing) roles. Often, individuals fill several roles. Individuals performing task roles attempt to keep the group focused on its goals.

Task roles include:

- *Initiator–contributor.* Redefines problems and offers solutions, clarifies objectives, suggests agenda items, and maintains time limits
- *Information seeker.* Pursues descriptive bases for the group's work
- *Information giver.* Expands information given by sharing experiences and making inferences
- *Opinion seeker.* Explores viewpoints that clarify or reflect the values of other members' suggestions
- *Opinion giver.* Conveys to group members what their pertinent values should be
- *Elaborator.* Predicts outcomes and provides illustrations or expands suggestions, clarifying how they could work
- *Coordinator.* Links ideas or suggestions offered by others
- *Orienter.* Summarizes the group's discussions and actions
- *Evaluator-critic.* Appraises the quantity and quality of the group's accomplishments against set standards
- *Energizer.* Motivates group to accomplish, qualitatively and quantitatively, the group's goals
- *Procedural technician.* Supports group activity by arranging the environment (e.g., scheduling meeting room) and providing necessary tools (e.g., ordering visual equipment)
- *Recorder.* Documents the group's actions and achievements

Nurturing roles facilitate the growth and maintenance of the group. Individuals assuming these roles are concerned with group functioning and interpersonal needs.

Nurturing roles include:

- *Encourager.* Compliments members for their opinions and contributions to the group
- *Harmonizer.* Relieves tension and conflict
- *Compromiser.* Suppresses own position to maintain group harmony
- *Gatekeeper.* Encourages all group members to communicate and participate
- *Group observer.* Takes note of group processes and dynamics and informs group of them
- *Follower.* Passively attends meetings, listens to discussions, and accepts group's decisions

**Status** is the social ranking of individuals relative to others in a group based on the position they occupy. Status comes from factors the group values, such as achievement, personal characteristics, the ability to control rewards, or the ability to control information. Status is usually enjoyed by members who most conform to group norms. Higher-status members often exercise more influence in group decisions than others.

**Status incongruence** occurs when factors associated with group status are not congruent, such as when a younger, less experienced person becomes the group leader. Status incongruence can have a disruptive impact on a group. For example, isolates are members who have high external status and different backgrounds from regular group members. They usually work at acceptable levels but are isolated from the group because they do not fit the group member profile. Sometimes status incongruence occurs because the individual does not need the group's approval and makes no effort to obtain it.

The most important role in a group is the leadership role. Leaders are appointed for most formal groups, such as command groups, teams, committees, or task forces. Leaders in informal groups tend to emerge over time and in relation to the task to be performed. Some of the factors contributing to the emergence of leadership in small groups include the ability to accomplish the group's goals, sociability, good communication skills, self-confidence, and a desire for recognition. Guidelines for performing this leadership role are discussed later in this chapter.

# Building Teams

**Team building** focuses on both task and relationship aspects of a group's functioning and is intended to increase efficiency and productivity. The group's work and problem-solving procedures, member–member relations, and leadership are analyzed, and exercises are prescribed to help members modify their patterns of interaction or processes of decision making.

### Assessment

The most important initial activities in team building are data gathering and diagnosis. Questions must be asked about the group's context (organizational structure, climate, culture, mission, and goals); characteristics of the group's work, including group members' roles, styles, procedures, job complexity; and the team, its problem-solving style, interpersonal relationships, and relations with other groups.

The following questions may be asked:

1. To what extent do the team's members understand and accept the goals of the organization?

2. What, if any, hidden agendas interfere with the group's performance? Hidden agendas are members' individual unspoken objectives that interfere with commitment or enthusiasm.

3. How effective is the group's leadership?

4. To what extent do group members understand and accept their roles?

5. How does the group make decisions?

6. How does the group handle conflict? Are conflicts dealt with through avoidance, forcing, accommodating, compromising, competing, or collaborating?

7. What personal feelings do members have about each other?

8. To what extent do members trust and respect each other?

9. What is the relationship between the team and other units in the organization?

Only after assessing and diagnosing problems can the leader take actions to improve team functioning (Hill, 2010).

### Team-Building Activities

Team-building activities, originally designed to improve interpersonal workplace relationships, have expanded to include meeting goals and accomplishing tasks (Salas et al., 2008). A recent study found that female students in medicine and nursing were more open-minded about cooperating with other health professions than were male medical or nursing students (Wilhelmsson et al., 2011). This is positive news for those involved in team building with women, less so with male participants.

Training sessions for team-building can be effective in helping participants acquire skills, but the results are short-lived if the skills are not reinforced on the job. To effectively maintain the team performance, learned behaviors should be measured and rewarded (Salas et al., 2008).

Team Strategies and Tools to Enhance Performance and Patient Safety (TeamSTEPPS) is a program developed by the Department of Defense and the Agency for Healthcare Research and Quality (AHRQ) to integrate teamwork into practice (Henriksen et al., 2008; King et al., 2008). TeamSTEPPS involves three phases:

- Assessing the need
- Training onsite
- Implementing and sustaining training

McKeon, Cunningham, and Detty Oswaks (2009) tested TeamSTEPPS in a health care setting and found that these safety-oriented skills can be taught and that nurses can learn to practice and evaluate high-reliability behaviors in practice.

Simulation-based training can also be used for team building (Rosen et al., 2008). Participants act out a simulated incident, receive feedback on their performance, and repeat the performance incorporating the learned behaviors. The program, LegacyMD (mentioned in Chapter 9) is an example (see Web resources for the URL). Rosen and colleagues (2008) found quality measures improved after simulation training.

Thoughtful team-building strategies allow group members to acknowledge the developmental process and respond to it in constructive ways. Team-building activities may also be used to facilitate the normal stages of group development (forming, storming, norming, performing, and adjourning or re-forming), an important process in managing teams.

In traditional work groups experiencing problems, team-building strategies may help improve performance. Numerous techniques and commercial resources are available.

A nurse manager may decide to assume personal responsibility for team building when the team is basically functional and simply needs some fine-tuning to deal more effectively with minor interpersonal issues or changing circumstances.

## Managing Teams

Managing teams differs from team building and depends on the task, group size and composition, productivity and cohesiveness, the group's development and growth, and the extent of shared governance in the organization.

## Task

The size of the group can influence its effectiveness, depending on the type of task: additive, disjunctive, divisible, or conjunctive (Steiner, 1972, 1976). The more people who work on an **additive task** (group performance depends on the sum of individual performance), the more inputs are available to produce a favorable result. For example, the game tug-of-war involves the combined effort of the team.

For a **disjunctive task** (the group succeeds if one member succeeds), the greater the number of people, the higher the probability that one group member will solve the problem. Consider the Olympics. The more athletes on one team, the greater the opportunity for a gold medal. Regardless of the event, a medalist from the United States team brings recognition to the country, and every citizen is able to share the honor.

With a **divisible task** (tasks that can break down into subtasks with division of labor), more people provide a greater opportunity for specialization and interdependence in performing the tasks. For instance, the construction of a car is a complex task. From design of the car to insertion of the last bolt, each individual involved has a specialized task. With a **conjunctive task** (the group succeeds only if all members succeed), more people increase the likelihood that one person can slow up the group's performance (e.g., a jury trial).

On many tasks, interdependence is important. There are three kinds:

- **Pooled interdependence**, in which each individual contributes but no one contribution is dependent on any other (e.g., a committee discussion)
- **Sequential interdependence**, in which group members must coordinate their activities with others in some designated order (e.g., an assembly line)
- **Reciprocal interdependence**, in which members must coordinate their activities with every other individual in the group (e.g., team nursing)

## Group Size and Composition

Groups with 5 to 10 members tend to be optimal for most complex organizational tasks, which require diversity in knowledge, skills, and attitudes and allow full participation. In larger groups, members tend to contribute less of their individual potential while the leader is called on to take more corrective action, do more role clarification, manage more disruption, and make recognition more explicit. Groups tend to perform better with competent individuals as members. However, coordination of effort and proper utilization of abilities and task strategies must occur as well. Homogeneous groups tend to function more harmoniously, whereas heterogeneous groups may experience considerable conflict.

## Productivity and Cohesiveness

**Productivity** represents how well the work group or team uses the resources available to achieve its goals and produce its services. If patient care is satisfactorily completed at the end of each shift in relation to the levels of staffing, supplies, equipment, and support services used, the group has been productive. Productivity is influenced by work-group dynamics, especially a group's cohesiveness and collaboration.

**Cohesiveness** is the degree to which the members are attracted to the group and how much they are willing to contribute. Cohesiveness is also related to homogeneity of interests, values, attitudes, and background factors. Strong group cohesiveness leads to a feeling of "we" as more important than "I" and ensures a higher degree of cooperation and interpersonal support among group members.

Group norms may support or subvert organizational objectives, depending on the level of group cohesiveness. High group cohesiveness may foster high or low individual performance, depending on the prevailing group norms for performance. When cohesiveness is low, productivity may vary significantly. Although groups, in general, tend toward lower productivity, nursing education and practice have especially high standards of performance that help to counter this tendency.

Groups are more likely to become cohesive when members:

- Share similar values and beliefs
- Are motivated by the same goals and tasks
- Must interact to achieve their goals and tasks
- Work in proximity to each other (on the same unit and on the same shift, for example)
- Have specific needs that can be satisfied by involvement in the group

Group cohesiveness is also influenced by the formal reward system. Groups tend to be more cohesive when group members receive comparable treatment and pay and perform similar tasks that require interaction among the members. Similarities in values, education, social class, gender, age, and ethnicity that lead to similar attitudes strengthen group cohesiveness.

Cohesiveness can produce intense social pressure. Highly cohesive groups can demand and enforce adherence to norms regardless of their practicality or effectiveness. In this circumstance, the nurse manager may have a difficult time influencing individual nurses, especially if the group norms deviate from the manager's values or expectations. For example, operating room nurses may be used to arriving at the time their shift starts and then changing into scrubs. The nurse manager, in contrast, may expect the staff to be changed and ready for work by the time the shift starts. In addition, group dynamics can affect absenteeism and turnover. Groups with high levels of cohesiveness exhibit lower turnover and absenteeism than groups with low levels of cohesiveness.

For most individuals, the work group provides one of the most important social contacts in life; the experience of working on an effective work team contributes significantly to one's professional confidence and to the quality of work life and job satisfaction. The work group often provides the primary motivation for returning to the job day after day even when employees are dissatisfied with the employing organization or other working conditions.

Work groups not only perform tasks but also provide the context in which novices learn basic skills and become socialized and experts engage in clinical mentorship, standard setting, quality improvement, and innovation. Work-group relations influence the satisfaction of staff with their jobs, the overall quality of work life, and the quality of the environment for patient care. Managers play key roles in guiding the tasks of work groups and ensuring efficient and effective performance; managers also encourage relationships among members of work teams that will promote coordination and cooperation.

## Development and Growth

Groups can also provide learning opportunities by increasing individual skills or abilities. The group may facilitate socialization of new employees into the organization by "showing them the ropes." The nurse manager must establish an atmosphere that encourages learning new skills and knowledge, creating a group-oriented learning environment by continuously encouraging group members to improve their technical and interpersonal skills and knowledge through training and development. Group cohesiveness and effectiveness improve as staff members take responsibility for teaching each other and jointly seeking new information or techniques.

## Shared Governance

Shared decision making is a hallmark of shared governance. That is, both managers and staff members participate in making decisions. Such participation can improve collaboration, staff retention, job satisfaction, productivity, and patient outcomes. Measuring the distribution of control, influence, power, and authority, Hess (2011) found that managers perceived staff to have more power in making decisions than staff perceived that they did. Workload issues offered opportunities for shared decision making in another study (MacPhee, Wardrop, & Campbell, 2010).

As a requirement for Magnet certification, shared governance increases staff involvement in the organization's functioning and future planning and, at the same time, increases staff allegiance to the organization.

# The Nurse Manager as Team Leader

Because staff nurses work in close proximity and frequently depend on each other to perform their work, the nurse manager's leadership is vital. A positive climate is one in which there is mutual high regard and in which group members safely may discuss work-related concerns, critique and offer suggestions about clinical practice, and comfortably experiment with new behaviors. Maintaining a positive work group climate and building a team is a complex and demanding leadership task.

## Communication

Communication is a central component of the nurse manager's leadership. The Joint Commission, the organization that accredits hospitals, found that poor interprofessional communication was the cause of nearly 70 percent of unexpected events causing death or serious injury (Joint Commission, 2011).

Effective nurse managers can facilitate communication in groups by maintaining an atmosphere in which group members feel free to discuss concerns, make suggestions, critique ideas, and show respect and trust. An important leadership function related to communication is gatekeeping, that is, keeping communication channels open, refocusing attention on critical issues, identifying and processing conflict, fostering self-esteem, checking for understanding, actively seeking the participation of all group members, and suggesting procedures for discussing group problems.

The manager's communication style also affects group cohesiveness. If the manager maintains a high degree of information power and controls not only what information is received but also who receives it, group performance may suffer. By interrupting, changing the subject, monopolizing the conversation, or ignoring the feedback, problems escalate and the leader remains uninformed and both individuals in the group and the group's ability to function suffer.

If, on the other hand, the manager shares information freely, encourages a high degree of mutual communication and participative problem solving, performance and job satisfaction improves. In participative groups, each individual has the opportunity, and is encouraged, to seek and share information and to communicate frequently with anyone and everyone in the group. Managers and staff alike check with each other to ensure that information is clear, to offer suggestions, and to provide feedback.

Handling conflict (Chapter 12) and change management (Chapter 5) are essential management skills as well (MacPhee & Bouthillette, 2008).

## Evaluating Team Performance

The manager may be accustomed to evaluating individual performance, but evaluating how well a team performs requires different assessments. Patient outcomes and team functioning are the criteria by which teams can be evaluated (Rosen et al., 2008). Outcome data, such as clinical pathway information, variances in critical paths, complication rates, falls, and medication errors, can help evaluate team performance.

Group functioning can be assessed by the level of work-group cohesion, involvement in the job, and willingness to help each other. Conversely aggression, competition, hostility, aloofness, shaming, or blaming are characteristics of poorly functioning groups. Stability of members is an additional measure of group functioning.

Influencing team processes toward the attainment of organizational objectives is the direct responsibility of the nurse manager. By publicizing team accomplishments, creating opportunities for team members to demonstrate new skills, and supporting social activities, the manager

## CASE STUDY 11-1

### INTRODUCING MULTIDISCIPLINARY TEAMS

Bruce Shapiro was promoted six months ago to nurse manager for the stroke rehabilitation unit of a nationally owned rehabilitation hospital. Patient care delivery systems have been under intensive review at the corporate level, and major changes in staffing are underway. Previously, physical and occupational therapists were staffed out of a separate department and reported to the director of physical therapy. Now all therapists will be unit based and report to the nurse manager. Documentation will now be team centered instead of being split among nursing, therapists, and other care providers.

Janice Simpson has been a physical therapist for 25 years and has been at the rehab hospital for the past 6 years. She worked as a shift leader for physical therapy until the new unit-based staffing was implemented. Janice has been assigned to the stroke rehab unit and will report to Bruce. She feels uncomfortable in her new role and is concerned about how she will fit in with the established nursing staff. Janice is also concerned that with the new documentation system, the physical therapy patient evaluations will not be included in determining patient goals.

Bruce is eager for Janice to join the staff of the stroke rehabilitation unit. He schedules individual meetings with Janice and the three other therapists who will be assigned to his unit. Bruce outlines the roles and expectations of staff on the unit and listens attentively to their questions and concerns. He also reviews the physical and occupational therapy job descriptions and reviews their respective documentation standards. At the monthly staff meeting, Bruce discusses the roles and responsibilities of the therapists with the nursing staff. A mentor is assigned to meet daily with each therapist for their first two weeks on the unit.

### Manager's Checklist

The nurse manager is responsible for:

- Understanding the new staffing policies and the impact on the unit
- Gaining knowledge related to physical and occupational therapy practice
- Easing the transition of new staff into the existing staff group and helping build trust and respect
- Educating all staff on the new staffing policies
- Ensuring that all therapists and nurses attend mandatory documentation training and audit patient records for compliance with new documentation standards
- Communicating with human resources if there are any questions regarding performance evaluation, scheduling, or compensation
- Reviewing the personnel files of new staff
- Establishing roles for the therapists in the unit governance structure
- Facilitating open communication with therapists and nurses to discuss concerns or suggestions
- Providing appropriate feedback to nursing management related to the new staffing changes

can increase the perceived value of group membership. Members of groups who have a history of success are attracted to each other more than those who have not been successful.

See how one nurse handled his new assignment as manager for an interprofessional team in Case Study 11-1.

# Leading Committees and Task Forces

Committees are generally permanent and deal with recurring problems. Membership on committees is usually determined by organizational position and role. **Formal committees** are part of the organization and have authority as well as a specific role. **Informal committees** are primarily for discussion and have no delegated authority. **Task forces** are ad hoc committees appointed for a specific purpose and a limited time. Task forces work on problems or projects that cannot be readily handled by the organization through its normal activities and structures. Task forces often deal with problems crossing departmental boundaries. They tend to generate recommendations and then disband.

Nurses are often selected for leadership roles on committees and task forces. In these leadership roles and as unit managers and team leaders, they conduct numerous meetings. The following section provides guidance for leading and conducting meetings.

## Guidelines for Conducting Meetings

Although meetings are vital to the conduct of organizational work, they should be held principally for problem solving, decision making, and enhancing working relationships. Other uses of meetings, such as socializing, giving or clarifying information, or soliciting suggestions must be thoroughly justified. Meetings should be conducted efficiently and should result in relevant and meaningful outcomes. Meetings should not result in damaged interpersonal relations, frustration, or inconclusiveness.

### Preparation

The first key to a successful meeting is thorough preparation. Preparation includes clearly defining the purpose of the meeting. The leader should prepare an agenda, determine who should attend, make assignments, distribute relevant material, arrange for recording of minutes, and select an appropriate time and place for the meeting. The agenda should be distributed well ahead of time, 7 to 10 days prior to the meeting, and it should include what topics will be covered, who will be responsible for each topic, what prework should be done, what outcomes are expected in relation to each topic, and how much time will be allotted for each topic.

Sometimes a "meeting before the meeting" is advisable (Sullivan, 2013). This is especially important if you are going into a meeting where you expect dissension. It may involve simply chatting with a few key people to identify any problems or issues they expect, or you may need to actually sit down with a key decision maker who has veto power. Also asking people you expect might have opposing points of view their opinion might be helpful as well.

### Participation

In general, the meeting should include the fewest number of stakeholders who can actively and effectively participate in decision making, who have the skills and knowledge necessary to deal with the agenda, and who adequately can represent the interests of those who will be affected by decisions made. Too few or too many participants may limit the effectiveness of a committee or task force.

### Place and Time

Meetings should be held in places where interruptions can be controlled and at a time when there is a natural time limit to the meeting, such as late in the morning or afternoon, when lunch or dinner make natural time barriers. Meetings should be limited to 50 to 90 minutes, except when members are dealing with complex, detailed issues in a one-time session. Meetings that exceed 90 minutes should be planned to include breaks at least every hour. Meetings should start and finish on time. Starting late positively reinforces latecomers, while penalizing those who arrive on time or early. If sanctions for late arrival are indicated, they should be applied respectfully and objectively. If it is the leader who is late, the cost of starting meetings late should be reiterated and an appropriate designee should begin the meeting on time.

### Member Behaviors

The behavior of each member may be positive, negative, or neutral in relation to the group's goals. Members may contribute very little, or they may use the group to meet personal needs. Some members may assume most of the responsibility for the group action, thereby enabling less participative members to avoid contributing.

Group members should:

- Be prepared for the meeting, having read pertinent materials ahead of time
- Ask for clarification as needed
- Offer suggestions and ideas as appropriate
- Encourage others to contribute their ideas and opinions
- Offer constructive criticism as appropriate

- Help the discussion stay on track
- Assist with implementation as agreed

These behaviors facilitate group performance. All attendees should be familiar with behaviors that they may employ to facilitate well-managed meetings. All meeting participants must be helped to understand that they share responsibility for successful meetings.

A leader can increase meeting effectiveness greatly by not permitting one individual to dominate the discussion; separating idea generation from evaluation; encouraging members to refine and develop the ideas of others (a key to the success of brainstorming); recording problems, ideas, and solutions on a white board or flip chart; checking for understanding; periodically summarizing information and the group's progress; encouraging further discussion; and bringing disagreements out into the open and facilitating their reconciliation. The leader is also responsible for drawing out the members' **hidden agendas** (personal goals or needs). Revealing hidden agendas ensures that these agendas either contribute positively to group performance or are neutralized. Guidelines for leading group meetings are provided in Box 11-1.

## Managing Task Forces

There are a few critical differences between task forces and formal committees. For example, members of a task force have less time to build relationships with each other, and, because task forces are temporary, there may be no desire for long-term positive relationships. Formation of a task force may suggest that the organization's usual problem-solving mechanisms have failed. This perception may lead to tensions among task force members and between the task force and other units in the organization. The various members of a task force usually come from different parts of the organization and, therefore, have different values, goals, and viewpoints. The leader will need to take specific action to efficiently familiarize task force members with each other and create bonds in relation to the task.

### Preparing for the First Meeting

Prior to the task force's first meeting, the leader must clarify the objectives in specific measurable outcomes, determine its membership, set a task completion date, plan how often and to whom the task force should report while working on the project, and ascertain the group's scope of authority, including its budget, availability of relevant information, and decision-making power. The task force leader should communicate directly and regularly with the administrator

---

## BOX 11-1 Guidelines for Leading Group Meetings

- Begin and end on time.
- Create a warm, accepting, and nonthreatening climate.
- Arrange seating to minimize differences in power, maximize involvement, and allow visualization of all meeting activities. (A U-shape is optimal.)
- Use interesting and varied visuals and other aids.
- Clarify all terms and concepts. Avoid jargon.
- Foster cooperation in the group.
- Establish goals and key objectives.
- Keep the group focused.
- Focus the discussion on one topic at a time.

- Facilitate thoughtful problem solving.
- Allocate time for all problem-solving steps.
- Promote involvement.
- Facilitate integration of material and ideas.
- Encourage exploration of implications of ideas.
- Facilitate evaluation of the quality of the discussion.
- Elicit the expression of dissenting opinions.
- Summarize discussion.
- Finalize the plan of action for implementing decisions.
- Arrange for follow-up.

or governing body that commissioned the task force's work so that ongoing clarification of its charge and progress can be tracked and adjusted.

Task force members should be selected on the basis of their knowledge, skills, personal concern for the task, time availability, and organizational credibility. They should also be selected on the basis of their interpersonal skills. Those who relish group activities and can facilitate the group's efforts are especially good members. The group leader should also plan to include one or two individuals who potentially may oppose task force recommendations in order to solicit their input, involve them in the decision-making process, and win their support. By holding personal conversations with task force members before the first meeting, the group leader can explore individual expectations, concerns, and potential contributions. It also provides the leader with an opportunity to identify potential needs and conflicts and to build confidence and trust.

### Conducting the First Meeting

The goal of the first meeting is to come to a common understanding of the group's task and to define the group's working procedures and relationships. Task forces must rely on the general norms of the organization to function. The task force leader should legitimize the representative nature of participation on the task force and encourage members to discuss the task force's process with the other members of the organization.

During the first meeting, a standard of total participation should be well established. The leader should remain as neutral as possible and should prevent premature decision making. Working procedures and relationships among the various members, subgroups, and the rest of the organization need to be established. The frequency and nature of full task force meetings and the number of subgroups must be determined. Ground rules for communicating must be established, along with norms for decision making and conflict resolution.

### Managing Subsequent Meetings and Subgroups

In running a task force, especially when several subgroups are formed, the leader should hold full task force meetings often enough to keep all members informed of the group's progress. Unless a task force is small, subgroups are essential. The leader must not be aligned too closely with one position or subgroup. A work plan should be developed that includes realistic interim project deadlines. The task force and subgroups should be held to these deadlines. The leader plays a key role in coaching subgroups and the task force to meet its deadlines.

The leader must also be sensitive to the conflicting loyalties sometimes created by belonging to a task force. One of the leader's most important roles is to communicate information to both task force members and the rest of the organization in a timely and regular fashion. The leader should solicit feedback from other key organizational representatives during the course of the task force's work.

### Completing the Task Force's Report

In bringing a project to completion, the task force should prepare a written report for the commissioning administrators that summarizes the findings and recommendations. Drafts of this report should be shared with the full task force prior to presentation. To identify any overlooked or sensitive information and reduce defensive reactions, it is especially important that the task force leader personally brief key administrators prior to presenting the report. This gives administrators a chance to read and respond to the report before making recommendations. The leader should consider involving a few task force members in the administrative presentation.

## Patient Care Conferences

Patient-related conferences are held to address the needs of individual patients or patient populations. The purpose of the conference determines the composition of the group. Patient-focused meetings are usually interprofessional and used for case management to discuss specific patient care problems. For example, an interprofessional team may form to discuss the failure of a rehabilitation regimen to help a home care patient and to develop new plans for intervention.

Often nurses are also involved in activities associated with improving the quality of care for various patient groups and their families. For example, a nurse manager might organize meetings with primary care physicians and other managers to discuss how to improve discharge planning, to explore strategies to reduce the length of inpatient stays, or to improve coordination with outpatient clinics.

The team leader of a patient care conference often may not be a manager with line responsibility to supervise, evaluate, or hire employees. Frequently in patient rounds, the nurse is the person who can lead the conversation because the nurse has spent the most amount of time with the patient. The team leader is, however, a coach, teacher, and facilitator. Thus, the team leader needs to have excellent leadership skills. The task of a team leader varies according to the task and the skill level of the team members.

Nurses may be members of teams as well as leaders. Understanding how groups and teams function (or do not) is essential to contribute to the organization, be successful in your position, and to garner satisfaction from your work.

## What You Know Now

- A group is an aggregate of individuals who interact and mutually influence each other.
- Groups may be classified as real or task, formal or informal, permanent or temporary.
- A team is a group of individuals with complementary skills, a common purpose and performance goals, and a set of methods for which they hold themselves accountable.
- Assessment of problems should precede team-building activities.
- Team-building now includes a focus on meeting goals and accomplishing tasks as well as improving interpersonal relationships.
- Team-building activities are more likely to be successful if skills are reinforced on the job.
- Managing teams depends on the task, group size and composition, productivity and cohesiveness, development and growth, and the extent of shared governance in the organization.
- The nurse manager's communication skills affect the team's productivity and performance.
- Managing meetings involves preparing thoroughly, facilitating participation, and completing the group's work.

## Tools for Building and Managing Teams

1. Notice how groups around you function. Use the best ideas with your own groups.
2. Watch effective leaders. Identify skills you could incorporate into your own leadership repertoire.
3. Recognize that you can develop good team leadership skills. Practice those discussed in the chapter.
4. At the next opportunity be prepared to follow the directions for leading meetings.
5. Make a development plan to enhance your leadership skills.

## Questions to Challenge You

1. Identify the groups that include you in your work or school. How are they different? Similar? Explain.
2. Describe an example of effective group leadership and an example of poor leadership.
3. Evaluate your own leadership performance. How could you improve?
4. Have you been involved in team building at work or school? Was it effective? Explain.
5. What roles do you usually play in a group meeting (or class)? What role would you like to play? Describe it.

**Pearson Nursing Student Resources**

Find additional review materials at
**www.nursing.pearsonhighered.com**

Prepare for success with additional NCLEX®-style practice
questions, interactive assignments and activities, Web links,
animations and videos, and more!

## Web Resources

TeamSTEPPS: http://teamstepps.ahrq.gov/
Legacy MD: http://legacymd.com

## References

Henriksen, K., Battles, J. B., Keyes, M. A., & Grady, M. L. (Eds.), (2008). *Advances in patient safety: New directions and alternative approaches (Vol. 3: Performance and tools)*. Rockville, MD: Agency for Healthcare Research and Quality.

Hess, R. G. (2011). Slicing and dicing shared governance. *Nursing Administration Quarterly, 35*(3), 235–241.

Hill, K. S. (2010). Building leadership teams. *Journal of Nursing Administration, 40*(3), 1031–1035.

Homans, G. (1950). *The human group*. New York: Harcourt.

Homans, G. (1961). *Social behavior: Its elementary forms*. New York: Harcourt.

Joint Commission on Accreditation of Healthcare Organizations. (2011). Root causes for sentinel events. Retrieved July 8, 2011 from http://www.jointcommission.org/Sentinel_Event_Statistics/

King, H. B., Battles, J., Baker, D. P., Alonso, A., Salas, E., Webster, J., Toomey, L., & Salisbury, M. (2008). TeamSTEPPS: Team strategies and tools to enhance performance and patient safety. Retrieved December 12, 2011 from http://www.ahrq.gov/downloads/pub/advances2/vol3/Advances-King_1.pdf

MacPhee, M., & Bouthillette, F. (2008). Developing leadership in nurse managers: The British Columbia Nursing Leadership Institute. *The Canadian Journal of Nursing Leadership, 21*(3), 64–75.

MacPhee, M., Wardrop, A., & Campbell, C. (2010). Transforming work place relationships through shared decision making. *Journal of Nursing Management, 18*(8), 1016–1126.

McKeon, L. M., Cunningham, P. D., & Detty Oswaks, J. S. (2009). Improving patent safety: Patient-focused, high-reliability team training. *Journal of Nursing Care Quality, 24*(1), 76–82.

Rosen, M. A., Salas, E., Wilson, K. A., King, H. B., Salisbury, M., Augenstein, J. S., Robinson, D. W., & Birnbach, D. J. (2008). Measuring team performance in simulation-based training: Adopting best practices for healthcare. *Simulation in Healthcare, 3*(1), 33–41.

Salas, E., DiazGranados, D., Weaver, S. J., & King, H. (2008). Does team training work? Principles for health care. *Academic Emergency Medicine, 15*(11), 1002–1009.

Steiner, I. D. (1972). *Group process and productivity*. New York: Academic Press.

Steiner, I. D. (1976). Task-performing groups. In J. W. Thibaut, J. T. Spence, & R. C. Carson (Eds.), *Contemporary topics in social psychology* (pp. 94–108). Morristown, NJ: General Learning Press.

Sullivan, E. J. (2013). *Becoming influential: A guide for nurses* (2nd ed.). Upper Saddle River, NJ: Prentice Hall.

Thompson, J. D. (1967). *Organizations in action*. New York: McGraw-Hill.

Wilhelmsson, M., Ponzer, S., Dahlgren, L. O., Timpka, T., & Faresjö, T. (2011). Are female students in general and nursing students more ready for teamwork and interprofessional collaboration in healthcare? *BMC Medical Education*. Retrieved July 8, 2011 from http://www.biomedcentral.com/1472-6920/11/15

# Handling Conflict

**Conflict**

**Interprofessional Conflict**

**Conflict Process Model**

ANTECEDENT CONDITIONS

PERCEIVED AND FELT CONFLICT

CONFLICT BEHAVIORS

CONFLICT RESOLVED OR SUPPRESSED

OUTCOMES

**Managing Conflict**

CONFLICT RESPONSES

FILLEY'S STRATEGIES

ALTERNATIVE DISPUTE STRATEGIES

## Learning Outcomes

*After completing this chapter, you will be able to:*

1. Describe why conflict can be positive or negative.
2. Discuss how conflict can help generate change.
3. Describe the components of conflict.
4. Identify different approaches that can be used to manage conflict.
5. Explain how to manage conflict.

## Key Terms

Accommodating
Avoiding
Collaboration
Competing
Competitive conflict
Compromise
Conflict
Confrontation

Consensus
Disruptive conflict
Felt conflict
Forcing
Integrative decision making
Lose–lose strategy
Mediation
Negotiation

Perceived conflict
Resistance
Resolution
Smoothing
Suppression
Win–lose strategy
Win–win strategy
Withdrawal

# Conflict

Conflict is a natural, inevitable condition in organizations, and a manager's communication frequently centers on conflict. It is often a prerequisite to change in people and organizations.

**Conflict** is defined as the consequence of real or perceived differences in mutually exclusive goals, values, ideas, attitudes, beliefs, feelings, or actions (a) within one individual (*intrapersonal conflict*), (b) between two or more individuals (*interpersonal conflict*), (c) within one group (*intragroup conflict*), or (d) between two or more groups (*intergroup conflict*). Conflict is dynamic. It can be positive or negative, healthy or dysfunctional.

A certain amount of conflict is beneficial to an organization. It can provide heightened sensitivity to an issue, further piquing the interest and curiosity of others. Conflict can also increase creativity by acting as a stimulus for developing new ideas or identifying methods for solving problems. Disagreements can help all parties become more aware of the trade-offs, especially costs versus benefits, of a particular service or technique.

Conflict also helps people recognize legitimate differences within the organization or profession and serves as a powerful motivator to improve performance and effectiveness as well as satisfaction. For example, during intergroup conflict, individual groups become more cohesive and task oriented, whereas communication between groups diminishes.

Competition occurs when two or more groups attempt the same goals and only one group can attain those goals. Filley (1975) defines **competitive conflict** as a victory for one side and a loss for the other side. The process by which the conflict is resolved is determined by a set of rules. The goals of each side are mutually incompatible, but the emphasis is on winning, not the defeat or reduction of the opponent. When one side has clearly won, competition is terminated.

**Disruptive conflict**, in contrast, does not follow any mutually acceptable set of rules and does not emphasize winning. The parties involved are engaged in activities to reduce, defeat, or eliminate the opponent. This type of conflict takes place in an environment charged with fear, anger, and stress.

# Interprofessional Conflict

Working in high-stress jobs, nurses often have conflicts with other health care professionals, administrators, or coworkers. A common example is conflict in the interprofessional team is feeling like each other's time isn't respected. To do multidisciplinary rounds, the doctor might want to meet at 1 P.M., the nurse at 1:30 P.M., the social worker at 10 A.M., etc. A time that works with the work flow of each job is important so that conflict doesn't arise over a person feeling that he or she isn't valued or respected.

Conflicts between physicians and nurses, however, dominate problems reported by both professions (Leever et al., 2010). For example, the physician may want to send the patient home today, while the nurse knows the patient is struggling to understand ordered medications. In addition, the physical therapist tells the nurse that the patient needs another day of practicing exercises before she can be safely discharged.

The nurse manager can teach staff how to handle interprofessional conversations to advocate for the patient, explaining the following:

- Use facts to support your point
- Speak from the vantage point of the patient
- Explain what will best help the patient
- Do not inject what you personally want

Interprofessional conflict is expected to escalate as the most effective and least expensive care is promoted (Webb, 2010). For example, nurse practitioners (NPs) already handle a considerable amount of routine care (e.g., minor injuries, sinusitis, sports exams) because of accessibility (often in retail clinics) and because of cost. Physicians and NPs may have conflicts over which profession should provide and—more importantly, be reimbursed—for this care.

How nurses handle conflict has been studied. The relationship between the nurse's personality type and how the person handles conflict was reported by Whitworth (2008). Using the Thomas Kilmann Mode Instrument (Thomas & Kilmann, 1974) the researcher found no statistical correlation between the two constructs. Whitworth suggested, however, that the environment may have more influence than personality factors.

Using the same instrument, Morrison (2008) examined nurses' emotional intelligence competencies and how nurses handle conflict. Emotional intelligence (Goleman, 2006) measures self-awareness, self-management, social awareness, and relationship management. In the nurses studied, higher emotional intelligence scores in all four measures correlated with collaborating, but negatively with accommodating.

Outcomes and conflict have also been studied. One study compared how groups managed conflict with their performance and satisfaction (Behfar et al., 2008). Researchers found that three conflict resolution styles more often led to positive performance and job satisfaction outcomes: focusing on content of the conflict rather than the delivery; explicitly discussing reasons for work assignments; and making assignments based on expertise rather than volunteering, default, or convenience. Cole, Bedeian, and Bruch (2011) found that transformational leader behavior and team performance was indirect, leading them to conclude that team empowerment improved performance.

## Conflict Process Model

Several authors have proposed models for examining conflict (Pondy, 1967; Filley, 1975; Thomas, 1976). All follow a generalized format for examining conflict. These models provide a framework that helps explain how and why conflict occurs and, ultimately, how one can minimize conflict or resolve it with the least amount of negative aftermath.

Conflict and its resolution develop according to a specific process (see Figure 12-1). This process begins with certain preexisting conditions (antecedent conditions). The parties are influenced by their feelings or perceptions about the situation (perceived or felt conflict), which initiates behavior, and conflict is exhibited. The conflict is either resolved or suppressed, and the outcome results in new attitudes and feelings between the parties.

**Figure 12-1** ● The conflict process.

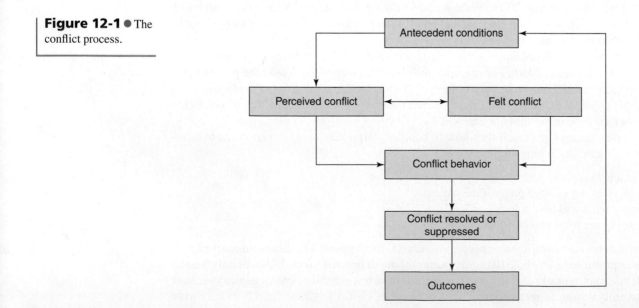

## Antecedent Conditions

Antecedent conditions are associated with increases in conflict. Antecedent conditions propel a situation toward conflict; they may or may not be the cause. In nursing, antecedent conditions include incompatible goals, differences in values and beliefs, task interdependencies (especially asymmetric dependencies, in which one party is dependent on the other but not vice versa), unclear or ambiguous roles, competition for scarce resources, differentiation or distancing mechanisms, and unifying mechanisms.

### Incompatible Goals

The most important antecedent condition to conflict is incompatible goals. As discussed in Chapter 2, goals are desired results toward which behavior is directed. Even though the common goal in health care organizations is to give quality patient care in a cost-effective manner, conflict in achieving these goals is inevitable because individuals often view this from different perspectives.

The dichotomy between health care providers and third-party payers is an example. Health care providers want to maximize the quality of care, whereas payers are concerned with minimizing costs.

A health care organization may have specific goals to achieve the best possible care for patients and control costs to stay within budget and, at the same time, to provide intrinsically satisfying jobs for its employees. These multiple goals will frequently conflict with each other, so they will have to be prioritized. Priority setting can be one of the most difficult but important activities a health care manager must face. Goals are important because they become the basis for allocating resources and thus become an important source (antecedent) of conflict in the organization.

Similarly, individuals themselves have multiple goals, and those goals may also conflict. Individuals allocate scarce resources, such as their time, on the basis of priority and, therefore, might achieve one goal at the expense of others. The inability to attain multiple (and mutually incompatible) goals—whether those goals are personal or organizational—can cause conflict.

### Role Conflicts

Roles are defined as other people's expectations regarding behavior and attitudes. Roles become unclear when one or more parties have related responsibilities that are ambiguous or overlapping. A manager might experience conflict between his or her responsibilities as an administrator and responsibilities as a staff member. Similarly, unclear or overlapping job descriptions or assignments may lead to conflict. For example, there could be conflict over such mundane issues as who has responsibility to deliver a patient to the radiology department—the nurse or the transport staff?

Task interdependence is another potential source of conflict. Nursing and housekeeping, for example, are interdependent. Housekeeping cannot completely clean a room until nursing has discharged the patient. Other examples of interdependence are the relationships among shifts and those between physicians and nurses. Interdependent relationships have the potential to initiate conflict.

### Structural Conflict

One conflict commonly seen in the health care environment is structural conflict. Structured relationships (manager to staff, peer to peer) provoke conflict because of poor communication, competition for resources, opposing interests, or a lack of shared perceptions or attitudes. The nurse manager following up on a patient complaint with corrective counseling or coaching with a staff nurse is an example of structural conflict. The staff member may dispute the complaint and become defensive. In this situation, the manager may impose positional power. Positional power is the authority inherent in a certain position—for example, the nurse administrator has greater positional power than a nurse manager.

### Competition for Resources

Competition for scarce resources can be internal (among different units in the organization) or external (among different organizations). Internally, competition for resources may involve assigning staff from one unit to another or purchasing high-technology equipment when another unit is desperate for staff.

Externally, health care organizations compete for finite external resources (e.g., designation as an accountable care organization for Medicare). Organizations are using a variety of means, such as developing new services and advertising, to try to capture the market in health care.

### Values and Beliefs

Differences in values and beliefs frequently contribute to conflict in health care organizations. Values and beliefs result from the individual's socialization experience. Conflicts between physicians and nurses, between nurses and administrators, or even between nurses with associate degrees versus those with baccalaureate degrees, often occur because of differences in values, beliefs, and experiences.

Distancing mechanisms or differentiation serve to divide a group's members into small, distinct groups, thus increasing the chance for conflict. This tends to lead to a "we–they" distinction. One of the more frequently seen examples is distancing between physicians and nurses. Opposition between intensive care nurses and nurses on medical floors, night versus day shifts, and unlicensed versus licensed personnel are also examples. Differentiation among subunits also occurs and is due to differences in structure. The administrative unit may be bureaucratic, the nursing unit structured on a more professional basis, and staff physicians on an even different structure. Nonstaff physicians may be relatively independent of the health care organization.

Unifying mechanisms occur when greater intimacy develops or when unity is sought. All nurses might be expected to reach consensus over an issue, but they might experience internal conflict if they are forced to accept a group position even though individually they may not be wholly committed to the decision. A nurse manager's friendship with a staff member may also lead to this type of conflict.

## Perceived and Felt Conflict

Perceived and felt conflict account for the conflict that may occur when the parties involved view situations or issues from differing perspectives, when they misunderstand each other's position, or when positions are based on limited knowledge. **Perceived conflict** refers to each party's perception of the other's position. **Felt conflict** refers to the negative feelings between two or more parties. It is characterized by mistrust, hostility, and fear.

To demonstrate how this process works, consider this situation. A nurse manager and a surgeon have worked together for years. They have mutual respect for each other's ability and skills, and they communicate frequently. When their subordinates clash, they are left with conflicting accounts of a situation, in which the only agreed-upon fact is that a patient received less-than-appropriate care. Now consider the same scenario if the nurse and doctor have never dealt with each other or if one feels that the other will not approach the problem constructively.

In the first situation (perceived conflict), their positive regard for each other's abilities makes the nurse and physician believe they can constructively solve the conflict. The nurse does not feel the physician will try to dominate, and the physician respects the nurse manager's leadership ability. With these preexisting attitudes, the physician and nurse can remain neutral while helping their subordinates solve the conflict.

If the nurse and physician were experiencing felt conflict, on the other hand, they might approach the situation differently. Each might assume the other will defend her or his subordinates at all costs and communication will be inhibited. The conflict is resolved by domination of the stronger person, either in personality or position. One wins; the other loses.

## Conflict Behaviors

Conflict behavior results from the parties' perceived or felt conflict. Behaviors may be overt or covert. Overt behavior may take the form of aggression, competition, debate, or problem solving. Covert behavior may be expressed by a variety of indirect tactics, such as scapegoating, avoidance, or apathy.

## Conflict Resolved or Suppressed

In the next stage of the process conflict is resolved or suppressed. **Resolution** occurs when a mutually agreed-upon solution is arrived at and both parties commit themselves to carrying out the agreement. **Suppression** occurs when one person or group defeats the other. Only the dominant side is committed to the agreement, and the loser may or may not carry out the agreement.

## Outcomes

The outcome affects how conflict will be addressed by the parties in the future. The optimal solution is to manage the issues in a way that will lead to a solution wherein both parties see themselves as winners and the problem is solved. This leaves a positive aftermath that will affect future relations and influence feelings and attitudes. In the example of conflict between the nurse manager and the physician, consider the difference in the aftermath and how future issues would be approached if both parties felt positive about the outcome, as compared to future interactions if one or both parties felt they had lost.

# Managing Conflict

Managing conflict is an important part of the nurse manager's job. Managers are often involved in conflict management on several different levels. They may be participants in the conflict as individuals, administrators, or representatives of a unit. In fact, they must often initiate conflict by confronting staff, individually or collectively, when a problem develops. They may also serve as mediators or judges to conflicting parties. There could be a conflict within the unit, between parties from different units, or between internal and external parties (for example, a university nursing instructor may have a conflict with staff on a particular unit).

Everyone must be realistic regarding the outcome. Often those inexperienced in conflict negotiation expect unrealistic outcomes. When two or more parties hold mutually exclusive ideas, attitudes, feelings, or goals, it is extremely difficult, without the commitment and willingness of all concerned, to arrive at an agreeable solution that meets the needs of both. Battles between Democrats and Republicans in Congress are an example.

Conflict management begins with a decision regarding if and when to intervene. Failure to intervene can allow the conflict to get out of hand, whereas early intervention may be detrimental to those involved, causing them to lose confidence in themselves and reduce risk-taking behavior in the future.

Some conflicts are so minor, particularly if they are between only two people, that they do not require intervention and would be better handled by the two people involved. Allowing them to resolve their conflict might provide a developmental experience and improve their abilities to resolve conflict in the future.

Sometimes it is best to postpone intervention purposely to allow the conflict to escalate, because increased intensity can motivate participants to seek resolution. You could escalate the conflict even further by exposing participants to each other more frequently without the presence of others and without an easy means of escape. Participants are then forced to face the conflict between them.

Giving participants a shared task or shared goals not directly related to the conflict may help them understand each other better and increase their chances to resolve their conflicts by themselves. Using such a method is useful only if the conflict is not of high intensity, if the participants are not highly anxious about it, and if the manager believes that the conflict will not decrease the efficiency of the unit in the meantime. When the conflict might result in considerable harm, however, the nurse manager must intervene.

If you decide to intervene in a conflict between two or more parties, you can apply mediation techniques, deciding when, where, and how the intervention should take place. Routine problems can be handled in either party's office, but serious confrontations should take place in a neutral location unless the parties involved are of unequal power. In this case, the setting should favor the disadvantaged participant, thereby equalizing their power.

The place should be one where distractions will not interfere and adequate time is available. Because conflict management takes time, the manager must be prepared to allow sufficient time for all parties to explain their points of view and arrive at a mutually agreeable solution. A quick solution that inexperienced managers often resort to is to impose positional power and make a premature decision. This results in a win–lose outcome, which leads to feelings of elation and eventual complacency for the winners, and loss of morale for the losers.

The following are basic rules on how to mediate a conflict between two or more parties:

1. Protect each party's self-respect. Deal with a conflict of issues, not personalities.

2. Do not put blame or responsibility for the problem on the participants. The participants are responsible for developing a solution to the problem.

3. Allow open and complete discussion of the problem from each participant.

4. Maintain equity in the frequency and duration of each party's presentation. A person of higher status tends to speak more frequently and longer than a person of lower status. If this occurs, the mediator should intervene and ask the person of lower status for response and opinion.

5. Encourage full expression of positive and negative feelings in an accepting atmosphere. The novice mediator tends to discourage expressions of disagreement.

6. Make sure both parties listen actively to each other's words. One way to do this is to ask one person to summarize the other person's comments before stating her or his own.

7. Identify key themes in the discussion and restate them at frequent intervals.

8. Encourage the parties to provide frequent feedback to each other's comments; each must truly understand the other's position.

9. Help the participants develop alternative solutions, select a mutually agreeable one, and develop a plan to carry it out. All parties must agree to the solution for successful resolution to occur.

10. At an agreed-upon interval, follow up on the progress of the plan.

11. Give positive feedback to participants regarding their cooperation in solving the conflict.

Conflict management is a difficult process, consuming both time and energy. Management and staff must be concerned and committed to resolving conflict by being willing to listen to others' positions and to find agreeable solutions.

## Conflict Responses

**Confrontation** is considered the most effective means for resolving conflicts. This is a problem-oriented technique in which the conflict is brought out into the open and attempts are made to resolve it through knowledge and reason. The goal of this technique is to achieve win–win solutions. Facts should be used to identify the problem. The desired outcome should be explicit. "This is the third time this week that you have not been here for report. According to hospital policy, you are expected to be changed, scrubbed, and ready for report in the lounge at 7:00 A.M." is an example.

Confrontation is most effective when delivered in private as soon as possible after the incident occurs. Employee respect and manager credibility are two important considerations when a situation warrants confrontation. A more immediate confrontation also helps both the employee and manager sort out pertinent facts. In an emotionally charged situation, however, it may be best for the parties to wait. Regardless of timing, the message is usually more effective if the manager listens and is empathetic.

**Negotiation** involves give-and-take on various issues among the parties. Its purpose is to achieve agreement even though consensus will never be reached. Therefore, the best solution is not often achieved. Negotiation often becomes a structured, formal procedure, as in collective bargaining (see Chapter 24). However, negotiation skills are important in arriving at an agreeable solution between any two parties. Staff learn to negotiate schedules, advanced practice nurses negotiate with third-party payers for reimbursement, insurance companies negotiate with vendors and hospitals for discounts, and clinic managers negotiate employment contracts with physicians. Although negotiation involves adept communication skills, its usefulness revolves around issues of conflict. Without differences in opinion, there would be no need for negotiation.

**Collaboration** implies mutual attention to the problem, in which the talents of all parties are used. In collaboration, the focus is on solving the problem, not defeating the opponent. The goal is to satisfy both parties' concerns. Collaboration is useful in situations in which the goals of both parties are too important to be compromised.

**Compromise** is used to divide the rewards between both parties. Neither gets what she or he wants. Compromise can serve as a backup to resolve conflict when collaboration is ineffective. It is sometimes the only choice when opponents of equal power are in conflict over two or more mutually exclusive goals. Compromising is also expedient when a solution is needed rapidly.

**Competing** is an all-out effort to win, regardless of the cost. Competing may be needed in situations involving unpopular or critical decisions. Competing is also used in situations in which time does not allow for more cooperative techniques.

**Accommodating** is an unassertive, cooperative tactic used when individuals neglect their own concerns in favor of others' concerns. Accommodating frequently is used to preserve harmony when one person has a vested interest in an issue that is unimportant to the other party. You may recall that Morrison (2008) found that nurses with higher emotional intelligence scores seldom used accommodating as a conflict response.

In situations where conflict is discouraged, suppression is often used. Suppression could even include the elimination of one of the conflicting parties through transfer or termination. Other, less effective techniques for managing conflict include withdrawing, smoothing, and forcing, although each mode of response is useful in given situations.

In **avoiding**, the participants never acknowledge that a conflict exists. Avoidance is the conflict resolution technique often used in highly cohesive groups. The group avoids disagreement because its members do not want to do anything that may interfere with the good feelings they have for each other.

**Withdrawal** from the conflict simply removes at least one party, thereby making it impossible to resolve the situation. The issue remains unresolved, and feelings about the issue may resurface inappropriately. If the conflict escalates into a dangerous situation, avoiding and withdrawing are appropriate strategies.

**Smoothing** is accomplished by complimenting one's opponent, downplaying differences, and focusing on minor areas of agreement, as though little disagreement existed. Smoothing may be appropriate in dealing with minor problems, but in response to major problems, it produces the same results as withdrawing.

**Forcing** is a method that yields an immediate end to the conflict but leaves the cause of the conflict unresolved. A superior can resort to issuing orders, but the subordinate will lack commitment to the demanded action. Forcing may be appropriate in life-or-death situations but is otherwise inappropriate.

**Resistance** can be positive or negative. It may mean a resistance to change or disobedience, or it may be an effective approach to handling power differences, especially verbal abuse.

## Filley's Strategies

Filley (1975) identified three basic strategies for dealing with conflict according to the outcome: win–lose, lose–lose, and win–win. In the **win–lose strategy**, one party exerts dominance, usually by power of authority, and the other party submits and loses. Forcing, competing, and negotiating are techniques likely to lead to win–lose competition.

Majority rule is another example of the win–lose outcome, especially within groups. It may be a satisfactory method of resolving conflict, however, if various factions vote differently on different issues and the group functions over time so that members win some and lose some. Win–lose outcomes often occur between groups. Frequent losing, however, can lead to the loss of cohesiveness within groups and diminish the authority of the group leader.

In the **lose–lose strategy**, neither side wins. The settlement reached is unsatisfactory to both sides. Avoiding, withdrawing, smoothing, and compromising may lead to lose–lose outcomes. One compromising strategy is to use a bribe to influence another's cooperation in doing something he or she dislikes. For example, the nurse manager may promise a future raise in an attempt to coerce a staff member to work an extra weekend.

Using a third party as arbitrator can also lead to a lose–lose outcome. Because an outsider may want to give something to each side, neither gets exactly what he or she desires, resulting in a lose–lose outcome. This is a common strategy in arbitration of labor-management disputes. Another strategy that may result in a lose–lose or win–lose outcome is resorting to rules. The outcome is determined by whatever the rules say, and confrontation is avoided.

The win–lose and lose–lose methods share some common characteristics:

1. The conflict is person-centered (we–they) rather than problem-centered. This is likely to occur when two cohesive groups that do not share common values or goals are in conflict.

2. Parties direct their energy toward total victory for themselves and total defeat for the other. This can cause long-term problems for the organization.

3. Each side sees the issue from her or his own point of view rather than as a problem in need of a solution.

4. The emphasis is on outcomes rather than definition of goals, values, or objectives.

5. Conflicts are personalized.

6. Conflict-resolving activities are not differentiated from other group processes.

7. There is a short-run view of the conflict; the goal is to settle the immediate problem rather than resolve differences.

The **win–win strategy** focuses on goals and attempt to meet the needs of both parties. Two specific win–win strategies are consensus and integrative decision making. **Consensus** involves attention to the facts and to the position of the other parties and avoidance of trading, voting, or averaging, where everyone loses something. The consensus decision is often superior to even the best individual one. This technique is most useful in a group setting because it is sensitive to the negative characteristics of win–lose and lose–lose outcomes. True consensus occurs when the problem is fully explored, the needs and goals of the involved parties are understood, and a solution that meets these needs is agreed upon.

**Integrative decision making** focuses on the means of solving a problem rather than the ends. This strategy is most useful when the needs of the parties are polarized. Integrative decision making is a constructive process in which the parties jointly identify the problem and their needs. They explore a number of alternative solutions and come to consensus on a solution. The focus of this group activity is to solve the problem, not to force, dominate, suppress, or compromise. The group works toward a common goal in an atmosphere that encourages the free exchange of ideas and feelings. Using integrative decision-making methods, the parties jointly identify the value needs of each, conduct an exhaustive search for alternatives that could meet the needs of each, and then select the best alternative. Like the consensus methods, integrative decision making focuses on defeating the problem, not each other.

## Alternative Dispute Strategies

Conflicts that have the potential to lead to legal action are often negotiated using alternative dispute resolution (ADR) (Sander, 2009). **Mediation** is a form of ADR that involves a third-party mediator to help settle disputes. Mediation agreements can satisfy all parties, cost less and take less time than legal remedies, and lead to improved interprofessional relationships (Gardner, 2010). Mediation has been used successfully in settling disputes in long-term care facilities (Rosenblatt, 2008).

ADR efforts have resulted in the creation of the International Institute of Conflict Prevention and Resolution, expanded state and federal legislation encouraging mediation, a dispute resolution division in the American Bar Association, and development of ADR courses in law schools. The use of ADR in public policy promises to increase in the coming years (Susskind, 2009).

See how one nurse manager handled a conflict between two members of her staff in Case Study 12-1.

## CASE STUDY 12-1

### CONFLICT MANAGEMENT

Mai Tran is the nurse manager of a 20-bed medical-surgical unit in a large university hospital. Her nursing staff is diverse in experience and educational background. Working in a teaching hospital, Mai believes that nurses should be open to new methods and work processes, with an emphasis on evidence-based practice.

Ken Robertson, RN, has worked for two years on the unit and is in his final semester of a master's program focusing on geriatric care. Eileen Holcomb, RN, has worked on the same unit for the past 28 years and was a graduate of the hospital's former diploma program. Ken recently completed a clinical rotation in dermatology and has worked with the skin care team at the hospital to develop new protocols for preventing skin breakdown. During a recent staff meeting, Ken presents the new protocols to the staff. Eileen makes several comments during the presentation that simply getting patients out of bed and making sure they have adequate nutrition is easier and less time-consuming than the new protocol. "All these new protocols are just a way to justify all those credentials behind a name," Eileen says, gathering a chorus of chuckles from some of the older nurses on the staff. Ken frowns at Eileen and responds, "As nurses become educated, we need to reflect a professional practice." Mai notices that several staff members are uncomfortable as the meeting ends.

Ken and Eileen continue to exchange sarcastic comments and glares over the next two shifts they work together. The obvious disagreement is affecting their coworkers, and gossiping is decreasing productivity on

the unit. Mai schedules individual meetings with Ken and Eileen to discuss their perspective. After reviewing the situation and determining that the issue is simply one of personality conflict, Mai brings Ken and Eileen together for a meeting in her office. Mai reviews the facts of the situation with them and shares her opinion that both have acted inappropriately. She states that their actions have affected not only their work, but that of the unit as a whole. She informs Ken and Eileen that they must act in a professional and respectful manner with each other or disciplinary action will be taken. She encourages them to work out any future problems in a cooperative manner and not to bring personal conflicts into the work environment.

### Manager's Checklist

The nurse manager is responsible for:

- Understanding how to manage conflict among staff members in a timely manner
- Understanding generational perceptions and how they impact group dynamics
- Understanding when disciplinary action is necessary
- Informing the human resource department of a potential personnel problem and the proposed solution
- Meeting with staff to help them resolve conflict
- Determining whether all staff should be educated on respect in the workplace
- Documenting interventions and outcomes as appropriate

Managing conflict is an essential skill for the manager and, indeed, all nurses. Avoiding unnecessary conflict or allowing conflict to fester and remain unresolved undermines the manager's effectiveness and can result in dissatisfied staff and turnover. Resolving conflict, on the other hand, can lead to better outcomes both with the immediate situation and encourage the manager to resolve conflict in the future.

More strategies for handling conflict can be found in Chapter 10, "Dealing with Difficult People and Situations," in *Becoming Influential: A Guide for Nurses* (Sullivan, 2013).

## What You Know Now

- Conflict is a dynamic process and the consequence of real or perceived differences between individuals or groups.
- Conflict can be positive and the first step in initiating change, or it may be negative and disruptive.
- Antecedent conditions that cause conflict include incompatible goals, role conflicts, structural conflict, competition for scarce resources, and differences in values and beliefs.
- A number of strategies exist to handle conflict; choosing the best one to use is based on the situation and the people involved.
- Learning to manage conflict is a requirement for all nurses and managers.

## Tools for Handling Conflict

1. Evaluate conflict situations to decide if and when to intervene.
2. Understand the antecedent conditions for the conflict and the positions of those involved.
3. Enlist others to help solve conflicts.
4. Select a conflict management strategy appropriate to the situation.
5. Practice the conflict management strategies discussed in the chapter and evaluate the outcomes.

## Questions to Challenge You

1. How are conflicts handled at work or school? Are leaders good conflict managers? Give an example to explain your answer.
2. Briefly describe a conflict in which you were involved. How did you handle yourself? How did the others involved? Did it turn out well? Explain.
3. What do you find to be the most difficult part of handling conflicts? Understanding others' positions? Devising a successful solution? Enlisting others' help? Encouraging participants to agree to a solution?
4. Study the chapter for help in improving your areas of weakness. Evaluate your performance.

**Pearson Nursing Student Resources**

Find additional review materials at
**www.nursing.pearsonhighered.com**

Prepare for success with additional NCLEX®-style practice questions, interactive assignments and activities, Web links, animations and videos, and more!

# References

Behfar, K. J., Peterson, R. S., Mannix, E. A., & Trochim, W. M. K. (2008). The critical role of conflict resolution in teams: A close look at the links between conflict type, conflict management strategies, and team outcomes. *Journal of Applied Psychology, 93*(1), 170–188.

Cole, M. S., Bedeian, A. G., & Bruch, H. (2011). Linking leader behavior and leadership consensus to team performance: Integrating direct consensus and dispersion models of group composition. *The Leadership Quarterly, 22*(2), 383–398.

Filley, A. C. (1975). *Interpersonal conflict resolution.* Glenview, IL: Scott, Foresman.

Gardner, D. (2010). Expanding scope of practice: Interprofessional collaboration or conflict? *Nursing Economics, 28*(4), 264–266.

Goleman, D. (2006). *Emotional intelligence: Why it can matter more than IQ.* New York: Bantam.

Leever, A. M., Hulst, M. V. D., Berendsen, A. J., Boendemaker, P. M., & Roodenburg, J. L. N. (2010). Conflicts and conflict management in the collaboration between nurses and physicians: A qualitative study. *Journal of Interprofessional Care, 24*(6), 612–624.

Morrison, J. (2008). The relationship between emotional intelligence competencies and preferred conflict-handling styles. *Journal of Nursing Management, 16*(8), 974–983.

Pondy, L. R. (1967). Organizational conflict: Concepts and models. *Administrative Science Quarterly, 12,* 296–320.

Rosenblatt, C. L. (2008). Using mediation to manage conflict in care facilities. *Nursing Management, 39*(2), 16, 17.

Sander, F. E. A. (2009). Ways of handling conflict: What we have learned, what problems remain. *Negotiation Journal, 25*(4), 533–537.

Sullivan, E. J. (2013). *Becoming influential: A guide for nurses* (2nd ed.). Upper Saddle River, NJ: Prentice Hall.

Susskind, L. (2009). Twenty-five years ago and twenty-five years from now: The future of public dispute resolution. *Negotiation Journal, 25*(4), 549–556.

Susskind, L. (2010). *Mediating values-based and identity-based disputes. The consensus building approach.* Retrieved July 12, 2011 from http://theconsensus-buildingapproach.blogspot.com/2010/04/mediating-values-based-and-identity.html

The Joint Commission. (2008, July 9). Behaviors that undermine a culture of safety. Retrieved October 15, 2010 from http://www.jointcommission.org/SentinelEvents/SentinelEventAlert/sea_40.htm

Thomas, K. W. (1976). Conflict and conflict management. In M. D. Dunnette (Ed.), *The handbook of industrial and organizational psychology.* Chicago: Rand McNally.

Thomas, K. W., & Kilmann, R. H. (1974). *Thomas-Kilmann Conflict Mode Instrument.* Tuxedo, NY: Xicom.

Webb, R. (2010). Healthcare reform and inevitable conflict: Smaller pie means smaller slices. Healthcare Neutral ADR Blog, Retrieved July 12, 2011 from http://www.healthcareneutraladrblog.com/2010/02/articles/commercial-healthcare-disputes/healthcare-reform-and-inevitable-conflict-smaller-pie-means-smaller-slices

Whitworth, B. S. (2008). Is there a relationship between personality type and preferred conflict-handling styles? An exploratory study of registered nurses in southern Mississippi. *Journal of Nursing Management, 16*(8), 921–932.

**Time Wasters**

TIME ANALYSIS

THE MANAGER'S TIME

**Setting Goals**

DETERMINING PRIORITIES

DAILY PLANNING AND SCHEDULING

GROUPING ACTIVITIES AND MINIMIZING
ROUTINE WORK

PERSONAL ORGANIZATION AND SELF-DISCIPLINE

**Controlling Interruptions**

PHONE CALLS, VOICE MAIL, TEXT MESSAGES

E-MAIL

DROP-IN VISITORS

PAPERWORK

**Controlling Time in Meetings**

**Respecting Time**

## Learning Outcomes

*After completing this chapter, you will be able to:*

1. Identify time wasters.
2. Identify goals.
3. Set priorities.
4. Group activities and minimize routine work.

5. Manage personal organization and self discipline.
6. Minimize time wasters.

## Key Terms

| | | |
|---|---|---|
| Goal setting | Job enlargement | Time waster |
| Interruption log | Time logs | To-do list |

Time management is a misnomer. No one manages time: What is managed is how time is used. In today's downsized health care organization, the pressure to do more in less time has increased. **Job enlargement** occurs when a flatter organizational structure causes positions to be combined and results in managers having more employees to supervise, a situation common today.

The managerial skills needed today are different from those in the past, according to a study by Gentry and colleagues (Gentry et al., 2008). Changes from the late 1980s until now include flatter organizational structures that result in more responsibilities shared throughout the organization and a greater use of electronic communications. Technology has changed how managers and staff interact. Geographic location is less important, as is time away from work. Being always connected can be both a time-saver and a time-stealer. Nonetheless, instant communication is here to stay.

Teams often do what managers formerly dictated, with the best decisions coming out of the team's cooperative efforts. Time management is equally important in teamwork as it is for individuals. Teams must plan and organize their work to meet deadlines. Efficiency is paramount.

Time can be used proactively or reactively (Carrick, Carrick, & Yurkow, 2007). If you focus your energy on people and events over which you have some direct or indirect control, you are using a proactive approach. If, on the other hand, you spend most of your time on what concerns you most about other people and events, your efforts are less apt to be effective. For example, you can set and follow your goals and priorities or you can spend your time worrying, blaming, or making excuses about what you do not accomplish. This chapter is designed to help you be proactive in targeting your use of time.

## Time Wasters

Why do we waste time? It is one of our most valuable resources, and yet everyone admits to wasting it. Box 13-1 answers this question by showing some of the constraints on an individual's ability to manage time effectively. These patterns of behavior must be understood and dealt with to be effective in managing time.

---

**BOX 13-1** Why We Fail to Manage Time Effectively

- We do what we like to do before we do what we don't like to do.
- We do things we know how to do faster than things we do not know how to do.
- We do things that are easiest before things that are difficult.
- We do things that require a little time before things that require a lot of time.
- We do things for which resources are available.
- We do things that are scheduled (for example, meetings) before nonscheduled things.
- We sometimes do things that are planned before things that are unplanned.
- We respond to demands from others before demands from ourselves.
- We do things that are urgent before things that are important.

- We readily respond to crises and emergencies.
- We do interesting things before uninteresting things.
- We do things that advance our personal objectives or that are politically expedient.
- We wait until a deadline approaches before we really get moving.
- We do things that provide the most immediate closure.
- We respond on the basis of who wants it.
- We respond on the basis of the consequences of our doing or not doing something.
- We tackle small jobs before large jobs.
- We work on things in the order of their arrival.
- We work on the basis of the squeaky-wheel principle (the squeaky wheel gets the grease).
- We work on the basis of consequences to the group.

In addition to these patterns of behavior, certain time wasters prevent us from effectively managing time. A **time waster** prevents a person from accomplishing the job or achieving the goal. Common time wasters include:

1. Interruptions, such as phone calls, text messages, and drop-in visitors

2. Meetings, both scheduled and unscheduled

3. Lack of clear-cut goals, objectives, and priorities

4. Lack of daily and/or weekly plans

5. Lack of personal organization and self-discipline

6. Lack of knowledge about how one spends one's time

7. Failure to delegate or working on routine tasks

8. Ineffective communication

9. Waiting for others and thus not using transition time effectively

10. Inability to say no

An experienced manager is often called on to help another new manager who requests help. It is always appropriate to mentor, teach, and guide others, but when you realize you are doing the person's work and your work is not getting done or is late, your time is wasted.

### Time Analysis

The first step is to analyze how time is being used. The second is to determine whether time use is appropriate to your role. You may find much of your time is taken up doing "busywork" rather than activities that contribute to a particular outcome. Job redesign places emphasis on ensuring that time is spent wisely and that the right individual is correctly assigned the responsibility for tasks.

**Time logs**, as shown in Box 13-2, are useful in analyzing the actual time spent on various activities. Select a typical week and keep a log of activities in 15 to 60 minute increments. Keep it simple. List columns for the time period and the activity. Review your log for what activities are essential and what can be delegated or eliminated. Alternatively, you can use a planner or appointment calendar in place of a separate log.

### BOX 13-2 Time Analysis Log

| Time | Activity | Purpose | Value |
|------|----------|---------|-------|
| 7:00–7:30 | Review e-mails received overnight; list work to accomplish during shift | To respond to people who have e-mailed and to plan what work must be done | Sets the plan for the day so as much work can be accomplished as possible |
| 7:30–8:30 | Be available for any night shift staff who need to talk with manager before leaving | Manager is accountable to all staff that work on unit. During this time, manager can have face-to-face interaction with night shift staff and follow up on any issues that present | Provides time for night shift staff to see and talk to manager and develop relationships and strong lines of communication |
| 8:30–10:00 | Budget planning meeting | Meet with VP of patient care and other managers to work on planning next fiscal year budget | Manager has input into the budget that he/she will work to meet during next fiscal year |

## The Manager's Time

A significant difficulty in moving from a staff nurse position to a leadership position is the need to develop different time-management and organizational skills. In a staff nurse role, the registered nurse has little, if any, free or uncommitted time. No planning is required, because every minute is taken. In contrast, when nurses move to a leadership position, they are responsible for defining how time will be spent. Learning to focus on setting goals, determining priorities, and evaluating time use is an important part of the analysis.

# Setting Goals

Nurses are accustomed to setting both long- and short-range goals, although typically such goals are stated in terms of what patients will accomplish rather than what the nurse will achieve. A critical component of time management is establishing one's own goals and time frames.

Goals are specific statements of outcomes that are to be achieved. They provide direction and vision for actions as well as a timeline in which activities will be accomplished. Defining goals and time frames helps reduce stress by preventing the panic people often feel when confronted with multiple demands. Although time frames may not be as fast as the nurse manager would like (the tendency is to expect change yesterday), necessary actions have been identified.

Individual or organizational goals encourage thinking about the future and what might happen, what one wants to happen, and what is likely to happen (Sullivan, 2013). **Goal setting** helps relate current behavior, activities, or operations to the organization's or individual's long-range goals. Without this future orientation, activities may not lead to the outcomes that will help achieve the goals and meet the ideals of the individual or organization. The focus should be to develop measurable, realistic, and achievable goals.

It is useful to think of individual or personal goals in categories, such as:

- Department or unit
- Interpersonal (at work)
- Professional
- Financial
- Family and friends (outside of work)
- Vacation and travel
- Physical
- Lifestyle
- Community
- Spiritual

This partial listing is a guide to stimulate thinking about goals. Think about long-term goals, lifetime goals, and short-term goals. These should be divided into job-related goals and personal goals. Job-related goals may revolve around unit or departmental changes, whereas personal goals may include personal life and community involvement.

Short-term goals should be set for the next 6 to 12 months, but need to be related to long-term goals. To manage time effectively, answer five major questions about these goals:

1. What specific objectives are to be achieved?

2. What specific activities are necessary to achieve these objectives?

3. How much time is required for each activity?

4. Which activities can be planned and scheduled for concurrent action, and which must be planned and scheduled sequentially?

5. Which activities can be delegated to staff?

Delegating tasks to others can be an efficient time-management tool. Delegation is the process by which responsibility and authority are transferred to another individual. It involves assigning tasks, determining expected results, and granting authority to the individual expected to accomplish these tasks. Delegation is perhaps the most difficult leadership skill for a nurse or a manager to acquire. Today, when more assistive personnel are being used to carry out the nurse's work and when the manager's span of control has expanded, appropriate delegation skills are essential for success. Chapter 10 discusses delegation in detail.

## Determining Priorities

To establish priorities, take into consideration both short- and long-term goals. Categorize them as:

- What you must do
- What you should do if possible
- What you could do if you have time to spare (Jones & Loftus, 2009)

Next determine the importance and urgency of each activity as shown in Table 13-1. Activities can be identified as:

- Urgent and important
- Important but not urgent
- Urgent but not important
- Busywork
- Wasted time

Activities that are both urgent and important must be completed. Activities that are important but not urgent may make the difference between career progression and maintaining the status quo. Urgent but not important activities must be completed immediately but are not considered important or significant. Busywork and wasted time are self-explanatory.

Additionally, others' emergencies or crisis can intrude on your priorities. Again, determine if these are truly urgent and important or if the person is overreacting to an immediate situation.

## Daily Planning and Scheduling

Once goals and priorities have been established, you can concentrate on scheduling activities. Prepare a **to-do list** each day, either after work hours the previous day or early before work on the same day. The list is typically planned by workday or workweek. If you have a combination of many responsibilities, a weekly to-do list may be more effective. Flexibility must be a major consideration in this plan; some time should remain uncommitted to allow you to deal with

**TABLE 13-1    Importance–Urgency Chart**

| Category of Time Use | Examples |
| --- | --- |
| Important and urgent | Replacing two call-offs and ensuring sufficient staffing for the upcoming shift. |
| Important, not urgent | Drafting an educational program for nurses on the changes in Medicare reimbursement. |
| Urgent, not important | Completing and submitting the "beds available" list for a disaster drill. |
| Busywork | Compiling new charts for future patient admissions. |
| Wasted time | Sitting by the phone waiting for return calls. |

emergencies and crises that are sure to happen. The focus is not on activities and events, but rather on the outcomes that can be achieved in the time available.

A system to keep track of regularly scheduled meetings (staff meetings), regular events (annual or quarterly report due dates), and appointments is also necessary. This system should be used when establishing the to-do list; it should include both a calendar and files.

The calendar might include information on the purpose of the meeting, who will be attending, and the time and place. Several commercial planning systems are available, including software for computers or smart phones. Any such system includes a daily, weekly, or monthly calendar; a to-do section; a memo or note section; and an address book with phone numbers. Separate files for projects, committees, or reports should be kept arranged by date.

## Grouping Activities and Minimizing Routine Work

Work items that are similar in nature and require similar environmental surroundings and resources should be grouped within divisions of the work shift. Set aside blocks of uninterrupted time for the really important tasks, such as preparing the budget.

Group routine tasks, especially those that are not important or urgent, during your least productive time. For example, list what you can do in five minutes, such as scan your e-mail, check text messages, confirm a meeting, or set up an appointment, or in ten minutes, such as return a phone call, scan a Website, or compose an e-mail. This helps you spend the small allotments of time productively.

Much time spent in transition or waiting can be turned into productive use. Commuting time can be used for self-development or planning work activities. We all have to wait sometimes: waiting for a meeting to start or to talk to someone are just two examples. Keep up with message boards on your phone's mail system or bring along materials to read or work on in case you are kept waiting. View waiting or transition time as an opportunity, especially to think.

If you are having difficulty completing important tasks and are highly stressed, especially as the day winds down, doing routine tasks for a while often helps reduce stress. Pick a task that can be successfully completed and save it for the end of the day. Reaching closure on even a routine task at the end of the day can reduce your sense of overload and stress.

Implementing the daily plan and daily follow-up is essential to managing your time. You should also repeat your time analysis at least semiannually to see how well you are managing your time, whether the job or the environment has changed, and if changes in planning activities are required. This can help prevent reverting to poor time-management habits.

## Personal Organization and Self-Discipline

Some other time wasters are lack of personal organization and self-discipline, including the inability to say no, having to wait for others, and excessive or ineffective paperwork. Effective personal organization results from clearly defined priorities based on well-defined, measurable, and achievable objectives. Because the nurse manager does not work alone, priorities and objectives are often related to those of many professionals, as well as to objectives of patients and their families.

How time is used is often a matter of resolving conflicts among competing needs. It is easy to become overloaded with responsibilities and with more tasks to do than can be accomplished in the time available. This is typical. There is never enough time for all the activities, situations, and events in which one might like to become involved. (Review the section on priority setting.)

To be effective, nurses and nurse managers must be personally well organized and possess self-discipline. This often includes being able to say no. Taking on too much work can lead to overload and stress. Being realistic about the amount of work to which you commit is an indication of effective time management. If a superior is overloading you, make sure that person understands the consequences of additional assignments. Be assertive in communicating your own needs to others.

An e-mail system without designated folders for automatic storage, a cluttered desk, working on too many tasks at one time, and failing to set aside blocks of uninterrupted time to do

## CASE STUDY 13-1

### TIME MANAGEMENT

For the past six years, Jane Schumann has been the manager of staff development for three hospitals in a Catholic health care system. After the health care system suffered record operating losses last fiscal year, many middle management positions were eliminated. Jane was retained, but had several other departments assigned to her. Now Jane is responsible for staff development, utilization review staff, in-house float pool, night nursing supervisors, agency staffing, coordination of student nurse clinical rotations, and training of all nursing staff for the new hospital information system at four different hospitals.

Jane has been overwhelmed with her new responsibilities. Wanting to establish trust and learn more about her staff, Jane has adopted an "open-door policy" resulting in many drop-in visits each day. She has been working much longer hours and most weekends. She has frequently had to fill in for night supervisors, stretching her workday to 18 hours. Her desk is stacked with paperwork and her voice mailbox is full of messages to be returned. On average, she returns 40 of the 60 e-mails received each day.

When Jane comes across information about a time-management seminar, she quickly signs up. At the seminar, Jane learns a number of strategies that she can use.

Back at work, she makes a plan. First, she makes a list of priorities for each of her departments and a time frame for completing each project. Then she completes daily plans for the next two weeks as well as a three-month plan for the upcoming quarter. Jane also determines who among her new staff members can assume additional responsibilities and notes which tasks can be delegated. She sorts through paperwork and establishes a filing system for each department. Jane decides that she will train her administrative assistant to file routine paperwork and route other paperwork to Jane or delegated personnel. Jane also decides that at each departmental meeting, she will establish specific times that she will be available for drop-in visitors. She schedules a meeting with the senior nursing executive to discuss the staffing implications for training nurses at the four hospitals to use the new hospital information system. Finally, she takes advantage of an upcoming four-day weekend to catch up on some well-deserved rest.

### Manager's Checklist

The nurse manager is responsible for:

- Prioritizing the workload
- Effectively delegating tasks and projects to others
- Respecting one's own time and the time of others
- Asking for help when appropriate

important tasks indicate a lack of personal self-discipline. Automate e-mails from specified senders, clear your desktop, and get out the materials you need to complete your highest-priority task and start working on it immediately. Focus on one task at a time, making sure to start with a high-priority one.

One manager who felt overwhelmed by all of her responsibilities used the strategies shown in Case Study 13-1 to help her solve her problems.

## Controlling Interruptions

An interruption occurs any time you must stop in the middle of one activity to give attention to something else. Interruptions can be an essential part of your job, or they can be a time waster. An interruption that is more important and urgent than the activity in which you are involved is a positive interruption: it deserves immediate attention. An emergency or crisis, for instance, may cause you to interrupt daily rounds.

Some interruptions interfere with achieving the job and are less important and urgent than current activities. Because the manager's role has expanded to a broader span of responsibility, more decision making is placed on teams and the staff. When a manager is interrupted to solve problems within the staff nurse's scope of accountability, the manager should not become responsible for solving the problem. Gently but firmly directing the individual to search for solutions will begin to break old patterns of behavior and help develop individual responsibility. Although it is time-consuming in the beginning, this practice eventually reduces the number of unnecessary interruptions.

Keeping an **interruption log** on an occasional basis may help. The log should show who interrupted, the nature of the interruption, when it occurred, how long it lasted, what topics were discussed, the importance of the topics, and time-saving actions to be taken. An example is shown in Box 13-3.

Analysis of these data may identify patterns for you to plan ways to reduce the frequency and duration of interruptions. They may also indicate that certain staff members are the most frequent interrupters and require individual attention to develop problem-solving skills.

## Phone Calls, Voice Mail, Text Messages

Phone calls are a major source of interruption, and the interruption log will provide considerable insight for the nurse manager regarding the nature of phone calls received. You will see how some people do not use the phone effectively. A ringing phone or beep from an incoming text is

---

**BOX 13-3    Interruption Log**

| Name | Purpose | Time | Topics | Importance | Actions |
|------|---------|------|--------|------------|---------|
| Joan, RN | Stopped in manager's office to talk | 10 minutes | Kids' baseball games, husband's new job | Not related to work activities, but helps build relationship with staff | Proactively plan time for occasional personal conversations with staff to build relationships; plan to eat lunch in breakroom one day per week with staff to have informal conversations |
| Bill, janitor | Ask manager if he/she has seen any furniture in hallways because a chair was missing from a patient room | 5 minutes | Patient's room furniture was missing | Patient rooms need a chair so the patient can get out of bed and have a place to sit. There is an issue with furniture that is sent for repair being misplaced when returned to the unit. | Ask the unit clerk to keep a log of all furniture sent off the unit for repair. When the furniture is returned, rather than putting it in the hallway until someone says a chair is needed in a room, the unit clerk proactively finds out where the chair belongs and takes it to that location. |
| Jason, nurse aide | Tells the manager that he has tried four different machines, but no one machine can measure blood pressure, temperature, and oxygen saturation | 15 minutes | When equipment fails, manager works with employee to call bio med department to get equipment in for repairs; four rental machines are brought to unit while others are being fixed | Staff need functioning equipment to do their jobs efficiently | Partner with bio med department to have unit equipment checked once per week to ensure each component of the machines is functioning properly |

highly compelling; few people can allow it to go unanswered. All of us receive numerous phone calls and texts, and some of them time wasters. Handling them effectively is a must:

- *Minimize socializing and small talk.* If you answer the phone with, "Hello, what can I do for you?" rather than, "Hello, how are you?" the caller is encouraged to get to business first. Be warm, friendly, and courteous, but do not allow others to waste time with inappropriate or extensive small talk. Calls placed and returned just prior to lunchtime, at the end of the day, and on Friday afternoons tend to result in more business and less socializing.
- *Plan calls.* The person who plans phone calls does not waste anyone's time, including that of the person called. Write down the topics you want to discuss before you make the call. That way, you will not need to call back to give additional information or ask a forgotten question.
- *Set a time for calls.* You may have a number of calls to return and make. It is best to set aside a time for routine phone calls, especially during your "downtime." Try not to interrupt what is being done at the moment. If an answer is necessary before a project can be continued, phone immediately; if not, phone for the information at a later time.
- *State the reason for the call and ask for preferred call times.* If a party is not available, explain why you are calling and provide several time frames when you will be available for a return call. Find out when the person you are calling is free. This makes it easier for him or her to be prepared for the call and helps prevent "phone tag."

Voice mail is an excellent way to send and receive messages when a real-time interaction is not essential. For example, one person or a large group of people can learn about an upcoming meeting in one voice mail message. They can phone their responses at their convenience (with no need to reach each other directly). Like other forms of communication, voice mail must be used appropriately.

Long messages or sensitive information is better conveyed one-on-one. Moreover, another person (e.g., unit clerk) may be responsible for taking voice mail messages off the system, so it is important to state the message in a professional manner, omitting personal or confidential information.

Text messages demand attention unless the phone is turned off. Even then, frequently glancing at the phone's screen alerts you to the message. Few of us can resist checking "just this one" message. Text messages are a combination of voice messages and e-mail, so establish a time to return them.

### E-Mail

#### Incoming Messages

E-mail can enhance time management or be a further time waster. E-mail minimizes the time you waste trying to contact individuals, enables you to contact many people simultaneously, and allows you to code the urgency of the message. Tone, however, is difficult to convey by e-mail. Therefore, it is better to use more personal forms of communication, such as the phone or in-person contact, for potentially sensitive or troublesome issues.

Checking e-mail too often can waste time. Each time you read a message, you are forced to think about it and you lose your focus on the task at hand. Turn off your e-mail alert and set specific times of day to check your in-box.

Also discourage people who forward you unwanted messages. Set your e-mail filter to direct these messages to your spam folder or tell the sender that you cannot receive personal messages at work (Merritt, 2009).

#### Outgoing Messages

Writing clear messages helps increase prompt and useful responses. Here are some tips:

- Direct messages only to the people involved (e.g., committee members) and copy others (e.g., the department chair).
- Title the subject line appropriately. For example, write "Meeting Friday morning" rather than "Information."

- Avoid salutations, if possible. "Dear" and "Hi" are often not needed on routine messages.
- Craft your message succinctly, but politely: "The division meeting will be held in conference room C at 9 A.M."

## Drop-In Visitors

Although often friendly and seemingly harmless, the typical "got-a-minute?" drop-in visit is rarely as short as that. Take charge of the visit by identifying the issue or question, arranging an alternative meeting, referring the visitor to someone else, or redirecting the visitor's problem-solving efforts.

If you are fortunate enough to have an office, you will find that open doors are open invitations for interruption. Although it is essential that you be available and accessible, you also need time to concentrate. Tell staff that you will be available for a specific block of time (a few hours at most) to address issues.

Of course, some interruptions are important and/or urgent. You must attend to those. For others, however, you can control the duration of the drop-in visitor (Jones & Loftus, 2009). Stand and remain standing. This appears gracious, yet is obvious enough to encourage a short visit. Before the person leaves, politely suggest that he or she visit during your office hours or send an e-mail to make a future appointment.

You can also control interruptions through the way you arrange your office furniture. You are asking for interruptions when you arrange your desk in a way that permits eye contact with passersby or drop-in visitors. A desk turned 90 or even 180 degrees from the door minimizes potential eye contact.

Encouraging people to make appointments to deal with routine matters also reduces interruptions. Regularly scheduled meetings with people who need to see you allow them to hold routine matters for those appointments. Meeting in someone else's office places you in charge of the time spent: it is easier to leave someone's office than to ask someone to leave yours.

## Paperwork

Health care organizations cannot function effectively without good information systems. In addition to phone calls and face-to-face conversations, nurses and managers spend considerable time writing and reading communications. Increasing government regulations, measures to avoid legal action, stronger privacy requirements, new treatments and medications, data processing, work processing, and electronics place pressure on everyone to cope with increasing paperwork (including electronic "paperwork").

1. *Plan and schedule paperwork.* Writing and reading reports, forms, e-mail, letters, and memos are essential elements of a job. They will, however, become a major source of frustration if their processing is not planned and scheduled as an integral part of daily activities. Learn the organization's information system and requirements, analyze the paperwork requirements of the position, and make significant progress on that part of the job daily.

2. *Sort paperwork for effective processing.* A system of file folders either for paper mail or e-mail can be very helpful. Here is a system to handle it:

   - Place all paperwork (or e-mail) requiring personal action in a red file or in an "action" folder on your computer's hard drive. Handle that according to its relative importance and urgency.
   - Place work that can be delegated in a separate file, and distribute it appropriately.
   - Place all work that is informational and related to present work in a yellow file folder or in an "informational" folder on your hard drive.
   - Place other reading material, such as professional journals, technical reports, and other items that do not relate directly to the immediate work, in a blue file folder or a "read" file.

The informational file contains materials that must be read immediately, whereas the reading file materials are not as urgent and can be read later.

Do not be afraid to throw things away or erase them from your computer's memory. Do not let them become clutter when they no longer have value. Use trash receptacles in the office and on the electronic system.

3. *Send every communication electronically.* Unless a paper memo, report, or letter is required, send your work electronically.

4. *Analyze paperwork frequently.* Review filing policies and rules regularly and purge files at least once each year. All standard forms, reports, and memos should be reviewed annually. Each should justify its continued existence and its present format. Do not be afraid to recommend changes and, when possible, initiate those changes.

5. *Do not be a paper shuffler.* "Handle a piece of paper only once" is a common adage, but impossible to follow if taken literally. Rather, each time you handle a piece of paper or e-mail message, take action to further process it. Paper shufflers are those who continually move things around on their desks or accumulate unread e-mails. They delay action unreasonably, and the problem mounts.

## Controlling Time in Meetings

Meetings consume much of the manager's time, and much of that time is wasted. To manage meetings follow these rules (Merritt, 2009):

- Do not meet simply because you always meet on Monday morning. If no meeting is needed, cancel it.
- Invite only key people to initial meetings. Others can be sent the minutes or invited to future meetings.
- Establish the meeting's goal and outcomes expected at the outset.
- Send information before the meeting so time is not spent reading it.
- Set a time limit for all meetings. Routine meetings should last no more than one hour. If more time is needed, schedule another meeting.
- Determine the agenda and keep to the topic.
- Follow-up with actions assigned.

## Respecting Time

The key to using time-management techniques is to respect one's own time as well as that of others. Using the above suggestions for time management communicates to those who interact with you that you expect them to respect your time. You, however, must reciprocate by respecting their time too. If you need to talk to someone, make an appointment, particularly for routine matters.

You should continually ask, "What is the best use of my time right now?" and should answer in three ways:

- For myself and my goals
- For my staff and their goals
- For the organization and its goals

Efforts to manage time may seem to take more time, but the reverse is true. Any activity that helps set goals, determine priorities, organize the workday, and minimize interruptions will pay off in increased efficiency and effectiveness.

## What You Know Now

- The first step in time management is to analyze how you use your time by keeping a time log.
- Determine priorities and set goals to establish daily planning and scheduling.
- Personal organization strategies help use time productively.
- An interruption log helps identify patterns that can be used to reduce unnecessary interruptions.
- Control phone calls by minimizing small talk, planning calls, setting aside time for calls, stating preferred call times, and using voice mail.
- To control interruptions by drop-in visitors, stand to meet visitors, encourage appointments, and arrange furniture to discourage unscheduled visitors.
- Written communication can also cause interruptions. These can be minimized by planning and scheduling paperwork and e-mails and using an effective filing system.
- People who respect their own time are likely to find others respecting it also.

## Tools for Managing Time

1. Recognize that there will never be enough time to accomplish everything you want.
2. Use a time log to identify and reduce time wasters.
3. Use a planning system to list goals, their priorities, and schedule the workday.
4. Set aside uninterrupted time to complete important tasks.
5. Group routine tasks and use short blocks of time to complete them.
6. Monitor interruptions and decide on ways to minimize them.

## Questions to Challenge You

1. What are your major time wasters? Keep a time log for one week. Compare how you thought you wasted time with what your time log revealed.
2. Write down your goals for the next week. What action steps can you take to realize your goals? At the end of the week, evaluate your progress. Then write down the next week's goals.
3. What is keeping you from accomplishing your goals? Think about how you can change the circumstances to better reflect your priorities.
4. Do you use a planner or other scheduling device? If not, investigate the choices and select the one that will work best for you. Then use it!
5. Think about how you handle interruptions. During the next week, try various strategies to minimize the effect of interruptions.

**Pearson Nursing Student Resources**

Find additional review materials at
**www.nursing.pearsonhighered.com**

Prepare for success with additional NCLEX®-style practice questions, interactive assignments and activities, Web links, animations and videos, and more!

## References

Carrick, L., Carrick, L., & Yurkow, J. (2007). A nurse leader's guide to managing priorities. *American Nurse Today, 2*(7), 40–41.

Gentry, W. A., Harris, L. S., Baker, B. A., & Leslie, J. B. (2008). Managerial skills: What has changed since the late 1980s. *Leadership & Organization Development Journal, 29*(2), 167–181.

Jones, L., & Loftus, P. (2009). *Time well spent: Getting things done through effective time management.* Philadelphia, PA: Kogan Page.

Merritt, C. (2009). *Too busy for your own good.* New York: McGraw Hill.

Sullivan, E. J. (2013). *Becoming influential: A guide for nurses* (2nd ed.). Upper Saddle River, NJ: Prentice Hall.

CHAPTER

# 14

# Budgeting and Managing Fiscal Resources

**The Budgeting Process**

**Approaches to Budgeting**

   INCREMENTAL BUDGET

   ZERO-BASED BUDGET

   FIXED OR VARIABLE BUDGETS

**The Operating Budget**

   THE REVENUE BUDGET

   THE EXPENSE BUDGET

**Determining the Salary (Personnel) Budget**

   BENEFITS

   SHIFT DIFFERENTIALS

   OVERTIME

   ON-CALL HOURS

   PREMIUMS

   SALARY INCREASES

   ADDITIONAL CONSIDERATIONS

**Managing the Supply and Nonsalary Expense Budget**

**The Capital Budget**

**Timetable for the Budgeting Process**

**Monitoring Budgetary Performance During the Year**

   VARIANCE ANALYSIS

   POSITION CONTROL

**Problems Affecting Budgetary Performance**

   REIMBURSEMENT PROBLEMS

   STAFF IMPACT ON BUDGET

## Learning Outcomes

*After completing this chapter, you will be able to:*

1. Describe how the budgeting process works.
2. Differentiate among types of budgets.
3. Demonstrate how to monitor and control budgetary performance.
4. Explain how to determine budget variance.
5. Describe how staff affect budgetary performance.

## Key Terms

Benefit time
Budget
Budgeting
Capital budget
Cost center
Direct costs
Efficiency variance
Expense budget
Fiscal year

Fixed budget
Fixed costs
Incremental (line-by-line) budget
Indirect costs
Nonsalary expenditure variances
Operating budget
Position control

Profit
Rate variances
Revenue budget
Salary (personnel) budget
Variable budget
Variable costs
Variance
Volume variances
Zero-based budget

Budgeting is the process of planning and controlling future operations by comparing actual results with planned expectations (Finkler & Kovner, 2007). A budget is a detailed plan that communicates these expectations and serves as the basis for comparing them to actual results. The budget shows how resources will be acquired and used over some specific time interval; its purpose is to allow management to project activities into the future so that the objectives of the organization are coordinated and met. It also helps ensure that the resources necessary to achieve these objectives are available at the appropriate time. Lastly, a budget helps management control the organization.

Budgeting is performed by business, government, and individuals. In fact, nearly everyone budgets, even though he or she may not identify the process as such. Even if a budget exists only in an individual's mind, it is nonetheless a budget. Anyone who has planned how to pay a particular bill at some time in the future—say, six months—has a budget. Although it is very simple, that plan accomplishes the essential budget functions. One now knows how much of a resource (money) is needed and when (in six months) it is needed. Note that the "when" is just as important as the "how much." The money has to be available at the right time.

Demands for patient safety, reimbursement changes with health care reform, technological advances, and the changing roles of health care providers require that budgets be constructed as accurately as possible and variances be as low as possible (Dunham-Taylor & Pinczuk, 2009). This is no small task. Attention to the budgeting process is the first step in understanding how to use resources most effectively.

## The Budgeting Process

A **budget** is a quantitative statement, usually in monetary terms, of the plans and expectations of a defined area over a specified period of time. Budgets provide a foundation for managing and evaluating financial performance. Budgets detail how resources (money, time, people) will be acquired and used to support planned services within the defined time period.

The budget process also helps ensure that the resources needed to achieve these objectives are available at the appropriate time and that operations are carried out within the resources available. The budgeting process increases the awareness of costs and also helps employees understand the relationships among goals, expenses, and revenues. As a result, employees are committed to the goals and objectives of the organization, and various departments are able to coordinate activities and collaborate to achieve the organization's objectives. Budgets also help management control the resources expended through an organizational awareness of costs. Finally, budget performance provides management with feedback about resources management and the impact on the budget.

**Budgeting** is a process of planning and controlling future operations by comparing actual results with planned expectations. Planning first involves reviewing established *goals* and *objectives* of both nursing and the organization. Goals and objectives help identify the organization's priorities and direct the organization's efforts. To plan, the organization must know the following:

- Demographics of the population served, community influences, and competitors
- Sources of revenue, especially with changes in reimbursement due to enactment of health care reform
- Statistical data, including:
  - Number of admissions or patient appointments
  - Average daily census
  - Average length of stay
  - Patient acuity
  - Projected occupancy or volume base for ambulatory or procedure-based units or home care visits

- Wage increases of market adjustments
- Price increases, including inflation rate, for supplies and other costs
- Costs for new equipment or technologies (e.g., wound vacs, sequential compression devices, monitoring equipment)
- Staff mix (e.g., RNs, LPNs, UAPs)
- Regulatory changes (e.g., legislation mandating nurse-to-patient ratios, state board of health regulations) for the budgetary period
- Organizational changes (e.g., decentralization of pharmacy or respiratory therapy services) that result in salary and benefit dollars being charged in portion to the unit

Management normally uses the past as the common starting point for projecting the future, but in today's volatile payment environment, the past may be a poor predictor of the future. This is one of the major drawbacks of the budgeting process. In a rapidly changing industry, basing budgets on historical data often requires readjustment during the actual budget period.

Controlling is the process of comparing actual results with the results projected in the budget. (See the section on monitoring performance during the year later in the chapter.) Two techniques for controlling budgetary performance are *variance analysis* and *position control*. By measuring the differences between the projected and the actual results, management is better able to make modifications and corrections. Therefore, controlling depends on planning.

## Approaches to Budgeting

Budgets may be developed in various formats depending on how the organization is structured. They may be considered as:

- *Cost centers.* Managers are responsible for predicting, documenting, and managing the costs (staffing, supplies) of the division.
- *Revenue centers.* Managers are responsible for generating revenues (previously by increasing patient volume, although health care reform may make the future of revenue-generating centers obsolete).
- *Profit centers.* Managers are responsible for generating revenues and managing costs so that the department shows a profit (revenues exceed costs).
- *Investment centers.* Managers are responsible for generating revenues and managing costs and capital equipment (assets).

Nursing units are typically considered to be cost centers, but they may also be viewed as revenue centers, profit centers, or investment centers. How the unit is considered is crucial in determining the manager's approach to budgeting.

Also, some nursing managers are responsible for service lines, and their staff are from multiple disciplines and departments. Other nurse managers are responsible for a single unit, such as a telemetry unit or the staff in a multiple-physician office.

The organization may choose various approaches, or combinations of approaches, for requesting departmental managers to prepare their budget requests. These approaches are incremental (line-by-line), zero-based, fixed, and variable.

### Incremental Budget

With an **incremental**, or **line-by-line, budget**, the finance department distributes a budget worksheet listing each expense item or category on a separate expense line. The expense line is usually divided into salary and nonsalary items. A budget worksheet is commonly used for mathematical calculations to be submitted for the next year. It may include several columns for the amount budgeted for the current year, the amount actually spent year-to-date, the projected total for the year based on the actual amount spent, increases and decreases in the expense amount for the new budget, and the request for the next year with an explanation attached.

The base or starting point for calculating next year's budget request may be either the previous year's actual results or projected expenditures for the current year. For salary expenses, the adjustment might be the average salary increase projected for next year. For nonsalary expenses, the finance department may provide an estimate of the average increase for supplies or opt to use a standard measure of cost increases, perhaps the consumer or medical price index projected for the next year.

To complete budget worksheets accurately, managers must be familiar with expense account categories. What type of expenses, such as instruments and minor equipment, are included under each line item? In addition, the manager has to keep abreast of different factors that have affected the expenditure level for each expense line during the current year. The projected impact of next year's activities will be translated into increases or decreases in expense levels of the nursing unit's expenditures for the coming year.

The advantage of the line-by-line budget method is its simplicity of preparation. The disadvantage of this method is that it discourages cost efficiency. To avoid budget cuts for the next year, an astute manager learns to spend the entire budget amount established for the current year, because this amount becomes the base for the next year.

### Zero-Based Budget

The **zero-based budget** approach assumes the base for projecting next year's budget is zero. Managers are required to justify all activities and programs as if they were being initiated for the first time. Regardless of the level of expenditure in previous years, every proposed expenditure for the new year must be justified under the current environment and its fit with the organization's objectives.

The advantage of zero-based budgeting is that every expense is justified. The disadvantage is that the process is time-consuming and may not be necessary. For that reason, organizations may not use this process every year. An adaptation of the zero-based budget is to start the budget with a lower base, for example, 80 percent of the current expenses. Managers then have to justify any budgetary expenses requested above the 80 percent base.

### Fixed or Variable Budgets

Budgets can also be categorized as fixed or variable. In a **fixed budget**, the budgeted amounts are set without regard to changes that may occur during the year, such as patient volume or program activities, that have an impact on the cost assumptions originally used for the coming year. In contrast, **variable budgets** are developed with the understanding that adjustments to the budget may be made during the year based on changes in revenues, patient census, utilization of supplies, and other expenses.

## The Operating Budget

The **operating budget**, also known as the annual budget, is the organization's statement of expected revenues and expenses for the coming year. It coincides with the **fiscal year** of the organization, a specified 12-month period during which the operational and financial performance of the organization is measured. The fiscal year may correspond with the calendar year—January to December—or another time frame. Many organizations use July 1 to June 30; the federal government begins its fiscal year on October 1. The operating budget may be further broken down into smaller periods of six months or four quarters; each quarter may be further separated into three one-month periods. The revenues and expenses are organized separately, with a bottom-line net profit or loss calculated.

### The Revenue Budget

The **revenue budget** represents the patient care income expected for the budget period. Most commonly, health care payers pay a predetermined rate based on discounts or allowances. In many cases, actual payment generated by a given service or procedure will not equal the charges that appear on the patient bill. Instead, the health care provider will be reimbursed based on a variety of methods. These include:

- Reimbursement of a predetermined amount, such as fixed costs per case (Medicare recipients);
- Negotiated rates, such as per diems (a specified reimbursement amount per patient, per day);
- Negotiated discounts; and
- Capitation (one rate per member, per month, regardless of the service provided).

Revenue projections for the next year are based on the volume and mix of patients, rates, and discounts that will prevail during the budget period. Projections are developed from historical volume data, impact of new or modified clinical programs, shifts from inpatient to outpatient procedures, and other influences. Today, however, these projections may not be viable, especially in the light of health care reform.

With implementation of accountable care organizations and medical homes, Medicare reimbursement is expected to change (Buerhaus, 2010). Instead of paying for inpatient services at a predetermined specific rate for each Medicare recipient based on the patient's diagnosis (DRGs), providers will be reimbursed for care of patient groups.

## The Expense Budget

The **expense budget** consists of salary and nonsalary items. Expenses should reflect patient care objectives and activity parameters established for the nursing unit. The expense budget should be comprehensive and thorough; it should also take into consideration all available information regarding the next year's expectations. Described in the next section are several concepts and definitions related to the budgetary process in a health care setting.

### Cost Centers

In health care organizations, nursing units are typically considered cost centers. A **cost center** is described as the smallest area of activity within an organization for which costs are accumulated. Cost centers may be revenue producing, such as laboratory and radiology, or non–revenue producing, such as environmental services and administration. Nursing managers are commonly given the responsibility for costs incurred by their department, but they have no revenue responsibilities.

In contrast, if managers are responsible for controlling both costs and revenues and if their financial performance is measured in terms of **profit** (the difference between revenues and expenses), then the manager is responsible for a profit center. Customarily, nursing is not directly reimbursed for its services. As stated previously, nursing costs today are included in the room charge although that may change as methods to match nurses' skills to patient needs improve.

### Classification of Costs

Costs are commonly classified as fixed or variable. **Fixed costs** are costs that will remain the same for the budget period regardless of the activity level of the organization, such as rental payments and insurance premiums. **Variable costs** depend on and change in direct proportion to patient volume and patient acuity, such as patient care supply expenses. If more patients are admitted to a nursing unit, more supplies are used, causing higher supply expenses.

Expenditures may also be direct or indirect. **Direct costs** are expenses that directly affect patient care. For example, salaries for nursing personnel who provide hands-on patient care are considered direct costs. **Indirect costs** are expenditures that are necessary but don't affect patient care directly. Salaries for security or maintenance personnel, for example, are classified as indirect costs.

# Determining the Salary (Personnel) Budget

The **salary budget**, also known as the **personnel budget**, projects the salary costs that will be paid and charged to the cost center in the budget period (see Table 14-1). Managing the salary budget is directly related to the manager's ability to supervise and lead the staff. Better managers tend to have more stable staff with fewer resources spent on supplementary staff, turnover, or absenteeism. In addition to anticipated salary expenses, factors such as benefits, shift differentials, overtime, on-call expenses, and bonuses and premiums may affect the salary budget as well.

## Benefits

After the number of required full-time equivalents (FTEs) is determined (see Chapter 16 on scheduling), it is also necessary to determine how many FTEs are necessary to replace personnel for **benefit time** (vacations, holidays, personal days, etc). This factor can be calculated by determining the average number of vacation days, paid holidays, personal days, bereavement days, or other days off with pay that the organization provides and the average number of sick days per employee as experienced by the cost center.

To determine FTEs required for replacement:

1. Determine hours of replacement time per individual.

2. Then determine FTE requirement.

| Benefit Time | Hours/shift | Replacement Hours |
|---|---|---|
| 15 vacation days | × 8 hours | = 120 |
| 8 holidays | × 8 hours | = 64 |
| 4 personal days | × 8 hours | = 32 |
| 5 sick days | × 8 hours | = 40 |
| | Total | = 256 |

**TABLE 14-1    Monthly Salary Budget and Year-to-Date Budget Comparison Report Fiscal Year Ending June 30**

| Position | June Actual Salary | June Budgeted Salary | June Variance | Year-to-Date Actual Salary | Year-to-Date Budgeted Salary | Year-to-Date Variance |
|---|---|---|---|---|---|---|
| Nurse Manager | $6,250 | $6,250 | $0 | $68,750 | $75,000 | $6,250 |
| Registered Nurses | 95,722 | 93,825 | (1,897) | 1,048,813 | 1,125,878 | 77,065 |
| Licensed Practical Nurses | 19,025 | 20,800 | 1,775 | 231,426 | 249,600 | 18,174 |
| Nursing Assistants | 14,886 | 13,200 | (1,686) | 159,500 | 158,400 | (1,100) |
| Unit Clerks | 5,483 | 5,495 | 12 | 60,391 | 65,273 | 4,882 |
| Float Pool RNs | 1,426 | 1,000 | (426) | 16,800 | 12,500 | (4,300) |
| **TOTAL SALARY:** | **$142,792** | **$140,570** | **($2,222)** | **$1,585,680** | **$1,686,651** | **$100,971** |

Divide replacement time by annual FTE base

$$\frac{256}{2,080} = 0.12$$

An FTE budget is calculated from the FTE calculations (Table 14-1). This budget provides the base for the salary budget. However, shift differentials, overtime, and bonuses or premiums may also affect budget performance and need to be considered.

### Shift Differentials

Some facilities use a set percentage to determine shift differential: 10 percent for evenings, 15 percent for nights, and 20 percent for weekends and holidays, for example. If the hourly rate is $18.00, for instance, then the cost for a nurse working evenings would be $18.00 plus $1.80 for each hour worked. On an eight-hour shift, the total cost would be $158.40, and for the year, $41,184. Other facilities use a set dollar amount per hour as the shift differential. For instance, evenings adds $2.50 per hour to base pay, night shift $4.00, and weekends $2.50 additional pay.

### Overtime

Fluctuations in workload, patient volume, variability in admission patterns, and temporary replacement of staff due to illness or time off all create overtime in the nursing unit. A projection of overtime for the next year can be calculated by determining by staff classification (RN, LPN, nursing assistant, and other employee classifications) the historical or typical number of hours of overtime worked and multiplying that number by 1.5 times the hourly rate. For example, if the average number of overtime hours paid in a unit for RNs is 35 hours per two-week pay period, and the average hourly rate is $18.00, the projected overtime cost for the year would be $24,570 for the RN category.

To determine overtime costs:

1.  Multiply average salary for classification      $18.00
    by factor      ×    1.50
    to obtain overtime rate      $27.00
2.  Multiply average overtime hours      35
    by overtime rate      ×   $27.00
    to obtain expenditure per pay period      $945.00
3.  Multiply number of pay periods      26
    by overtime expenditure      ×$945.00
    to obtain annual overtime costs      $24,570.00

Clearly, overtime can rapidly deplete finite budget dollars allocated to a nursing unit. The nurse manager should explore options to overtime, such as using part-time or per diem workers in order to keep the cost per hour more in line with the regular hourly rates. A competent manager certainly would also evaluate unit productivity to decrease overtime.

### On-Call Hours

If the nursing unit uses a paid on-call system, the approximate number of hours that employees are put on call for the year should be estimated and that cost added to the budget. Typically under the on-call system, staff members are requested to be available to be called back to work if patient need arises, and the number of hours on call are paid at a flat rate per hour.

### Premiums

Some organizations offer premiums for certifications or clinical ladder steps. In this situation, a fixed dollar amount may be added to the base hourly rate of eligible personnel; for example, an additional $1.00 per hour paid for professional certifications. This would result in the hourly rate of the employee being adjusted from a base of $18.00 to $19.00. In this case, if the employee is full time and works 2,080 hours a year (40 hours a week multiplied by 52 weeks a year), the annual new salary would be $39,520, or $19.00 multiplied by 2,080.

### Salary Increases

Merit increases and cost-of-living raises also need to be factored into budget projections. These increases are usually calculated on base pay. For example, if a three percent cost-of-living raise is projected and the base salary for an RN is $40,000, then the new base becomes $41,200.

### Additional Considerations

Other important factors to consider when developing the salary budget are changes in technology, clinical supports, delivery systems, clinical programs or procedures, and regulatory requirements. Changes in patient care technology or the introduction of new equipment may influence the number, skill, or time that unit personnel may spend in becoming trained to use the new equipment and, later, operating and maintaining it. If significant, the projected number of additional labor hours for the new budgetary period should be incorporated into the request.

The Joint Commission, the organization that accredits health care organizations, evaluates an institution to determine whether it is adhering to the level of staffing required to maintain a safe patient care environment (Joint Commission, 2011). For example, the institution may have established a standard for critical care units and some other specialty units that a minimum of two staff members are required at all times, regardless of patient number or acuity. Additionally, some states have mandated staffing levels.

Departments such as environmental services, dietary, escort, or laboratory may provide the nursing unit with support in performing certain tasks, such as transporting patients or specimens. Any change in the level of support they provide should be reviewed, and the effect of such change on the unit's staffing levels should be quantified for the next year's budget request. Changes in staffing can place new demands on the unit. Therefore, orientation and additional workload needs should also be considered.

In addition, changes might be made to the way the organization charges costs. For example, some direct or indirect costs formerly charged under other divisions might now be allocated to the various units. You might find your unit charged its fair share of the heating or security budget. Major changes, of course, are planned ahead of time but some changes occur during the budget year, and the unit might be expected to absorb those additional costs within its original budget.

# Managing the Supply and Nonsalary Expense Budget

The supply and nonsalary expense budget identifies patient-related supplies needed to operate the nursing unit. In addition to supplies, other operating expenses—such as office supplies, rental fees, maintenance costs, and equipment service contracts—may also be paid out of the nursing unit's nonsalary budget.

An analysis of the current expense pattern and a determination of its applicability for the next budget period should be performed first. Any projected changes in patient volume, acuity, and patient mix should also be considered because they will affect next year's supply use and other nonsalary expenses. As an example, if patient days for a particular type of patient are projected to multiply and cause a five percent increase in the use of intravenous solutions, this increase should be addressed in the budget request by requesting an additional five percent for intravenous solution supplies for the next year.

Increases due to an inflation rate index, or at a rate estimated by the finance or purchasing department, are included as part of the budget request. A simple way of calculating the effect of a price increase is to take the estimated total ending expense for the year and multiply it by the inflationary factor.

To determine projected price increases:

| Multiply current total line item expense | $12,758 |
|---|---|
| by inflation factor plus 1.0 | $\times 1.05$ |
| | $13,396 |

Increases in expenses, such as maintenance agreements and rental fees, should also be incorporated as part of the budget request. The introduction of new technology and changes in programs and regulatory requirements may require additional resources for supplies as well as increased salaries.

## The Capital Budget

The **capital budget** is an important component of the plan to meet the organization's long-term goals. This budget identifies physical renovations, new construction, and new or replacement equipment planned within a specified time period. Organizations define capital items based on certain conditions or criteria. Usually, capital items must have an expected performance of one year or more and exceed a certain dollar value, such as $500 or $1,000.

The capital budget is limited to a specified amount, and decisions need to be made how best to allocate available funds. Priority is given to those items needed most. Not all items that fall under capital budget will necessarily get funding in a given year.

Today, few nurse managers are asked to prepare a capital budget because most organizations are buying through consortiums or negotiated agreements with one supplier. Many health care organizations have departments that coordinate bringing in selected vendors and items and limit choices to that equipment. The nurse manager would then be responsible for reporting what needs exist, helping select and determine the amount of equipment needed. The capital pool is expensed out across all units that use the equipment.

The impact of the new equipment on the unit's expenses, such as the number of staff needed to run the equipment, use of supplies, and maintenance costs, needs to be considered as part of the operating budget, however. Likewise, the need for additional nursing and nonnursing personnel to operate the new equipment, additional workload, and training of personnel should be quantified for the next year's budget.

## Timetable for the Budgeting Process

Depending on the size and complexity of the organization, the budgeting process takes between three and six months. The process begins with the first-level manager. The individual at this level of management may or may not have formalized budget responsibilities, but he or she is key to identifying needed resources for the upcoming budget period.

The manager seeks information from staff about areas of needed improvement or change and reviews unit productivity and the need for updated technology or supplies. The manager uses this information to prepare the first draft of the budget proposal.

Depending on the levels of organizational management, this proposal ascends through the managerial hierarchy. Each subsequent manager evaluates the budget proposal, making adjustments as needed. By the time the budget is approved by executive management, significant changes to the original proposal usually have been made.

The final step in the process is approval by a governing board, such as a board of directors or designated shareholders. Typically, the budget process timetable is structured so that the budget is approved a few months before the beginning of the new fiscal year.

Clearly articulating budgetary needs is essential for the manager to be successful in budget negotiations. Senior management must prioritize budget requests for the entire organization, and they base those decisions on strong supporting documentation. Nurse managers should not expect to receive all of their budget requests, but they need to be prepared to defend their priorities.

## Monitoring Budgetary Performance During the Year

The difference between the amount that was budgeted for a specific revenue or cost and the actual revenue or cost that resulted during the course of activities is known as the **variance**. Variance might occur in the actual cost of delivering patient care for a certain expense line item in a specified period of time. Nurse managers are commonly asked to justify the reason for variances and present an action plan to reduce or eliminate these variances.

Managers receive reports summarizing the expenses for the department (see Table 14-1). In the past, monthly reports on paper were sent to managers, but technology makes such a system obsolete today. Reports can be compiled and communicated rapidly, allowing managers to adjust quicker.

The reports show expense line items with the budgeted amount, actual expenditure, variance from budget, and the percentage from the budgeted amount that such variance represents. These reports often also show the comparison between actual year-to-date results and the year-to-date budget.

To assess variance:

- Identify items that are over or under budgeted amounts
- Find out why the variance occurred (e.g., a one-time event or an ongoing occurrence)
- Keep notes on what you have learned in preparation for next year's budget
- Examine the payroll and note overtime or use of agency personnel
- Validate the use of overtime or additional personnel and keep a note for your files

Keeping notes throughout the year will help prevent the annual budget process from becoming an overwhelming challenge. Trying to reconstruct what happened and why during the past 12 months is unlikely to present a complete and accurate picture of events and makes creating a future budget more difficult.

### Variance Analysis

In the daily course of events, it is unlikely that projected budget items will be completely on target in all situations. One of the manager's most important jobs is to manage the financial resources for the department and to be able to respond to variances in a timely fashion.

When expenses occur that differ from the budgeted amounts, organizations usually have an established level at which a variance needs to be investigated and explained or justified by the manager of the department. This level may be a certain dollar amount, such as $500, or it may be a percentage, such as a five percent or ten percent increase above the budget.

In determining causes for variance, the nurse manager must review the activity level of the unit for the same period. There may have been increases in census or patient acuity that generated additional expense in salary and supplies.

Also, in many situations, variances might not be independent of one another. Variances may result from expenses that follow a seasonal pattern and occur only at determined times in the year (renewal of a maintenance agreement is one example). Expenses may also follow a tendency or trend either to increase or to decrease during the year. Even if the situation is outside the manager's usual responsibility or control, the manager needs to understand and be able to identify the cause or reason for the variance.

To determine when a variance is favorable or unfavorable, it is important to relate the variance to its impact on the organization in terms of revenues and expenses. If more earnings came in than expected, the variance is favorable; if less, the variance is negative. Likewise, if less was spent than expected, the variance is favorable; if more was spent, the variance is negative.

For instance, the nurse manager might receive the following expense report:

| Budgeted Expenditures | Actual Expenditures | Variance (in $) | Percent (in %) |
|---|---|---|---|
| $34,560 | $36,958 | (2,398) | (6.9) |

This expense variance is considered unfavorable because the actual expense was greater than the budget. In this example, more money was spent on medical/surgical supplies than was projected in the budget.

If the variance percentage of the actual budget amount is not presented in the reports, it can be calculated as follows:

$$\frac{\$2,398}{\$34,560} = 0.069$$

Divide the dollar variance by the budget amount, then multiply by 100:

$$0.069 \times 100 = 6.9\% \text{ over budget}$$

### Salary Variances

With salary expenditures, variances may occur in volume, efficiency, or rate. Typically these factors are related and have an impact on each other. **Volume variances** result when there is a difference in the budgeted and actual workload requirements, as would occur with increases in patient days. An increase in the actual number of patient days will increase the salary expense, resulting in an unfavorable volume variance. Although the variance is unfavorable, concomitant increases in revenues for the organization should be apparent. Thus, the impact to the organization should be welcomed, even though it generated higher salary costs at the nursing unit level.

**Efficiency variance**, also called quantity or use variance, reflects the difference between budgeted and actual nursing care hours provided. Patient acuity, nursing skill, unit management, technology, and productivity all affect the number of patient care hours actually provided versus the original number planned or required. At the same time, if the census had been higher than expected, it would be understandable if more hours of nursing care were provided and paid. A favorable efficiency, or fewer nursing care hours paid, could suggest that patient acuity was lower than projected, that staff was more efficient, or that higher-skilled employees were used. An unfavorable efficiency may be due to greater patient acuity than allowed for in the budget, overstaffing of the unit, or the use of less experienced or less efficient employees.

**Rate variances**, also known as price or spending variance, reflect the difference in budgeted and actual hourly rates paid. A favorable rate variance may reflect the use of new employees who were paid lower salaries. Unfavorable rate variance may reflect unanticipated salary increases or increased use of personnel paid at higher wages, such as agency personnel.

### Nonsalary Expenditure Variances

A **nonsalary expenditure variance** may be due to changes in patient volume, patient mix, supply quantities, or prices paid. New, additional, or more expensive supplies used at the nursing unit because of technology changes or new regulations could also influence expenditure totals.

## Position Control

Another monitoring tool used by nurse managers is the position control. The **position control** is used to compare actual numbers of employees to the number of budgeted FTEs for the nursing unit. The position control is a list of approved, budgeted FTE positions for the nursing cost center. The positions are displayed by category or job classification, such as nurse manager, RNs, LPNs, and so on. The nurse manager updates the position control with employee names and FTE factors for each individual with respect to personnel changes, new hires, and resignations that take place during the year.

# Problems Affecting Budgetary Performance

## Reimbursement Problems

The manager may be called upon to help with problems of reimbursement. Here are some examples:

- *Insurance company disputes charges for a patient stay and refuses to pay them.* The insurance company thinks patient should have been discharged a day sooner and refuses to pay for last day of stay because a good clinical reason to be in the hospital isn't documented.

  **Here are three alternative solutions:**

  1. Ask the physician to elaborate on the clinical reasons why the patient necessitated another day stay in the hospital and submit that documentation to the insurance company.
  2. Negotiate the charge with the insurance company and take a settlement on payment that is agreeable to both parties.
  3. Have an internal utilization review group go through the patient's chart and extract lab values, clinical presentation symptoms, testing, etc., that were done on day of stay being disputed and submit to insurance company as an appeal to denial to pay, demonstrating necessity to stay.

- *Patient disputes charges during stay and refuses to pay them.* The patient gets a PICC line (invasive procedure, longer term intravenous line) placed for IV antibiotics to be infused for one to two weeks. The PICC line is placed because one to two weeks of antibiotics is not something typically a peripheral IV line would be used for because they don't hold up as well and can't infiltrate or the patient could get phlebitis. Then, after the PICC line is placed, two days later the doctor decides to discontinue IV antibiotics and remove the PICC line. The patient refuses to pay for the PICC line because it wasn't used for one to two weeks as the doctor had originally said and feels he should not pay for the doctor's "change of mind."

  **Here are three alternative solutions:**

  1. Meet with the patient to discuss his case and explain that with his initial clinical presentation, the physician's decision to place the PICC line was reasonable and the hospital will not waive charges.
  2. Agree to negotiate charge with the patient because the PICC line was placed with reasonable and prudent judgment but was not utilized as long as was initially discussed with the patient.
  3. Agree to drop charges for PICC line placement.

- *Patient is not able to obtain resources needed when discharged.* A patient is ready for discharge to home but is on an expensive antibiotic. Even with insurance, she can't afford the co-pay of $200. So the health care team has to try to find a resource to help the patient pay for the antibiotic or find a replacement drug.

### Staff Impact on Budget

Staff can acutely affect the organization's finances. Misuse of sick time, excessive overtime or turnover, and wasteful use of resources can result in negative variance. The manager plays a key role in explaining the unit's goals, the organization's financial goals, and how each individual is responsible for helping the organization meet those goals.

#### Improving Performance

Organizations have implemented a number of different programs and incentives for increasing employee awareness and minimizing costs. Techniques to decrease absenteeism and turnover may be instituted (see Chapter 20). Displaying equipment costs on supply stickers or requisitions and indicating medication costs on medication sheets increase staff awareness of costs. Participation in quality improvement and action teams also serves to inform staff of cost factors. Bonuses based on net gains have been shared with employees, in addition to cost-of-living raises.

When one staff member wants to take time off, the shift still must be covered. Nurse managers must hire enough staff to cover the unit even when people are on vacation without using excessive overtime. Float pool or PRN staff (staff scheduled on an as-needed basis) are often used to cover staff time off. Managers must plan how to cover each employee's nonproductive time (vacation, sick, education, etc.) in the least expensive way.

---

## CASE STUDY 14-1

### BUDGET MANAGEMENT

Byron Marshall is a nurse manager for the surgical services department of a private orthopedic hospital. Byron has received notice from the vice president of clinical services that next year's budget is due to her for review at the end of the month. Byron has kept careful records during the previous 12 months for use in preparing the surgical services department budget.

Each month, Byron has received and reviewed monthly reports of revenue and expense for his department. He validated each month's budget targets, carefully noting areas that didn't meet budget projections. For example, when April pharmacy charges were 15 percent above budget projections, Byron noted that surgery volume was up 30 percent over the previous year, accounting for the increase in preanesthesia drug charges. Nursing salaries were also over budget for the year, but again, increased surgery volume had resulted in the addition of two full-time surgery technicians to the department. When summer vacations resulted in agency staffing in the OR, Byron saved copies of the approval from the vice president and the human resources department and noted the total cost to his department.

Byron will use the budget information for the past 12 months to project the next fiscal year's budget for his department. Information from the human resources department provides data for cost of living and merit increases in salary, while materials management has projected a 20 percent across-the-board increase in surgical supplies and pharmaceutical charges. Byron will also request replacement of two OR tables and three gurneys as part of the capital budget. These items had been requested by staff during the last department meeting when Byron asked for changes and improvements in the budget. Budget discussion is part of each staff meeting and Byron provides copies of actual budget numbers to the staff each month. He has found that showing revenue and expense reports to staff increases compliance with overtime expenses and supply usage.

With monthly preparation, good record keeping, and accurate analysis, Byron is confident that his budget presentation will be on time and on target.

### Manager's Checklist

The nurse manager is responsible for:

- Learning and understanding the responsibilities of financial planning for the department
- Reviewing monthly revenue and expense reports for accuracy and completeness
- Understanding and tracking the reasons why particular areas did not meet the budget
- Communicating to staff the importance of fiscal responsibility
- Planning for capital items on an ongoing basis
- Identifying and incorporating increasing or decreasing expenses into the department budget
- Preparing and presenting a complete departmental budget to administration

## Magnet Hospital Performance

In Magnet-certified hospitals, staff are taught about budgeting and how the unit's money "works." Bedside staff make excellent, informed decisions about what resources should be used and understand the give and take of budget management. Bedside staff are empowered to make decisions that impact how they work. For example, the charge nurse on the unit takes phone calls about unit staffing. The float pool might have an additional aide coming in to work who is not assigned yet. The charge nurse takes the phone call from the staffing office to ask if the unit needs another aide and makes the decision.

Another example includes flexing staff for needs on the unit. The charge nurse, along with the coworkers, decide whether someone can be sent home on a slow day or if another staff member should be called in if the unit is excessively busy.

Managing fiscal resources is a challenge for all nurse managers. This is even more true today as legislation and regulation of health care reform is implemented. Close attention to costs, balanced by awareness of quality and patient safety, is essential.

Case Study 14-1 illustrates how one nurse manager handled his budget.

## What You Know Now

- A budget is a quantitative statement, usually written in monetary terms, of plans and expectations over a specified period of time.
- The operating or annual budget is the organization's statement of expected revenues and expenses for the coming year.
- The revenue budget represents the patient care revenues expected for the budget period based on volume and mix of patients, rates, and discounts that will prevail during the same period of time.
- Nursing units are typically considered cost centers, but may be considered revenue centers, profit centers, or investment centers.
- Nurse managers may be responsible for service lines and staff from multiple disciplines and departments.
- Nurse managers have input into capital expenses and are responsible for salary and operating costs related to new equipment.
- A full-time equivalent (FTE) is a full-time position that can be equated to 40 hours of work per week for 52 weeks, or 2,080 hours per year.
- The position control is a list of approved, budgeted FTEs that compares the budgeted number of FTEs by classification (RN, LPN), shift, and status to the actual available employees of the unit.
- Variance is the difference between the amount that was budgeted for a specific revenue or cost and the actual revenue or cost that resulted during the course of activities.
- Monitoring the budget throughout the year requires attention to variances and the reasons they occurred.

## Tools for Budgeting and Managing Resources

1. Understand the budgeting process in your organization.
2. Determine the number of full-time equivalents necessary to staff the unit.
3. Compute the salary and nonsalary budget, including salary increases and various additional factors.
4. Monitor variances over the budget period and identify negative variances, keeping notes in your files.
5. Understand that factors out of your control, such as changes in technology or indirect or direct costs that may be assigned to your budget, affect your budget and its performance.
6. Encourage staff to monitor resource use, including time and supplies.

## Questions to Challenge You

1. Do you have a budget for your personal and professional income and expenses? If so, how well do you manage it? If not, begin next month to track your income and expenses for one month. See if you are surprised at the results.

2. How well does your organization manage its resources? Can you make suggestions for improvement?
3. Are there tasks or functions in your work that you believe are redundant, unnecessary, or repetitive or that could be done by a lesser-paid employee? Explain.
4. Does your organization waste salary or nonsalary resources? If not, think of ways that organizations could waste resources. Describe them.

**Pearson Nursing Student Resources**

Find additional review materials at
**www.nursing.pearsonhighered.com**

Prepare for success with additional NCLEX®-style practice questions, interactive assignments and activities, Web links, animations and videos, and more!

## References

Buerhaus, P. I. (2010). Health care payment reform: Implications for nurses. *Nursing Economics, 28*(1), 49–54.

Dunham-Taylor, J., & Pinczuk, J. Z. (2009). *Financial management for nurse managers: Merging the heart with the dollar.* Burlington, MA: Jones & Bartlett.

Finkler, S. A., & Kovner, C. T. (2007). *Financial management for nurse managers and executives* (3rd ed.). St. Louis, MO: Saunders.

Joint Commission. (2011). Comprehensive accreditation manual for hospitals: The official handbook. Retrieved July 28, 2011 from http://www. jcrinc.com/ Accreditation-Manuals/ PCAH11/2130/

Welton, J. M., Zone-Smith, L., & Bandyopadhyay, D. (2009). Estimating nursing intensity and direct cost using the nurse-patient assignment. *Journal of Nursing Administration, 39*(6), 276–284.

# Recruiting and Selecting Staff

## Learning Outcomes

*After completing this chapter, you will be able to:*

1. Describe how to recruit applicants.
2. Discuss how to select candidates.
3. Describe how to interview prospective candidates.
4. Distinguish between appropriate and inappropriate questions to ask during an interview.
5. Determine how to make a hiring decision.
6. Discuss the legal issues involved in hiring.

## Key Terms

Four Ps of marketing
Age Discrimination Act
Americans with Disabilities Act
Behavioral interviewing
Bona fide occupational
   qualification (BFOQ)

Business necessity
Interrater reliability
Interview guide
Intrarater reliability
Negligent hiring
Personnel decisions

Position description
Validity
Work sample questions

# The Recruitment and Selection Process

Recruiting and selecting staff who will contribute positively to the organization is crucial in the fast-paced world of health care and in the face of ever-increasing nursing shortages (U.S. Department of Labor, 2011). The direct costs of recruiting, selecting, and training an employee who must later be terminated because of unsatisfactory performance is expensive and unnecessary. The hidden costs may be even more expensive and include poor quality of work, disruption of morale, and patients' ill will and dissatisfaction, which may contribute to later liability.

The purpose of the recruitment and selection process is to match people to jobs. Responsibility for selecting nursing personnel in health care organizations is usually shared by the human resources (HR) department, which may include a nurse recruiter, and nursing management. First-line nursing managers are the most knowledgeable about job requirements and can best describe the job to applicants. HR performs the initial screening and monitors hiring practices to be sure they adhere to legal stipulations.

Before recruiting or selecting new staff, those responsible for hiring must be familiar with the position description. The **position description** (see Box 15-1) describes the skills, abilities, and knowledge required to perform the job.

The position description should reflect current practice guidelines and include:

- Principal duties and responsibilities involved in a particular job
- Tasks required to carry out those duties
- Personal qualifications (skills, abilities, knowledge, and traits) needed for the position
- Competency-based behaviors (perhaps)

# Recruiting Applicants

The purpose of recruitment is to locate and attract enough qualified applicants to provide a pool from which the required number of individuals can be selected. Even though recruiting is primarily carried out by HR staff and nurse recruiters, nurse managers and nursing staff play an important role in the process. Recruiting is easier when current employees spread the recruiting message, reducing the need for expensive advertising and reward methods.

The best recruitment strategy is the organization's reputation among its nurses. Aiken and colleagues (Aiken et al., 2008) found that a positive hospital care environment not only reduced patient mortality but improved nurses' perception of the work setting. Brady-Schwartz (2005) found that nurses in Magnet hospitals demonstrated higher levels of job satisfaction than those in non-Magnet hospitals. It follows that satisfied nurses are more likely to speak highly of the organization.

Individual nurse managers also affect how well the unit is able to attract and retain staff. A nurse manager who is able to create a positive work environment through leadership style and clinical expertise will have a positive impact on recruitment efforts, because potential staff members will hear about and be attracted to that area (e.g., hospital unit, home health team). In contrast, an autocratic manager is more likely to have a higher turnover rate and less likely to attract sufficient numbers of high-quality nurses.

Any recruiting strategy includes essentially four elements:

1. Where to look
2. How to look
3. When to look
4. How to sell the organization to potential recruits

Each of these elements may be affected by market competition, nursing shortages, reputation, visibility, and location.

## BOX 15-1 Position Description: Registered Nurse Adult Medical Intensive Care Unit (MICU)

### Job Overview

The medical intensive care unit registered nurse is responsible for direct patient care of adults admitted to the MICU for management of complex life-threatening illness. The RN reports directly to the MICU nurse manager.

### Qualifications

- Current licensure in good standing in the state of practice.
- Minimum of one year previous adult ICU experience within the past three years or two years telemetry experience within the past three years.
- Current BLS mandatory, ACLS or TNCC preferred. ACLS must be obtained with six months of employment.

### Responsibilities

- Performs complete, individualized patient assessment within unit time frames and determines patient care priorities based on assessment findings.
- Completes additional patient assessments as required, based on patient status, protocols, and/or physician orders.
- Administers medications and appropriate treatments as ordered by the physician accurately and within specified time frames.
- Initiates and maintains an individualized patient plan of care for each patient, using nursing interventions as appropriate.
- Provides ongoing education to the patient and the patient's family.
- Documents patient assessments, medication and therapy administration, patient response to treatments, and interventions in an accurate and timely manner.
- Initiates emergency resuscitation procedures according to ACLS protocols.
- Maintains strict confidentiality of all information related to the patient and the patient's family.
- Provides nursing care in a manner that is respectful and sensitive to the needs of the patient and the patient's family and protects their dignity and rights.
- Communicates changes in patient condition to appropriate staff during the shift.
- Maintains (or obtains within six months of initial hire) certification in ACLS.
- Completes unit-based training modules for critical care competency on an annual basis.

### Where to Look

For most health care organizations, the best place to look is in their own geographic area. During nursing shortages, however, many organizations conduct national searches. This effort is frequently futile because most nurses look for jobs in their local area. If the agency is in a major metropolitan area, a search may be relatively easy; if it is located in a rural area, however, recruitment may need to be conducted in the nearest city. Organizations tend to recruit where past efforts have been the most successful. Most organizations adopt an incremental strategy whereby they recruit locally first and then expand to larger and larger markets until a sufficient applicant pool is obtained.

Because proximity to home is a key factor in choosing a job, recruitment efforts should focus on nurses living nearby. The state board of nursing can provide the names of registered nurses by zip code to allow organizations to target recruitment efforts to surrounding areas. Also, personnel officers in large companies or other organizations in the area can be asked to assist in recruiting nurse spouses of newly hired employees.

Collaborative arrangements with local schools of nursing offer opportunities for recruitment. Providing preceptors or mentors for students during their clinical rotation or offering externships or residencies encourages postgraduation students to consider employment in the organization. Nurses who work with students play a key role in recruitment. Students are more likely to be attracted to the organization if they see nurses' work valued and appreciated and perceive a positive impression of the work group.

Employing students as aides may provide another recruitment tool because it allows students to learn first hand about the organization and what it has to offer. In turn, the organization can evaluate the student as a potential employee post-graduation. Some organizations provide assistance with student loan payments if the student continues to work after graduation. Of major importance to new graduates is the orientation program. Graduates look for an orientation that provides successful transition into professional practice. Other top factors they consider are the reputation of the agency, benefits, promotional opportunities, specialty area, and nurse–patient ratio.

### How to Look

Posting online on general job search sites (e.g., www.monster.com) or on nurse-specific job referral sites (www.nurse.com) is a common practice. Professional associations such as Sigma Theta Tau International (http://stti.monster.com) and the American Nurses Association (www. nursingworld.org/careercenter) offer job search services. Specialty organizations, such as the American Organization of periOperative Nurses (http://www.aorn.org) could be used for a surgical nurse position.

Employee referrals, advertising in professional journals, attendance at professional conventions, job fairs, career days, visits to educational institutions, employment agencies (both private and public), and temporary help agencies are all recruiting sources. Advertising in professional journals, Websites, newspapers, or on public access TV can be an effective recruiting tool as well.

During extreme nursing shortages, some organizations offer bonuses to staff members who refer candidates and to the recruits themselves. Direct applications and employee referrals are quick and relatively inexpensive ways of recruiting people, but these methods also tend to perpetuate the current cultural or social mix of the workforce. It is both legally and ethically necessary to recruit individuals without regard to their race, ethnicity, gender, or disability. In addition, organizations can benefit from the diversity of a staff composed of people from a wide variety of social, experiential, cultural, generational, and educational backgrounds.

On the other hand, nurses referred by current employees are likely to have more realistic information about the job and the organization and, therefore, their expectations more closely fit reality. Those who come to the job with unrealistic expectations may experience dissatisfaction. In an open labor market, these individuals may leave the organization, creating high turnover. When nursing jobs are less plentiful or the economy is in a recession, dissatisfied staff members tend to stay in the organization because they need the job, but they are not likely to perform as well as other employees.

### When to Look

The time lag in recruiting is a concern to nursing because of the shortage. Positions in certain locations (e.g., rural areas) or specialty areas (e.g., critical care) may be especially difficult to fill. Careful planning is necessary to ensure that recruitment begins well in advance of anticipated needs.

### How to Promote the Organization

A critical component of any recruiting effort is marketing the organization and available positions to potential employees. The nursing division and/or HR should develop a comprehensive marketing plan. Generally, four strategies are included in marketing plans and are called the **four Ps of marketing**:

1. Product
2. Place
3. Price
4. Promotion

The consumer is the key figure toward which the four concepts are oriented, and in the recruiting process, the consumer is the potential employee.

*Product* is the available position(s) within the organization. Consider several aspects of the position and organization, such as:

- Professionalism
- Standards of care
- Quality
- Service
- Respect

*Place* refers to the physical qualities and location, such as:

- Accessibility
- Scheduling
- Parking
- Reputation
- Organizational culture

*Price* includes:

- Pay and differentials
- Benefits
- Sign-on bonuses
- Insurance
- Retirement plans

*Promotion* includes:

- Advertising
- Public relations
- Direct word of mouth
- Personal selling (e.g., job fairs, professional meetings)

Developing an effective marketing message is important. Sometimes the tendency is to use a "scatter-gun" approach (recruit everywhere), sugarcoat the message, or make it very slick. A more balanced message, which includes honest communication and personal contact, is preferable. Overselling the organization creates unrealistic expectations that may lead to later dissatisfaction and turnover.

Realistically presenting the job requirements and rewards improves job satisfaction, in that the new recruit learns what the job is actually like. Promising a nurse every other weekend off and only a 25 percent rotation to nights on a severely understaffed unit and then scheduling the nurse off only every third weekend with 75 percent night rotations is an example of unrealistic job information. It is important to represent the situation honestly and describe the steps that management is taking to improve situations that the applicant might find undesirable. He or she can then make an informed decision about the job offer.

## Cross-Training as a Recruitment Strategy

In today's rapidly changing health care environment, the patient census fluctuates rapidly, and staffing requirements must be adjusted appropriately. These conditions may bring about layoffs and daily cancellations and contribute to low morale. Offering cross-training to potential employees may increase the applicant pool.

Cross-training has the benefits of increasing morale and job satisfaction, improving efficiency, increasing the flexibility of the staff, and providing a means to manage fluctuations in the census. It gives nurses, such as those in obstetrics and neonatal areas, an opportunity to provide more holistic care. On the other hand, some nurses do not want to be cross-trained, and thus requiring cross-training could reduce retention.

If cross-training is used, care should be taken to provide a didactic knowledge base in addition to clinical training. How broadly to cross-train is an important decision, because training in too many areas may overload the nurse and reduce the quality of care. (See Chapter 17 on the use of floating to improve retention.)

## Selecting Candidates

Once an applicant makes contact with the organization, HR reviews the application and may conduct a preliminary interview (see Table 15-1). If the applicant does not meet the basic needs of the open position or positions, he or she should be so informed. Rejected applicants may be qualified for other positions or may refer friends to the organization and thus should be treated with utmost courtesy.

Reference checks and managerial interviews are next. In most cases, the interview is last, but practices may vary. Even if an applicant receives poor references, it is prudent to carry out the interview so that the applicant is not aware that the reference checking led to the negative decision. In addition, applicants may feel they have a right to "tell their story" and may spontaneously provide information that explains poor references.

The nurse manager should participate in the interview process because he or she is:

- Best able to assess applicants' technical competence, potential, and overall suitability
- Able to answer applicants' technical, work-related questions more realistically.

In some organizations, the candidate's future coworkers also participate in the interview process to assess compatibility.

The nurse manager must keep others involved in the selection process informed. The manager is usually the first to be aware of potential resignations, requests for transfer, and maternity or family medical leaves that require replacement staff. The manager is also aware of changes in the work area that might necessitate a redistribution of staff, such as the need for a night rather than a day nurse. Communicating these needs to HR promptly and accurately helps ensure effective coordination of the selection process.

---

**TABLE 15-1    Selection Process**

1. Review application (nurse manager and HR)

2. Conduct screening interview (HR).

3. Contact references (HR).

4. Conduct second interview (nurse manager).

5. Compare applicants (nurse manager/nursing department).

6. Make hire/no hire decision (nurse manager/nursing department).

7. Perform background check (HR).

8. Make phone offer, conditional on clean drug test within 24 hours (nurse manager).

9. With clean drug test, offer is official.

# Interviewing Candidates

The most common selection method, the interview, is an information-seeking mechanism between an individual applying for a position and a member of an organization doing the hiring. After the applicant's initial screening with HR, the nurse manager usually conducts an interview.

The interview is used to clarify information gathered from the application form, evaluate the applicant's responses to questions, and determine the fit of the applicant to the position, unit, and organization. In addition, the interviewer should provide information about the job and the organization. Finally, the interview should create goodwill toward the employing organization through good customer relations.

An effective interviewer must learn to solicit information efficiently and to gather relevant data. Interviews typically last between one and one and a half hours, and include an opening, an information-gathering and information-giving phase, and a closing. The opening is important because it is an attempt to establish rapport with the applicant so she or he will provide relevant information.

Gathering information, however, is the core of the interview. Giving information is also important because it allows the interviewer to create realistic expectations in the applicant and sell the organization, if that is needed. However, this portion of the interview should take place after the information has been gathered so that the applicant's answers will be as candid as possible. The interviewer should answer any direct questions the candidate poses. Finally, the closing is intended to provide information to the candidate on the mechanics of possible employment.

## Principles for Effective Interviewing

### Developing Structured Interview Guides

Unstructured interviews present problems: if interviewers fail to ask the same questions of every candidate, it is often difficult to compare them. The interview is most effective when the information on the pool of interviewees is as comparable as possible. Comparability is maximized via a structured interview supported by an interview guide. An **interview guide** is a written document containing questions, interviewer directions, and other pertinent information so that the same process is followed and the same basic information is gathered from each applicant. The guide should be specific to the job, or job category.

Instead of the traditional interview questions, such as "tell me about yourself, what are your strengths and weaknesses, and why do you want to work for us," specific questions that target job-related behaviors are more common today. **Behavioral interviewing**, also called competency-based interviewing, uses the candidate's past performance and behaviors to predict behavior on the job. The questions are based on requirements of the position. Examples of specific behaviors expected of staff nurses and related sample questions are found in Table 15-2.

In addition, you can develop additional questions based on the specific job. For example, you may want to add questions on teamwork and collaboration as they relate to the position. Box 15-2 lists job-related questions for a medical telemetry unit position that candidates could be asked.

Interview guides reduce interviewer bias, provide relevant and effective questions, minimize leading questions, and facilitate comparison among applicants. Space left between the questions on the guide provides room for note taking, and the guide also provides a written record of the interview. An example of an interview script is shown in Box 15-3.

### Preparing for the Interview

Most managers do not adequately prepare for the interview, which should be planned just like any business undertaking. All needed materials should be on hand, and the interview site should be quiet and pleasant. If others are scheduled to see the applicant, their schedules should be checked to make sure they are available at the proper time. If coffee or other refreshments are to be offered, advance arrangements need to be made. Lack of advance preparation may lead to insufficient interviewing time, interruptions, or failure to gather important information. Other problems include losing focus in the interview because of a desire to be courteous or because

| TABLE 15-2 | Examples of Behavioral Interview Questions |
|---|---|
| **Behavior** | **Sample Question** |
| Decision making | What was your most difficult decision in the last month, and why was it difficult? |
| Communication | What do you think is the most important skill in successful communication? |
| Adaptability | Describe a major change that affected you and how you handled it. |
| Delegation | How do you make the decision to delegate? Describe a specific situation. |
| Initiative | What have you done in school or in a job that went beyond what was required? |
| Motivation | What is your most significant professional accomplishment? |
| Negotiation | Give an example of a negotiation situation and your role in it. |
| Planning and organization | How do you schedule your time? What do you do when unexpected circumstances interfere with your schedule? |
| Critical thinking | Describe a situation in which you had to make a decision by analyzing information, considering a range of alternatives, and selecting the best choice for the circumstances. |
| Conflict resolution | Describe a situation in which you had to help settle a conflict. |

## BOX 15-2   Job Related Questions for Medical Telemetry Unit

**Describe your actions in the following situations.**

1. You are documenting your patient's heart rhythms in his medical record for the shift. A peer is sitting near you and doing the same. You see that RN document the patient's heart rhythm as sinus rhythm, when you know the patient has had a trial fibrillation the whole shift.

2. The physician is rounding on your patient. The patient has had an elevated blood pressure of 160/90 despite already having received all of her antihypertensive medications for the day. The patient has reported to you that she is also experiencing a headache. You tell the doctor about the blood pressure reading and the patient's headache. You request that the physician order another medication to help lower the patient's blood pressure. The physician says to you, "Oh, she'll be fine" and begins to walk away.

3. You are caring for an elderly woman. Her daughter is at her bedside. The patient has been having recurrent flare-ups of congestive heart failure and has been readmitted to the hospital three times in the last month. Each time she returns, the swelling in her extremities and her difficulty breathing is worse than the time before. The physician rounds on the patient and her daughter and shares that the health care team will work to help her, but it appears that her heart is getting weaker again, and the congestive heart failure is going to continue to get harder to manage. After the doctor leaves, you enter the room. The patient is sleeping and the daughter is quietly crying.

4. You run to the room of a patient where the code blue alarm has been activated. Your team is doing CPR and attaching the code cart to the patient. You put on gloves and step in to help. As you approach the bed of the patient, you look at the patient's wrist and see a do not resuscitate bracelet on his arm.

5. You are caring for a patient with paranoid schizophrenia and a heart dysrhythmia. It is time to administer his 9 A.M. meds. When you enter the room with the medications that the patient takes to prevent ventricular tachycardia, he begins screaming, "No, I won't take those medications, you're trying to poison me!"

6. You are caring for a patient who is recovering from a myocardial infarction. You have been talking to her about her new cardiac diet and what she can do to be healthy when she leaves the hospital. You discuss eating low amounts of salt, a well-rounded diet rich in fruits and vegetables, and avoiding fried and sugary foods. Later in the day, you pass the patient's room and see her eating fried chicken and French fries that her family brought.

| BOX 15-3 | Interview Script for Hiring |
|---|---|

1. Why did you choose to become a nurse?
2. Why would you like to work at this hospital?
3. What about this patient specialty interests you?
4. Tell me about your previous work experiences.
5. How do your previous work experiences prepare you for this job?
6. How would your previous coworkers describe you?
7. What does teamwork mean to you?
8. Tell me about a time when you were successful because of great teamwork.
9. Tell me about a time you experienced a lack of teamwork. Describe what happened.
10. Describe a situation in which you had a conflict with a patient or family member. What happened?
11. Tell me about a time you had a conflict with a coworker or teacher. Explain what happened.
12. Tell me about a time you were working with someone who wasn't putting his or her full effort forward, and it was impacting patient care. What did you do?
13. What makes you most nervous about coming to this job?
14. What do you find exciting about coming to this job?
15. What are you most proud of professionally?
16. What is something about you that makes you better than any other candidate for this job?
17. What are you looking for from your manager?
18. What do you plan to do in the next five and ten years of nursing and beyond? What are your goals?
19. What questions do you have about this job?

the interviewee is particularly dominant. This typically keeps the interviewer from obtaining the needed information.

In general, when time is limited, it is better to use part of it for planning rather than spend it all on the interview itself. Before the interview, the interviewer should review job requirements, the application and résumé, and note specific questions to be asked. Planning should be done on the morning of the interview or the evening before for an early morning interview. If you are sure that time will be available, planning is best done immediately before an interview or between interviews. Unfortunately, a busy manager may have to deal with unexpected crises between interviews and may not be able to use the time to plan the next interview.

A cardinal rule is to review the application or résumé before beginning the interview. If the interviewee arrives with the résumé or application in hand, ask him or her to wait for a few minutes while you review the material. In doing a quick review, look for the following four things:

1. Clear discrepancies between the applicant's qualifications and the job specifications. If you find them, then only a brief interview may be necessary to explain why the applicant will not be considered. (If a preliminary screening is performed by the HR, such applicants should not be referred to nurse managers.)

2. Specific questions to ask the applicant during the interview.

3. A rapport builder (something you have in common with the applicant) to break the ice at the beginning of the interview.

4. Areas where you need more information. Remember that the résumé is prepared by the applicant and is intended to market an applicant's assets to the organization. It does not give a balanced view of strengths and weaknesses. So, examine the résumé critically for gaps.

The setting of the interview is important in order to provide a relaxed, informal atmosphere. Both you and the applicant should be in comfortable chairs, as close together as comfortably possible. No table or desk should separate you. If you are using an office, arrange the chairs so that the applicant is at the side of the desk. There should be complete freedom from distracting phone calls and other interruptions. If the view is distracting, do not seat the applicant so that she or he can look out a window.

### Opening the Interview

Begin the interview on time. Give a warm, friendly greeting, introduce yourself, and ask the applicant for her or his preferred name. Try to minimize your status; do not patronize or dominate. The objective is to establish an open atmosphere so applicants reveal as much as possible about themselves. Establish and maintain rapport throughout the interview by talking about yourself, discussing mutual interests such as hobbies or similar experiences, and using nonverbal cues, such as maintaining eye contact. Finally, start the interview by outlining what will be discussed and setting a limit on the meeting time.

Be careful not to form hasty first impressions. Interviewers tend to be influenced by first impressions of a candidate, and such judgments often lead to poor decisions. First impressions may degrade the quality of the interview; interviewers may search for information to justify their first impressions, good or bad. If you have gotten a negative first impression and thus decide not to hire a potentially successful candidate, you have wasted an hour or so and possibly lost a good recruit. If, you hire an unsuccessful candidate based on a positive first impression, problems may continue for months. Conversely, your personal characteristics may influence the applicant's decisions. You create first impressions with your tone of voice, eye contact, personal appearance, grooming, posture, and gestures.

Take notes, using the structured interview guide. Explain that you are doing this in order to remember more about what is discussed in the interview, and tell the candidate that you hope he or she does not mind. There are various ways to ask questions, but ask only one at a time. When possible, ask open-ended questions, such as those listed in Table 15-1. Open-ended questions cannot be answered with a yes, no, or one-word answer and usually elicit more information about the applicant (Parrish, 2006). Closed questions (e.g., what, where, why, when, how many) should only be used to elicit specific information.

**Work sample questions** are used to determine an applicant's knowledge about work tasks and his or her ability to perform the job. It is easy to ask a nurse whether she or he knows how to care for a patient who has a central intravenous line in place. A yes answer does not necessarily prove the candidate's ability, so you might ask some very specific questions about central lines. Avoid leading questions, in which the answer is implied by the question (e.g., "We have lots of overtime. Do you mind overtime?"). You may also want to summarize what has been said, use silence to elicit more information, repeat the applicant's statements back to him or her to clarify an issue, or indicate acceptance by urging the applicant to continue.

### Giving Information

Before reaching the information-giving part of the interview, consider whether the candidate is promising enough to warrant spending a lot of time on this. Unless the candidate is clearly unacceptable, be careful not to communicate a negative impression, because your evaluation of the candidate may change when the entire packet of material is reviewed or if more promising candidates decline the job offer. You must also know what information you should give, and what is being provided by others. Detailed benefit or compensation questions are usually answered by HR. If you cannot answer a promising candidate's questions, arrange for someone to contact the candidate later with that information.

### Closing the Interview

You may want to summarize the applicant's strengths at the end of the interview. Make sure to ask the applicant whether she or he has anything to add or ask about the job and the organization. You may also want to mention the candidate's weaknesses, particularly if they are objective and clearly related to the job (such as lack of experience in a particular field). Mentioning a perception of a subjective weakness, such as poor supervisory skills, may lead to legal problems. Wrap up by thanking the applicant and completing any notes that you have been taking.

## Involving Staff in the Interview Process

Today's trend toward decentralization of decision making may lead to sharing interview responsibilities with staff. Involving staff in interviews helps strengthen teamwork, improves work-group effectiveness, increases staff involvement in other unit activities, and increases the likelihood of selecting the best candidate for the position.

If staff are involved in interviews, several steps must be taken to protect the integrity of the interview process. An organized orientation to interviewing should be given that includes:

- Federal, state, and local laws and regulations governing interviewing, as well as any collective-bargaining agreements that may affect the process
- Tips on handling awkward interviewing situations
- Time for rehearsing interviewing skills; like the manager, staff should follow a structured interview guide to help standardize the process

*Graham Nelson is nurse manager of a dialysis center. Training a new renal dialysis nurse is an expensive process. To reduce turnover among nursing staff, Graham includes peer interviews as part of the overall interview process. Peer interviews can help ensure that potential employees will interact well with existing staff and ensure a cultural fit with the dialysis team. Additionally, an interviewee can gain a better understanding of the day-to-day workflow of the center.*

## Interview Reliability and Validity

Numerous research studies have been performed on the reliability and validity of employment interviews. In general, agreement between two interviews of the same measure by the same interviewer (**intrarater reliability**) is fairly high, agreement between two interviews of the same measure by several interviewers (**interrater reliability**) is rather low, and the ability to predict job performance (**validity**) of the typical interview is very low. Research has also shown that:

1. Structured interviews are more reliable and valid.

2. Interviewers who are under pressure to hire in a short time or meet a recruitment quota are less accurate than other interviewers.

3. Interviewers who have detailed information about the job for which they are interviewing exhibit higher interrater reliability and validity.

4. The interviewer's experience does not seem to be related to reliability and validity.

5. There is a decided tendency for interviewers to make quick decisions and therefore be less accurate.

6. Interviewers develop stereotypes of ideal applicants against which interviewees are evaluated. Individual interviewers may hold different stereotypes, which decreases interrater reliability and validity.

7. Race and gender may influence interviewers' evaluations.

The greatest weakness in the selection interview may be the tendency for the interviewer to try to assess an applicant's personality characteristics. Although it is difficult to eliminate such subjectivity, evaluations of applicants are often more subjective than they need to be. Information collected during an interview should answer three fundamental questions:

1. Can the applicant perform the job?

2. Will the applicant perform the job?

3. Will the candidate fit into the culture of the unit and the organization?

The best predictor of the applicant's future behavior in these respects is past performance. Previous work and other experience, past education and training, and current job performance should be considered rather than personality characteristics, which even psychologists cannot measure very accurately.

# Making a Hire Decision

### Education, Experience, and Licensure

Education and experience requirements for nurses have long been important screening factors and bear a close relationship to work sample tests. Educational requirements are a type of job knowledge sample because they tend to ensure that applicants have at least a minimal amount of knowledge necessary for the job.

Educational preparation is particularly important for nurses. For example, nurses who are graduates of associate degree and diploma programs are prepared to care for individuals in structured settings and use the nursing process, the decision-making process, and their management skills in the care of those individuals. Baccalaureate graduates can provide nursing care for individuals, families, groups, and communities using the nursing and decision-making processes. Baccalaureate graduates are also prepared for beginning community health positions and possess the leadership and management skills needed for entry-level management positions.

Avoid making assumptions about the type of experience and number of years of experience that an applicant has. Factors such as job requirements, patient acuity, clinic populations, autonomy, and degree of specialization vary from organization to organization. Therefore, careful interviewing is needed to determine the applicant's knowledge and skill level.

References and letters of recommendation are also used to assess the applicant's past job experience, but there is little evidence that these have any validity. Because few people write unfavorable letters of recommendation, such letters do not really predict job performance. Criticisms are likely to be mild and may be reflected by the lack of positive language. Letters with any criticism should be verified with a telephone call, if possible, to avoid overreacting to an unusually honest author.

To avoid legal problems, many organizations only include employment dates, salary, and whether the applicant is eligible for rehire in letters of recommendation. Many organizations do not allow supervisors to write letters of recommendation. Negative references may be viewed as a potential for slander or other legal recourse. Almost every organization will at least verify position title and dates of employment, which helps detect the occasional applicant who falsifies an entire work history. Unfortunately, leaving out a position from a work history is more common than including a position not actually held. The only way to detect such omissions is to ask that candidates list the year and month of all their educational and work experiences. Caution is necessary when asking about time between jobs; be careful not to inquire about marital or family status.

In almost every selection situation, an applicant fills out an application form that requests information about previous experience, education, and references. As application forms are reviewed, the critical question to be asked is whether the applicant has distorted responses, either intentionally or unintentionally. Studies indicate that there is usually little distortion, at least not on the easily verifiable information. Applicants may stretch the truth a bit, but rarely are there complete falsehoods. Relative to other predictors, the application form may be one of the more valid predictors in a selection process.

Licensure status can be verified online with the state board of nursing. Because results of the computerized NCLEX-RN® examination are available in 7 to 10 days, most organizations wait for new graduates to obtain a license before starting employment.

### Integrating the Information

When comparing candidates, first weigh the qualities required for the job in order of importance, placing more emphasis on the most important elements. Second, weigh the qualities desired on the basis of the reliability of the data. The more consistent the observation of behavior from different elements in the selection system, the more weight that dimension should be given. Third, weigh job dimensions by trainability—consider the amount of education, experience, and additional training the applicant can reasonably be expected to receive, and consider the likelihood that the behavior in that dimension can be improved with training. Dimensions most likely to be learned in training (e.g., using new equipment) should be given the least weight so that more weight is placed on dimensions less likely to be learned in training (e.g., being emotionally able to care for terminally ill children).

Attempt to compare data across individuals in making a decision. It is more accurate to make decisions based on a comparison of several persons than to make a decision for each individual after each interview. Analysis of the entire applicant pool requires good interview records but lessens the impact of early impressions on the hiring decision because the interviewer must consider each job element across the entire pool.

### Making an Offer

Before an offer is made, most organizations obtain permission to do criminal background checks. After the interview, if the nurse manager wants to offer a position to a candidate, HR is notified. HR then does a thorough background check on the candidate to confirm reported criminal history, licensure, and employment history. After that clears, the candidate is called and offered the position, with the condition that a drug screen completed within 24 hours of the phone offer is clean. If so, the offer is official.

In addition, organizations are liable for the character and actions of the employees they hire. To satisfy this requirement, the employer must check applicants' backgrounds before hiring in regard to licensure, credentials, and references. Failure to do so constitutes **negligent hiring** if that employee harms a patient, visitor, or another employee.

## Legality in Hiring

As a result of Title VII of the Civil Rights Act of 1964, the Equal Pay Act of 1963, the Age Discrimination Act of 1967, and Title I of the Americans with Disabilities Act of 1990 and its amendments of 2009, recruitment and selection activities are subject to considerable scrutiny regarding discrimination and equal employment opportunity. Title VII of the Civil Rights Act specifically prohibits discrimination in any **personnel decision** on the basis of race, color, sex, religion, or national origin. "Any personnel decision" includes not only selection but also entrance into training programs, performance appraisal results, termination, promotions, compensation, benefits, and other terms, conditions, and privileges of employment.

The Act applies to most employers with more than 15 employees, although there are several exemptions—among them, a **bona fide occupational qualification (BFOQ)**, a business necessity, and the validity of the procedure used to make the personnel decision. Discrimination is allowed on the basis of national origin (citizenship or immigration status), religion, sex, and age; for instance, if that discrimination can be shown to be a "bona fide occupational qualification reasonably necessary for the normal operation of a business." Examples include a woman playing a female part in a play, a Sunday school teacher of a certain religion, or a female correctional counselor at a women's prison. Claims of "customer preference" for female flight attendants or gross gender characteristics such as "women cannot lift over 30 pounds" have not been supported as BFOQs.

A BFOQ allows an organization to exclude members of certain groups (such as all men or all women) if the organization can demonstrate that a selection method is a **business necessity**. A business necessity is likely to withstand a legal challenge only in the unusual instances when a selection method that discriminates against a protected group is necessary to ensure the safety of workers or customers.

The Equal Employment Opportunity Commission (EEOC) is charged with enforcing and interpreting the Civil Rights Act and has issued Uniform Guidelines on Employee Selection Procedures (43 Federal Register, 1978). The guidelines specify the kinds of methods and information required to justify the job relatedness of selection procedures. These guidelines are not described in detail here; however, the methods of selection discussed in this chapter do follow their specifications. Remember that the law does not say one cannot hire the best person for the job. What it says is that race, color, sex, religion, disability, national origin, or any other protected factor must not be used as selection criteria. As long as the decision is not made on the basis of protected status, one is complying with the Equal Employment Opportunity (EEO) law.

EEO law and successive court decisions have had three major impacts on selection procedures. First, organizations are more careful to use predictors and techniques that can be shown not to discriminate against protected classes. Second, organizations are reducing the use of tests, which may be difficult to defend if they screen out a large number of minority applicants. Third, organizations are relying heavily on the interview process as a selection device. Interviews are also subject to EEO and other regulations.

Table 15-3 presents appropriate questions to ask in an interview. The basic rule of thumb for interviewing is when you are in doubt about a question's legality, ask, How is this question related to job performance? If it can be proved that only job-related questions are asked, EEO law will not be violated.

The **Age Discrimination Act** prohibits discrimination against applicants and employees over the age of 40. Questions in recruitment and selection that are appropriate with respect to age are also presented in Table 15-3.

### TABLE 15-3 Preemployment Questions

| | Appropriate to Ask | Inappropriate to Ask |
|---|---|---|
| Name | Applicant's name. Whether applicant has school or work records under a different name. | Questions about any name or title that indicate race, color, religion, sex, national origin, or ancestry. Questions about father's surname or mother's maiden name. |
| Address | Questions concerning place and length of current and previous addresses. | Any specific probes into foreign addresses that would indicate national origin. |
| Age | Requiring proof of age by birth certificate after hiring. Can ask if applicant is over 18. | Requiring birth certificate or baptismal record *before* hiring. |
| Birthplace or national origin | | Any question about place of birth of applicant or place of birth of parents, grandparents, or spouse. Any other question (direct or indirect) about applicant's national origin. |
| Race or color | Can request *after* employment as affirmative action data. | Any inquiry that would indicate race or color. |
| Sex | | Any question on an application blank that would indicate sex. |
| Religion | | Any questions to indicate applicant's religious denomination or beliefs. A recommendation or reference from the applicant's religious denomination. |
| Citizenship | Questions about whether the applicant is a U.S. citizen; if not, whether the applicant intends to become one. Questions regarding whether applicant's U.S. residence is legal; requiring proof of citizenship *after* hiring. | Questions of whether the applicant, parents, or spouse are native born or naturalized. Requiring proof of citizenship *before* hiring. |

**TABLE 15-3    Continued**

| | Appropriate to Ask | Inappropriate to Ask |
|---|---|---|
| Photographs | May require after hiring for identification purposes only. | Requesting a photograph *before* hiring. |
| Education | Questions concerning any academic, professional, or vocational schools attended. | Questions specifically asking the nationality, racial, or religious affiliation of any school attended. |
| | Inquiry into language skills, such as reading and writing of foreign languages. | Inquiries as to the applicant's mother tongue or how any foreign language ability was acquired (unless it is necessary for the job). |
| Relatives | Name, relationship, and address of a person to be notified in case of an emergency. | Any unlawful inquiry about a relative or residence mate(s) as specified in this list. |
| Children | | Questions about the number and ages of the applicant's children or information on child-care arrangements. |
| Transportation | | Inquiries about transportation to or from work (unless a car is necessary for the job). |
| Organization | Questions about organization memberships and any offices that might be held. | Questions about any organization an applicant belongs to that may indicate the race, age, disabilities, color, religion, sex, national origin, or ancestry of its members. |
| Physical condition/ disabilities | Questions about being able to meet the job requirements, with or without some accommodation. | Questions about general medical condition, state of health, specific diseases, or nature/severity of disability. |
| Military service | Questions about services rendered in armed forces, the rank attained, and which branch of service. | Questions about military service in any armed forces other than the United States. |
| | Requiring military discharge certificate *after* being hired. | Requesting military service records *before* hiring. |
| Work schedule | Questions about the applicant's willingness to work the required work schedule. | Questions about applicant's willingness to work any particular religious holiday. |
| References | General and work references not relating to race, color, religion, sex, national origin or ancestry, age, or disability. | References specifically from clergy (as specified above) or any other persons who might reflect race, age, disability, color, sex, national origin, or ancestry of applicant. |
| Financial | | Questions about banking, credit rating, outstanding loans, bankruptcy, or having wages garnished. |
| Other qualifications | Any question that has direct reflection on the job to be applied for. | Any non-job-related inquiry that may present information permitting unlawful discrimination. Questions about arrests or convictions (unless necessary for job, such as security clearance). |

## CASE STUDY 15-1

### SELECTING STAFF

Jack Turner is nurse manager of the emergency department in a large metropolitan area hospital. He has four full-time RN positions open in his department. There are three nursing programs located in the city: a state university program, a community college program, and an RN-to-BSN completion program.

Jack recently participated in a nursing job fair hosted by his hospital. The event was well attended by nursing students, and he received several promising résumés of soon-to-be graduate nurses. Jack notes that one of the applicants, Sabrina Ashworth, will graduate next month with a BSN. She has been working for the past year as a nursing assistant in the ER of another local hospital. In addition to her ER work, Sabrina has a high grade point average and indicates a strong interest in trauma and critical care. Jack contacts the human resource department to set up an interview with Sabrina.

Sabrina agrees to an interview for an RN position in the ER department. Jack schedules a conference room adjacent to the ER for the interview. Prior to Sabrina's arrival, he reviews her résumé and application, noting her educational background, previous work history, and recent volunteer trip to Mexico to assist with a vaccination program. Jack has assembled a packet for Sabrina, including a job description and materials from human resources that outline the application process.

The interview begins promptly. Jack warmly greets Sabrina and establishes rapport. He follows the interview guide provided by the human resource department. Jack informs Sabrina that he will be taking notes during the interview process. After reviewing her educational and work history, Jack asks Sabrina several situational questions related to work in the ER. He also allows time for Sabrina to ask questions about the RN position. Jack also has two RN staff members give Sabrina a tour of the ER department. Finally, Jack outlines the next steps in the application process and indicates that he will follow up with Sabrina in 7 to 10 days.

Following the interview, Jack works with the human resource department and asks for transcript and reference checks for Sabrina. After verifying her transcript and receiving positive references, Jack extends an offer to Sabrina, which she accepts.

### Manager's Checklist

The nurse manager is responsible for:

- Understanding the organization's human resource policies and procedures related to selecting staff
- Working closely with the human resource department to facilitate the selection and hiring of qualified staff
- Knowing state and federal regulations related to the application and interview process
- Preparing for the interview process
- Conducting the interview
- Following up with applicants in a timely manner

The **Americans with Disabilities Act** that took effect in July 1990 prohibits discrimination based on an individual's disability. A disability is defined as a physical or mental impairment that substantially limits one or more of the major life activities, or has a record of such impairment (e.g., attended a school for the deaf), or is regarded as having such an impairment (e.g., uses a cane to walk). A qualified individual is one who, with or without reasonable accommodation, can perform the essential functions of the position under consideration.

The Act was amended in 2009 (U.S. Department of Justice, 2009). The definition of a disability was broadened in several ways beneficial to employees: The amended Act includes disabilities not previously covered (e.g., epilepsy, diabetes, bipolar disorder). The amendments expand the definition of major life activities to include major bodily functions (e.g., immune system, brain functions) and eliminate the ameliorative effects of mitigating measures from consideration (e.g., medication, prosthetics).

Employers with 15 or more employees are required to make accommodations to the known disability of a qualified applicant if it will not impose "undue hardship" on the operation of the business. Reasonable accommodations may include making existing facilities used by employees readily accessible to and usable by individuals with disabilities; job restructuring; part-time or modified work schedules; reassignment to a vacant position; acquiring or modifying equipment or devices; adjusting or modifying examinations, training materials, or policies; and providing qualified readers and interpreters.

The 2009 amendments included some employer-friendly provisions as well. Reverse discrimination claims by nondisabled individuals are not in violation of the Act. Although the pool of individuals covered in the amendments is expanded, the reasonable accommodation features remain the same, as do existing exclusions for criminal behavior and current drug use.

Recruiting and selecting the most appropriate staff is one of the most important jobs in an organization. Candidates whose qualifications fit the job requirements are more likely to be productive and to remain on the job. The tendency, especially during times of shortages, is to short-cut the process, but this is ill advised. The effort to attract and select the best candidates pays off over time for the organization.

One nurse manager used the recommendations in this chapter to hire a nurse as shown in Case Study 15-1.

## What You Know Now

- The selection of staff is a critical function that requires matching people to jobs, and responsibility for hiring is often shared by HR and nurse managers.
- Position description is fundamental to all selection efforts because it defines the job.
- Recruitment is the process of locating and attracting enough qualified applicants to provide a pool from which the required number of new staff members can be chosen.
- Selection processes should be job related and most often include screening application forms, résumés, medical examinations, reference and background checks, and interviews.
- Interviewing is a complex skill that is intended to obtain information about the applicant and to give the applicant information about the organization.
- Successful interviews require planning, implementation, and follow-up in order to make the best decisions.
- Developing a structured interview guide is a critical element in interviewing.
- Selection decisions are subject to provisions in the Civil Rights Act of 1964, Equal Pay Act of 1963, the Age Discrimination Act of 1967, and the Americans with Disabilities Act of 1990 as amended in 2009.

## Tools for Recruiting and Selecting Staff

1. Conduct or modify a job description as needed.
2. Coordinate recruitment efforts with the human resource department.
3. Ensure that your area of responsibility sends the message you want (see Box 15-1).
4. Prepare adequately for interviews.
5. Conduct interviews following recommendations presented in the chapter.
6. Process the information obtained in interviews and reference and background checks to make a final decision.

## Questions to Challenge You

1. What approach does your organization use to recruit employees? Is it effective? How could the process be improved?
2. Imagine that a potential candidate asks you to describe your present workplace. What would you say?
3. Have you ever participated in a staff interview, either as a candidate or as a member of the staff? Describe your experience. Would you do anything differently now that you've read the chapter?
4. Cross-training has been used as a recruitment strategy. What are the pros and cons of using this strategy?
5. Consider the last interview you had for a job or school. Did the interviewer follow the principles discussed in this chapter? Explain.

**Pearson Nursing Student Resources**
Find additional review materials at
**www.nursing.pearsonhighered.com**
Prepare for success with additional NCLEX®-style practice
questions, interactive assignments and activities, Web links,
animations and videos, and more!

## Web Resources

Job search websites:
Monster.com: www.monster.com
Nurse.com: www.nurse.com
Sigma Theta Tau International Honor Society of Nursing: http://stti.monster.com
Nurse's CareerCenter: www.nursingworld.org/careercenter

## References

Aiken, L. H., Clarke, S. P., Sloane, D. M., Lake, E. T., & Cheney, T. (2008). Effects of hospital care environment on patient mortality and nurse outcomes. *Journal of Nursing Administration, 38*(5), 223–229.

Brady-Schwartz, D. C. (2005). Further evidence on the Magnet Recognition Program: Implications for nursing leaders. *Journal of Nursing Administration, 35*(9), 397–403.

Parrish, F. (2006). How to recruit, interview, and retain employees. *Dermatology Nursing, 18*(2), 179–180.

U. S. Department of Justice. (2009). Americans with disabilities act of 1990, as amended. Retrieved July 25, 2011 from http://www.ada.gov/pubs/ada.htm

U. S. Department of Labor, Bureau of Labor Statistics. (2011). Statistics on registered nurses. Retrieved July 25, 2011 from http://www.dol.gov/wb/factsheets/Qf-nursing-05.htm

# Staffing and Scheduling

## Staffing

PATIENT CLASSIFICATION SYSTEMS

DETERMINING NURSING CARE HOURS

DETERMINING FTEs

DETERMINING STAFFING MIX

DETERMINING DISTRIBUTION OF STAFF

## Scheduling

CREATIVE AND FLEXIBLE STAFFING

AUTOMATED SCHEDULING

SUPPLEMENTING STAFF

## Learning Outcomes

*After completing this chapter, you will be able to:*

1. Determine staffing needs.
2. Demonstrate how to use patient classification systems to calculate nursing care hours necessary.
3. Calculate FTEs.

4. Determine the appropriate staffing mix and distribution of staff.
5. Describe the various ways to schedule staff.
6. Explain how to supplement staff when needed.

## Key Terms

Baylor plan
Block staffing
Demand management
Full-time equivalent (FTE)

Nursing care hours (NCHs)
Patient classification systems (PCSs)
Pools
Self-scheduling

Staffing
Staffing mix

S taffing and scheduling is an important responsibility of the nurse manager and a critical aspect of providing nursing care. Higher nurse staffing levels reduce mortality in hospitalized patients (Schilling et al., 2010; Needleman et al., 2011). Furthermore, failing to match patient needs to nurses' skills also increases patient mortality (Needleman et al., 2011).

The impact of California's mandated nurse staffing supports these findings. Not only did higher nurse staffing levels translate into lower mortality, but hospitals reported better nurse retention rates as a result (Aiken et al., 2010). In addition, Magnet hospitals report higher nurse staffing levels (Hickey et al., 2010) and improved teamwork (Kalisch & Lee, 2011).

## Staffing

The goal of **staffing** is to provide the appropriate numbers and mix of nursing staff (nursing care hours) to match actual or projected patient care needs (patient care hours) to provide effective and efficient nursing care. There is no single or perfect method to achieve this. In addition, variability in patient census requires continuous fine-tuning.

A hospital unit may experience a steady census during the seven days of the week or a higher census from Monday to Friday. Its patient days may be distributed evenly during the year, or it may consistently experience peaks in occupancy in certain months (seasonality pattern) such as during an outbreak of influenza. Outpatient clinics may be busier on days when specialists are available or vaccines are offered. Staffing is a challenge in all health care settings.

To determine the number of staff needed, managers must examine workload patterns for the designated unit, department, or clinic. For a hospital, this means determining the level of care, average daily census, and hours of care provided 24 hours a day, seven days a week.

Both the Joint Commission, hospitals' accrediting body, and the American Nurses Association identify staffing requirements. The Joint Commission (2011) requires that the right number of competent staff be provided to meet patients' needs based on organization-selected criteria. The American Nurses Association (ANA) (Manojlovich, 2009) specifies requirements for staffing systems as shown in Box 16-1.

### Patient Classification Systems

**Patient classification systems (PCSs)**, sometimes referred to as patient acuity systems, use patient needs to objectively determine workload requirements and staffing needs. To be most effective, patient classification data are collected midpoint for every shift by the unit nursing staff and analyzed before the next shift to ensure appropriate numbers and mix of nursing staff.

Ideally, this system would accurately predict the number and skill level of nurses needed for the next shift. But much can go amiss. Some nurses may call in sick; the nurses scheduled may not have the skill set necessary for a new admission, for example; or, most important, the patient's condition may change.

---

### BOX 16-1    Requirements for Staffing Systems

A reliable and valid staffing plan must:

- Be created with input from direct-care registered nurses
- Be based on the number of patients and patient-acuity level with consideration of patient admissions, discharges, and transfers on each shift
- Reflect the level of preparation and experience of those providing care

- Reflect staffing levels recommended by specialty organizations
- Provide that an RN not be forced to work in a unit without having established that he or she is able to provide professional care on such a unit

Adapted from Manojlovich, M. (2009). Seeking staffing solutions. *American Nurse Today, 4*(3), 26.

Picard and Warner (2007) suggest fine-tuning PCS systems to predict the demand for nursing expertise several days in advance. They complain that basing staffing on immediate patient needs is short-sighted and often results in failure as mentioned above. Their system, called **demand management**, uses best-practices staffing protocols to predict and control the demand for nurses based on patient outcomes. Based on historical data, a patient progress pattern typifies expected patient outcomes throughout a stay. Deviations are tracked and staffing adjusted accordingly. This system allows the manager to staff into the next few days with more assurance than predicting from one shift to the next. Whatever system is used, the next step is to determine the necessary nursing care hours.

## Determining Nursing Care Hours

Patient workload trends are analyzed for each day of the week (each hour in critical care) or for a specific patient diagnosis to determine staffing needs, known as **nursing care hours (NCHs)**. For example, if 26 patients with the following acuities required 161 nursing care hours, then an average of 6.19 nursing hours per patient per day (NHPPD) are required. NHPPD are calculated by dividing the total nursing care hours by the total census (number of patients).

There are no specific standards for NCHs for any type of patient or patient care unit. NCHs may vary on the average from five to seven hours of care for patients on medical and/or surgical units, to 10 to 24 hours of care for patients in critical care units, to 24 to 48 hours of care for selected patients, such as new, severely burned patients.

| Number of Patients | Acuity Level | Associated Hours of Care | Total Hours of Care |
|---|---|---|---|
| 3 | I | 2 | 6 |
| 10 | II | 6 | 60 |
| 11 | III | 7 | 77 |
| 2 | IV | 9 | 18 |
| *Total* 26 | | | *161* |

## Determining FTEs

Positions are defined in terms of a **full-time equivalent (FTE)**. One FTE equals 40 hours of work per week for 52 weeks, or 2,080 hours per year. In a two-week pay period, one FTE would equal 80 hours. For computational purposes, one FTE can be filled by one person or a combination of staff with comparable expertise. For example, one nurse may work 24 hours per week, and two other nurses may each work 8 hours per week. Together, the three nurses fill one FTE (24 + 8 + 8 = 40).

Several methods are available for determining the number of FTEs required to staff a unit 24 hours a day, seven days a week. One technique incorporates information regarding the hours of work for the staff for two weeks, average daily census, and hours of care. The average daily census can be determined by dividing the total patient days (obtained from daily census counts for the year) by the number of days in the year.

■ **EXAMPLE**

$$\text{Total patient days} = \frac{9490}{365} = 26 \text{ patients per day}$$

*Data*

Number of hours worked per FTE in two weeks = 80
Number of days of coverage in two weeks = 14
Average daily census = 26
Average nursing care hours (from PCS) = 6.15

*Formula*

$$x = \frac{\text{average nursing care hours} \times \text{days in staffing period} \times \text{average patient census}}{\text{hours of work per FTE in two weeks}}$$

$$x = \frac{6.15 \times 14 \times 26}{80} = \frac{2238.6}{80} = 27.98, \text{ or } 28 \text{ FTFEs}$$

A second technique uses nursing care hours and annual hours of work provided by one FTE:

*Data*

Number of hours worked per FTE in one year $= 2080$
Total nursing care hours (from PCS) $= 161$

*Formula*

$$x = \frac{\text{Total nursing care hours} \times \text{days in a year}}{\text{Total annual hours per one FTE}}$$

$$x = \frac{161 \times 365}{2080} = \frac{58,765}{2080} = 28.25, \text{ or } 28 \text{ FTEs}$$

One person working full-time usually works 80 hours (10 eight-hour shifts) in a two-week period. However, to staff an eight-hour shift takes 1.4 FTEs, one person working 10 eight-hour shifts (1.0 FTE) and another person working four eight-hour shifts (0.4 FTE) in order to provide for the full-time person's two days off every week. For 12-hour shifts, it takes 2.1 FTEs to staff one 12-hour shift each day, each week; two people each working three 12-hour shifts and one person working one 12-hour shift each week (0.9 FTE = 0.9 FTE = 0.3 FTE = 2.1 FTEs). Therefore, the same number of FTEs is required to staff a unit for 24 hours a day for two weeks, regardless of whether the staff are all on 8-hour shifts (1.4 FTEs × 33 shifts = 4.2 FTEs) or 12-hour shifts (2.1 FTEs × 32 shifts = 4.2 FTEs).

## Determining Staffing Mix

The same data used to determine FTEs are used to identify **staffing mix**. For example, for patient care needs involving general hygiene care, feeding, transferring, or turning patients, licensed practical nurses (LPNs) or unlicensed assistive personnel (UAPs) can be used. For patient care needs involving frequent assessments, patient education, or discharge planning, RNs will be needed because of the skills required. A high RN-skill mix allows for greater staffing flexibility. Again, information on typical or usual patient needs is obtained by using trends from the patient classification system.

## Determining Distribution of Staff

For many patient care units, the distribution of staff varies from shift to shift and by days of the week. Patient census on a surgical unit will probably fluctuate throughout the week, with a higher census Monday through Thursday and a lower census over the weekend. In addition, some surgical units may have more complex cases earlier in the week and short-stay surgical cases later in the week. Surgical patients may have a shorter length of stay (LOS) than many medical patients. The patient census on a medical unit rarely fluctuates Monday through Friday, but may be less on weekends, when diagnostic tests are not done.

The workload on many units also varies within the 24-hour period. The care demands on a surgical unit will be heaviest early in the morning hours prior to the start of the surgical schedule; mid-morning, when the unit receives patients from critical care units; late in the afternoon, when patients return from the postanesthesia recovery unit; and in the evening hours, when same-day surgical patients are discharged.

Critical care units may have greater care needs in the mornings when transferring patients to medical or surgical units and in the early afternoon hours when admitting new surgical cases.

Medical units usually have the heaviest care needs in the morning hours, when patients' daily care needs are being met and physicians are making rounds. On skilled nursing and rehabilitation units, care needs are greatest before and immediately after mealtimes and in the evening hours; during other times of the day, patients are often away from the unit and involved in various therapeutic activities.

In contrast with the medical, surgical, critical care, and rehabilitation units that have definite patterns of patient care needs, labor-and-delivery and emergency department areas cannot predict when patient care needs will be most intense. Thus, labor-and-delivery and emergency department areas must rely on block staffing to ensure that adequate nursing staff are available at all times.

Here's what a nurse manager told a new nurse candidate when asked about the nurse to staff ratio:

> *"On the surgical step-down floor, we most typically staff at a one-RN-to-four-patient ratio. We also plan to have a charge nurse who is not taking patients to assist staff with extra tasks and needs. On occasion, a nurse may have three patients or five patients. We always work to be flexible, looking at the acuity of the patients and the competencies of the staff who are working. During each shift, we reassess every four hours and as needed to ensure assignments are still appropriate and patient needs haven't significantly changed, necessitating a reassignment of patients. We also have nurse aides on this floor. They help with vital signs, bed changes, baths, and ambulation. There is most typically one aide for every 8 to 12 patients. Also, a unit clerk answers the phones and greets guests. This team dynamic creates for great patient care."*

**Block staffing** involves scheduling a set staff mix for every shift. However, there may be trends in peak workload hours in emergency departments, when additional staff (RN, UAP, or secretary) beyond the block staff are necessary. Examples of peak workload hours within the emergency department may be from 6:00 P.M. to 10:00 P.M. to accommodate patient needs after physicians' offices close, or from 12:00 A.M. to 3:00 A.M. to accommodate alcohol-related injuries. All these needs in patterns of care must be known when staffing requirements and work schedules are established. Data reflecting peak workload times must be continuously monitored to maintain the appropriate levels and mix of staff.

# Scheduling

## Creative and Flexible Staffing

Nurse shortages and current restrictions in salary budgets have made creative and flexible staffing patterns necessary and probably everlasting. Combinations of 4-, 6-, 8-, 10-, and 12-hour shifts and schedules that have nurses working six consecutive days of 12-hour shifts with 13 days off, and staffing strategies, such as weekend programs and split shifts, are common.

Flexible staffing patterns can be a major challenge and, in some cases, a mathematical challenge. However, once a schedule is established and agreed to by the nurse manager and the staff, it can become a cyclic schedule for an extended period of time, such as 6 to 12 months. This allows staff members to know their work schedule many months ahead of time.

The use of 8-hour and 12-hour shifts is fairly straightforward. Problems with combined staffing patterns may include:

- The perception that nurses don't work full-time when they work several days in a row and then are off for several days in a row
- Disruption in continuity of care if split shifts are used (7:00 to 11:00 A.M.; 11:00 A.M. to 3:00 P.M.; 3:00 P.M. to 7:00 P.M.; 7:00 P.M. to 1:00 A.M.; 1:00 A.M. to 7:00 A.M. shifts)
- Immense challenges for nurse managers to communicate with all staff in a timely manner

Advantages of using combined staffing patterns are that it:

- Better meets patient care needs during peak workload times
- Improves staff satisfaction
- Maximizes the availability of nurses

Ten-hour shifts provide greater overlap between shifts to permit extra time for nurses to complete their work; for this reason, they may increase salary expenditures. There are a few specialty units in which 10-hour shifts would be cost-efficient: postanesthesia recovery areas, operating departments, and emergency departments are examples.

### Self-staffing and Scheduling

Some hospitals have instituted self-staffing. This is an empowerment strategy that allows unit staff the authority to use their backup staffing options if the patient workload increases or if unscheduled staff absences occur. Likewise, staff can and must go home early if the patient workload decreases.

**Self-scheduling** allows the staff to create and manage the schedule. Self-scheduling can be positive for the staff and for the manager, but attention must be paid to balancing unit needs with individual requests (Bailyn, Collins, & Song, 2007). Whether the schedule is determined by the manager or by staff, the schedule can be transparent for all staff by posting it online (also see section on automated scheduling). In this way, the organization can demonstrate fairness in scheduling and leverage staff expertise in an equitable manner.

### Shared Schedule

A new tool currently in use is a shared schedule. Two people share one full-time schedule by splitting the day of 12 hours into half days of 6.5 hours each, alternating morning and afternoon shift. This allows nurses who might not be able to work the full 12 hours to share the shift.

### Open Shift Management

Open shift management is an innovative technique to allow an organization's staff to self-schedule additional shifts (Bantle, 2007). With the schedule posted online, as described above, staff members can select assignments and shifts that fit their expertise and accommodate their personal schedules. This strategy is especially valuable to health care systems with several hospitals in which nurses from one hospital can select assignments at any of the others. The organization itself could establish an internal staffing pool (see next section).

Case Study 16-1 shows how one hospital used open scheduling to decrease its use of agency staff and improve staff morale.

### Weekend Staffing Plan

Hospitals can no longer arbitrarily staff patient care units on weekends or at nights with marginal numbers or levels of qualified staff. The acuity of patients in hospitals, including medical and surgical patients, mandates staffing units on the weekends by the same principles used for weekdays. Thorough trend analysis of patient data can provide the justification necessary to appropriately decrease the number of RNs, at least for some levels, because of differences in patient care needs throughout the day.

A creative method for weekend staffing is the **Baylor plan**. Developed at Baylor University Medical Center, nurses agree to work only 12-hour shifts on the weekend and are paid for a standard work week. Numerous hospitals have adopted this model for weekend staffing (Cedar Community Hospital, 2011; St. Vincent's Hospital, 2011).

## Automated Scheduling

Technology today makes automated scheduling feasible (Douglas, 2010). Matching patient demand to nurse staffing is better done by automated systems than by individuals. To aid in scheduling decisions, data should include patient information, nurse characteristics, and hospital

## CASE STUDY 16-1

### SCHEDULING

Tori Abraham and Jillian Moore are both nurse managers of general med/surg units at separate hospitals that are part of a large metropolitan health care system. Staffing among the med/surg units has been problematic due to increased patient volume and cost control measures enacted by the health care corporation. Staff members have complained numerous times that extra shifts are only offered to part-time employees and that premium pay shifts are given to those with more seniority. As the holidays approach, staff tension increases as a lottery system has traditionally been used to assign shifts for major holidays. Additionally, since employees are free to transfer within any of the eight metropolitan hospitals, there has been significant turnover on the med/surg units as employees decide to transfer to ambulatory care and same day surgery facilities.

Tori and Jillian have volunteered to be part of a new scheduling system for their health care system. Nurses and nursing assistants will be able to view open shifts on each unit and e-mail Tori or Jillian with requests to staff shifts for which they are qualified. By allowing staff to have greater control over which additional shifts and at which facility they prefer to work, the nurse managers hope to decrease agency staffing and increase employee satisfaction. Additional units are expected to come online, which will also allow staff to have experience on oncology, skilled nursing, and orthopedic patients. The education department will provide a database of employee certifications to managers to ensure that staff wishing to work away from their home units are qualified for the job.

After 90 days of using the new open shift scheduling system, Tori and Jillian are pleased with the results. Agency staff use has decreased by 60 percent, and staff members report they are happier with the ability to schedule their own additional shifts as well as work at a different facility without having to transfer. Holiday staffing has been easier, as those employees who prefer to work premium pay for holidays are able to self-schedule. Tori and Jillian present their findings to the chief nursing officer and will be part of the team implementing systemwide use of open shift scheduling.

### Manager's Checklist

The nurse manager is responsible for:

- Understanding the scheduling and staffing needs for his or her areas of responsibility
- Analyzing the economic impact of using agency staffing for open shifts and the financial impact on budget
- Ensuring adequate staffing for safe and appropriate patient care
- Communicating with staff members regarding concerns or frustrations over scheduling and staffing
- Using creative problem solving to address scheduling and staffing issues
- Improving employee job satisfaction and patient care skills

data (Frith, Anderson, & Sewell, 2010). Automated systems improve patient care outcomes because nurses spend more time with the patients who need the most nursing care. In addition, using nurses' time appropriately improves financial outcomes as well (Barton, 2011).

Data are often displayed on a dashboard. A dashboard is a computer display of real-time data collected from various sources and categorized for use in decision making.

## Supplementing Staff

When there is a need for additional staff because of scheduled or unscheduled absences, increased workload demands, or existing staff vacancies, the nurse manager or staffing person must find additional staff. Options include using PRN staff (staff scheduled on an as-needed basis), part-time staff, internal float pools, or outside agency nurses.

Supplemental staff are needed when workload increases beyond that which the existing staff can manage, staff absences and resignations occur, and staff vacancies exist. Chronic staffing problems need to be addressed in a proactive manner involving the nurse manager, the chief nurse executive, and the nursing personnel on the unit with the problem. Strategies for dealing with turnover and for managing absenteeism are discussed in Chapter 20.

### Internal Pools

Acute staffing problems can be addressed by establishing internal float pools using nursing staff and unlicensed assistive personnel (UAPs). Internal float **pools** of nurses can provide supplemental staffing at a substantially lower cost than external agency nurses. In addition, internal staff are familiar with the organization. All staff participating in the internal float pool must be adequately trained for the type of patient care they will be giving.

Internal float pools can be centralized or decentralized. A centralized pool is the most efficient. A pool of RNs, LPNs, UAPs, and unit clerks are available for placement anywhere in the institution. However, it may be difficult to place the person with the correct skills for a particular unit at the needed time.

In decentralized pools, a staff member usually works only for one nurse manager or on only one unit. The advantages of decentralized pools include better accountability, improved staffing response, and improved continuity of care. Critical care units, operating rooms, maternal–child units, and other highly specialized or technical areas tend to use a decentralized system.

In addition, staff can receive cross-training in preparation for assignment to another unit. A critical-care nurse might be cross-trained for the step-down unit, for example. Dual-unit positions could be established in the recruiting phase to give the organization the maximum flexibility in scheduling and the employee an opportunity to acquire additional skills.

### External Pools

For some institutions, agency nurses become part of the regular staff contracted to fill vacancies for a specified period of time (e.g., a nurse on maternity leave). However, most agency nurses are used as supplemental staff. All agency nurses require orientation to the facility and unit, and they must work under the supervision of an experienced in-house nurse. Management must verify valid licensure, ensure that either the agency or agency nurse has current malpractice insurance, and develop a mechanism to evaluate the agency nurse's performance. Although an agency nurse may meet an urgent staffing need, continuity of care may be compromised and there may be some staff resentment because these nurses may earn two to three times the salary of in-house nurses.

Concern about the quality of agency nurses appears to be unfounded, according to a study analyzing adverse events in Pennsylvania hospitals (Aiken, Xue, Clarke, & Sloane, 2007). Rather, adverse outcomes resulted from deficits in the hospital environments, not from the quality of the agency nurse assigned there.

Ensuring that sufficient staff are available and that they are scheduled appropriately is a demanding task and one that is constantly in flux. Nevertheless, such activities are critical to achieving positive patient outcomes and providing safe, effective, and cost-conscious staffing.

## What You Know Now

- The goal of staffing and scheduling is to provide an adequate mix of nursing staff to match patient care needs.
- The Joint Commission requires that organizations determine criteria for nurse staffing and provide adequate numbers of competent staff to meet that criteria.
- Patient classification systems use patient needs to determine workload requirements and staffing needs.
- Scheduling involves assigning available staff in a way that patient care needs are met.
- Flexible and creative staffing and scheduling techniques are increasingly necessary.
- Self-staffing and scheduling, including open shift management, is an option in which nursing staff participate in designing the schedule and accept responsibility for ensuring attendance.
- Automated scheduling improves patient outcomes and uses fiscal resources appropriately.

## Tools for Handling Staffing and Scheduling

1. Familiarize yourself with the current patient classification, acuity system, or automated system in use.
2. Determine the nursing care hours needed.

3. Determine FTEs needed.
4. Create or modify a schedule that best meets your patients' needs.
5. Supplement staff as needed.
6. Consider self-staffing if appropriate.

## Questions to Challenge You

1. What has been your experience with staffing? Use any work setting where you are or have been an employee. How well did it work? Was there adequate coverage to meet the needs of the organization? Explain.
2. Using the formulas for calculating FTEs in the chapter, create your own examples and work the problems from them. Were you able to compute needed FTEs? Now calculate the hours needed when nursing staff work 8-hour or 12-hour shifts.
3. On occasion, there are more staff available than are needed. As a nurse manager, how would you handle this? How might the staff respond?
4. No one is ever completely satisfied with the schedule. How would you handle a staff member who repeatedly asks to have his schedule changed?

### Pearson Nursing Student Resources
Find additional review materials at
**www.nursing.pearsonhighered.com**

Prepare for success with additional NCLEX®-style practice questions, interactive assignments and activities, Web links, animations and videos, and more!

## References

Aiken, L. H., Xue, Y., Clarke, S., & Sloane, D. M. (2007). Supplemental nurse staffing in hospitals and quality of care. *Journal of Nursing Administration, 37*(7/8), 335–342.

Aiken, L. H., Sloane, D. M., Cimiotti, J. P., Clarke, S. P., Flynn, L., Seago, J. A., Spetz, J., & Smith, H. L. (2010). Implications of the California nurse staffing mandate for other states. *Health Services Research, 45*(3), 904–921.

Bailyn, L., Collins, R., & Song, Y. (2007). Self-scheduling for hospital nurses: An attempt and its difficulties. *Journal of Nursing Management, 15*(1), 72–77.

Bantle, A. (2007). Automated workforce tracking keeps you flexible. *Nursing Management, 38*(9), 29.

Barton, N. S. (2011). Matching nurse staffing to demand. *Nursing Management, 42*(2), 37–39.

Cedar Community Hospital. (2011). Baylor weekend staffing program. Retrieved July 29, 2011 from http://www.cedarcommunity.org/opportunities_92_2341037709.pdf

Douglas, K. (2010). Digital dashboards and staffing: A perfect match. *American Nurse Today, 5*(5), 52–53.

Frith, K. H., Anderson, F., & Sewell, J. P. (2010). Assessing and selecting date for a nursing services dashboard. *Journal of Nursing Administration, 40*(1), 10–16.

Hickey, P., Gauvreau, K., Connor, J., Sporing, E., & Jenkins, K. (2010). The relationship of nurse staffing, skill mix, and Magnet recognition to institutional volume and mortality for congenital heart surgery. *Journal of Nursing Administration, 40*(5), 226–232.

Joint Commission. (2011) Comprehensive accreditation manual for hospitals: The official handbook. Retrieved July 28, 2011 from http://www.jcrinc.com/Accreditation-Manuals/PCAH11/2130/

Kalisch, B. J., & Lee, K. H. (2011). Nurse staffing levels and teamwork: A cross-sectional study of patient care units in acute care hospitals. *Journal of Nursing Scholarship, 43*(1), 82–88.

Manojlovich, M. (2009). Seeking staffing solutions. *American Nurse Today, 4*(3), 25–27.

Needleman, J., Buerhaus, P., Pankratz, S., Leibson, C. L., Stevens, S. R., & Harris, M. (2011). Nurse staffing and inpatient hospital mortality. *New England Journal of Medicine, 364*(11), 1037–1045.

Picard, B., & Warner, M. (2007). Demand management: A methodology for outcomes-driven staffing and patient flow management. *Nurse Leader, 5*(2), 30–34.

Schilling, P. L., Campbell, D. A., Englesbe, M. J., & Davis, M. M. (2010). A comparison of in-hospital mortality risk conferred by high hospital occupancy, differences in nurse staffing levels, weekend admission, and seasonal influenza.

*Medical Care, 48*(3), 224–232.

St. Vincent's Hospital. (2011). Baylor staffing plan agreement. Retrieved July 28, 2011 from http://intranet.stv.org/documents/docmanager/nursingservices/display/formnumber8720_/87200350baylors/8720-0350BaylorStaffing-PlanAgreement.pdf

# Motivating and Developing Staff

## Learning Outcomes

*After completing this chapter, you will be able to:*

1. Describe how motivation and ability affect job performance.
2. Discuss how different theories explain motivation.
3. Explain how orientation, preceptors, and on-the-job instruction can help motivate staff.
4. Describe the benefits of nurse residency programs, career advancement strategies, and leadership development on motivation.
5. Discuss why succession planning is essential to the future.

## Key Terms

Content theories
Equity theory
Expectancy theory
Extinction
Goal-setting theory
Horizontal promotion

Motivation
On-the-job instruction
Operant conditioning
Orientation
Preceptor
Process theories

Punishment
Reinforcement theory
    (behavior modification)
Shaping

Acontinual and troublesome question facing managers today is why some employees perform better than others. Making decisions about who performs what tasks in a particular manner without first considering individual behavior can lead to irreversible, long-term problems.

Each employee is different in many respects. A manager needs to ask how such differences influence the behavior and performance of the job requirements. Ideally, the manager performs this assessment when the new employee is hired. In reality, however, many employees are placed in positions without the manager having adequate knowledge of their abilities and/or interests. This often results in problems with employee performance, as well as conflict between employees and managers. Employee performance literature ultimately reveals two major dimensions as determinants of job performance: motivation and ability (Hersey, Blanchard, & Johnson, 2007).

## A Model of Job Performance

Nurse managers spend considerable time making judgments about the fit among individuals, job tasks, and effectiveness. Such judgments are typically influenced by both the manager's and the employee's characteristics. For example, ability, instinct, and aspiration levels—as well as age, education, and family background—account for why some employees perform well and others poorly. Based on these factors, a model that considers motivation and ability as determinants of job performance is presented in Table 17-1.

This performance model identifies six categories likely to be viewed as important:

1. Daily job performance

2. Attendance

3. Punctuality

4. Adherence to policies and procedures

5. Absence of incidents, errors, and accidents

6. Honesty and trustworthiness

Although there is conceptual overlap in these categories, separate designation of each helps emphasize their importance.

When using this model, carefully consider several factors. First, the health care organization should establish and communicate clear descriptions of daily job performance so that deviations from expected behaviors can be easily identified and documented. Second, behaviors

---

**TABLE 17-1    A Simplified Model of Job Performance**

| Motivation | And | Ability | = | Employee Performance |
|---|---|---|---|---|
| Compensation | | Responsibilities | | Daily job performance |
| Benefits | | Education—basic/advanced | | Attendance |
| Job design | | Continuing education | | Punctuality |
| Leadership style | | Skills/abilities | | Adherence to policies and procedures |
| Recruitment and selection | | | | Absence of incidents/errors/accidents |
| Employee needs/goals/abilities | | | | Honesty and trustworthiness |

considered troublesome in one department may be acceptable in another department. Finally, some behaviors are viewed as serious only when repeated (e.g., being late to work), whereas others are classified as troublesome following only one incident (e.g., a medication error with severe consequences).

## Employee Motivation

**Motivation** describes the factors that initiate and direct behavior. Because individuals bring to the workplace different needs and goals, the type and intensity of motivators vary among employees. Nurse managers prefer motivated employees because they strive to find the best way to perform their jobs. Motivated employees are more likely to be productive than are nonmotivated workers. This is one reason that motivation is an important aspect of enhancing employee performance.

## Motivational Theories

Historically, motivational theories were concerned with three things:

1. What mobilizes or energizes human behavior

2. What directs behavior toward the accomplishment of some objective

3. How such behavior is sustained over time

The usefulness of motivational theories depends on their ability to explain motivation adequately, to predict with some degree of accuracy what people will actually do, and, finally, to suggest practical ways of influencing employees to accomplish organizational objectives. Motivational theories can be classified into at least two distinct groups: content theories and process theories.

### Content Theories

**Content theories** emphasize individual needs or the rewards that may satisfy those needs. There are two types of content theories: instinct and need. Instinct theorists characterized instincts as inherited or innate tendencies that predisposed individuals to behave in certain ways. These theories were attacked for their difficulty in pinpointing the specific motivating behaviors and the acute awareness of the variability in the strengths of instincts across individuals. In addition, the development of need theories supported the concept that motives were learned behaviors.

### Process Theories

Whereas content theories attempt to explain why a person behaves in a particular manner, **process theories** emphasize how the motivation process works to direct an individual's effort into performance. These theories add another dimension to the manager's understanding of motivation and help predict employee behavior in certain circumstances. Examples of process theories are reinforcement theory, expectancy theory, equity theory, and goal-setting theory.

**Reinforcement theory**, also known as **behavior modification**, views motivation as learning (Skinner, 1953). According to this theory, behavior is learned through a process called **operant conditioning,** in which a behavior becomes associated with a particular consequence. In operant conditioning, the response–consequence connection is strengthened over time—that is, it is learned.

Consequences may be positive, as with praise or recognition, or negative. Positive reinforcers are used for the express purpose of increasing a desired behavior.

*Kyle, a staff nurse, offered a creative idea to redesign work flow on the unit. His manager supported the idea and helped Kyle implement the new process. In addition, the manager praised Kyle for the extra effort and publicly recognized him for the idea. Kyle was encouraged by the outcome and sought other solutions to work-flow problems.*

Negative reinforcers are used to inhibit an undesired behavior. **Punishment** is a common technique.

> *To get Rose to chart adequately, the manager required her to come to his office daily with her patient charts, and they reviewed her charting together. She was required to do this until she achieved an acceptable level of charting. Rose found the task laborious and humiliating. As a result, Rose was soon charting appropriately.*

Because punishment is negative in character, an employee may fail to improve and also may avoid the manager and the job, as well. The effects of punishment are generally temporary. Undesirable behavior will be suppressed only as long as the manager monitors the situation and the threat of punishment is present. Conversely, positive reinforcement is the best way to change behavior.

**Extinction** is another technique used to eliminate negative behavior. By removing a positive reinforcer, undesired behavior is extinguished.

> *Consider the case of Jasmine, a chronic complainer. To curb this behavior, her manager chose to ignore her many complaints and not try to resolve them. Initially, Jasmine complained more, but eventually she realized her behavior was not getting the desired response and stopped complaining.*

A problem with operant conditioning (behavior modification) is that there is no sure way to elicit the desired behavior so that it can be reinforced. In addition, staff and the manager may view consequences differently.

> *Take Thad, for example. As a new employee, Thad conscientiously completed critical paths for his assigned patients. When the manager recognized Thad for his good work, his peers began to exclude him from the group. Although the manager was attempting positive reinforcement, Thad quit completing critical paths because he felt the manager had alienated him from his coworkers.*

Another procedure is **shaping**. Shaping involves selectively reinforcing behaviors that are successively closer approximations to the desired behavior. When people become clearly aware that desirable rewards are contingent on a specific behavior, their behavior will eventually change.

Behavior modification works quite well, provided that rewards can be found that, in fact, employees see as positive reinforcers, and provided that supervisory personnel can control such rewards or make them contingent on performance. This does not mean that all rewards work equally well or that the same rewards will continue to function effectively over a long time. If someone is praised four or five times a day every day, the praise would soon begin to wear thin: it would cease to be a positive reinforcer. Care must be taken not to over do a good thing.

Like reinforcement theory, **expectancy theory** (Vroom, 1964) emphasizes the role of rewards and their relationship to the performance of desired behaviors. Expectancy theory regards people as reacting deliberately and actively to their environment.

> *In an effort to improve the amount of delegation by the nurses on her unit, Andrea approached the situation from an expectancy theory perspective. She identified that the nurses wanted to assign more duties to assistive personnel but were reluctant because of concerns about liability. Once Andrea was able to clarify liability issues, the nurses were eager to delegate tasks that could be performed by nonlicensed staff in order to devote more time to their professional responsibilities.*

Expectancy theory also considers multiple outcomes. Consider the possibility of a promotion to nurse manager. Even though a staff nurse believes such a promotion is positive and is a desirable reward for competent performance in patient care, the nurse also realizes that there are possibly some negative outcomes (e.g., working longer hours, losing the close camaraderie enjoyed with other staff members). These outcomes may influence the staff nurse's decision.

Similarly, **equity theory** suggests that a person perceives that one's contribution to the job is rewarded in the same proportion that another person's contribution is rewarded. Job contributions include such things as ability, education, experience, and effort, whereas rewards include job satisfaction, pay, prestige, and any other outcomes an employee regards as valuable (Adams, 1963, 1965).

Unlike expectancy theory and equity theory, **goal-setting theory** suggests that it is not the rewards or outcomes of task performance per se that cause a person to expend effort, but rather the goal itself (Locke, 1968).

> *Timothy was new to a home care hospice program. An important skill in care with the terminally ill is therapeutic communication. Timothy and his manager recognized that he needed help to improve his skills in communicating with these patients and their families. His manager asked him to write two goals related to communication. Timothy expressed a desire to attend a communications workshop and also indicated he would try at least one new communication technique each week. Within a month, Timothy's therapeutic communication skills had already improved. As a result, Timothy was more satisfied with his position, his patients received more compassionate care, and Timothy found his work more rewarding.*

Each theory of work motivation contributes something to our understanding of, and ultimately our ability to influence, employee motivation.

## Manager as Leader

The manager serves as a role model, exemplifying leadership qualities that reflect the organization's values, mission, and vision and plays a key role in staff members' job satisfaction and retention (Failla & Stichler, 2008). Additionally, the manager can create conditions that enhance employee motivation (Doucette, 2009) and provide opportunities and encouragement for staff development (Urquhart, 2009).

## Staff Development

### Orientation

Getting an employee started in the right way is essential. A well-planned **orientation** reduces the anxiety that new employees feel when beginning the job. In addition, socializing the employee into the workplace contributes to unit effectiveness by reducing dissatisfaction, absenteeism, and turnover (see Chapter 20).

Orientation is a joint responsibility of both the organization's staff development personnel and the nursing manager. In most organizations, the new staff nurse completes the orientation program, whereupon the nurse manager (or someone appointed to do this) provides an on-site orientation. Staff development personnel and unit staff should have a clear understanding of their respective, specific responsibilities so that nothing is left to chance. The development staff should provide information involving matters that are organization-wide in nature and relevant to all new employees, such as benefits, mission, governance, general policies and procedures, safety, quality improvement, infection control, and common equipment. The nurse manager should concentrate on those items unique to the employee's specific job.

New employees often have unrealistically high expectations about the amount of challenge and responsibility they will find in their first job. If they are assigned fairly undemanding, entry-level tasks, they feel discouraged and disillusioned. The result is job dissatisfaction, turnover, and low productivity.

So, one function of orientation is to correct any unrealistic expectations. The nurse manager needs to outline specifically what is expected of new employees. Such realistic job previews help prevent early departures from the organization and, possibly, the nursing profession.

Socializing new employees can sometimes be difficult because of the anxiety people feel when they first come on the job. They simply do not hear all of the information they are given. They spend a lot of energy attempting to integrate and interpret the information presented, and consequently they miss some of it. So repetition may be necessary the first few days or weeks on the job. Ongoing follow-up is important.

*Trina Prescott, RN, joined the pediatric oncology unit of a large university teaching hospital. Her nurse manager, Lily Yuen, scheduled a lunch with Trina 30 days after she started. Lily had a relaxed conversation with Trina about the first 30 days of her employment. Trina expressed how much she enjoyed her new job, but that she still felt uncomfortable accessing implanted vascular ports without assistance. Lily makes a note to schedule one-on-one teaching for Trina with a nurse from the IV team. Scheduling a lunch with new employees approximately 30 to 60 days into their employment has improved new employee retention and increased open communication between Lily and her staff.*

## On-the-Job Instruction

The most widely used educational method is **on-the-job instruction**. This often involves assigning new employees to experienced nurse peers, preceptors, or the nurse manager. The learner is expected to learn the job by observing the experienced employee and by performing the actual tasks under supervision.

On-the-job instruction has several positive features, one of which is its cost-effectiveness. New nurses learn effectively at the same time they are providing care. Moreover, this method reduces the need for outside instructional facilities and reliance on professional educators. Transfer of learning is not an issue because the learning occurs on the actual job. However, on-the-job instruction often fails because there is no assurance that accurate and complete information is presented, and the instructor may not know learning principles. As a result, presentation, practice, or feedback may be inadequate or omitted.

On-the-job instruction fulfills an important function; however, staff members involved may not view it as having equal value to more standardized and formal classroom instruction.

To implement effective on-the-job instruction, the following are suggested:

1. Employees who function as educators must be convinced that educating new employees in no way jeopardizes their own job security, pay level, seniority, or status.

2. Individuals serving as educators should realize that this added responsibility will be instrumental in attaining other rewards for them.

3. Pair teachers and learners to minimize any differences in background, language, personality, attitudes, or age that may inhibit communication and understanding.

4. Select teachers on the basis of their ability to teach and their desire to take on this added responsibility.

5. Staff nurses chosen as teachers should be carefully educated in the proper methods of instruction.

6. Formalize assignments so that nurses do not view on-the-job instruction as happenstance or second-class instruction.

7. Rotate learners to expose each one to the specific know-how of various staff nurses or education department teachers.

8. Employees serving as teachers should understand that their new assignment is by no means a chance to get away from their own jobs but that they must build instructional time into their workload.

9. The efficiency of the unit may be reduced when on-the-job instruction occurs.

10. The learner must be closely supervised to prevent him or her from making any major mistakes and carrying out procedures incorrectly.

## Preceptors

One method of orientation is the **preceptor** model, which can be used to assist new employees and to reward experienced staff nurses. The preceptor model provides a means for orienting and socializing the new nurse as well as providing a mechanism to recognize exceptionally competent staff nurses. Staff nurses who serve as preceptors are selected based on their clinical competence, organizational skills, ability to guide and direct others, and concern for the effective orientation of new nurses.

The primary function of the preceptor is to orient the new nurse to the unit. This includes proper socialization of the new nurse within the group as well as familiarizing her or him with unit functions. The preceptor teaches any unfamiliar procedures and helps the new nurse develop any necessary skills. The preceptor acts as a resource person on matters of unit functions as well as policies and procedures. The preceptorship is for approximately three weeks, although the time may vary depending to the nurse's individual learning needs or the organization's policies.

New nurses may need to use their preceptors as counselors as they make their transition to the unit. If new nurses experience discrepancy between their educational preparation or their expectations and the realities of working in the unit, the preceptor's role as counselor can prove invaluable in helping them cope with "reality shock."

The preceptor also serves as a staff nurse role model demonstrating work-related tasks, how to set priorities, solve problems and make decisions, manage time, delegate tasks, and interact with others. In addition, the preceptor evaluates the new nurse's performance and provides both verbal and written feedback to encourage development.

The staff development department's function is to teach the experienced nurse the role of a preceptor, principles of adult education applicable to learning needs, how to teach necessary skills, how to plan teaching, how to evaluate teaching and learning objectives, and how to provide both formal and informal feedback.

## Mentoring

Mentoring is another strategy to improve retention. Mentors take a greater role than preceptors in developing staff. Precepting usually is associated with orientation of staff, whereas mentoring occurs over a much longer period and involves a bigger investment of personal energy. Mentoring is suggested as a strategy to retain new graduates (Butler & Felts, 2006).

A mentor is a wiser and more experienced person who guides, supports, and nurtures a less experienced person. Mentors are usually the same sex as the protégé, eight to fifteen years older, highly placed in the organization, powerful, and willing to share their experiences. They are not threatened by the mentee's potential for equaling or exceeding them. Mentees are selected by mentors for several reasons: good performance, loyalty to people and the organization, a similar social background or a social acquaintance with each other, appropriate appearance, an opportunity to demonstrate the extraordinary, and high visibility.

Mentor–mentee relationships seem to advance through several stages. The initiation stage usually lasts six months to a year, during which the relationship gets started. The mentee stage is that in which the mentee's work is not yet recognized for its own merit, but rather as a byproduct of the mentor's instruction, support, and encouragement. The mentor thus buffers the mentee from criticism.

A breakup stage may occur from six months to two years after a significant change in the relationship, usually resulting from the mentee taking a job in another department or organization so that there is a physical separation of the two individuals. It also can occur if the mentor refuses to accept the mentee as a peer or when the relationship becomes dysfunctional for some reason. The lasting friendship stage is the final phase and will occur if the mentor accepts the mentee as a peer or if the relationship is reestablished after a significant separation. The complete mentoring process usually includes the last stage.

### Coaching

Coaching is a strategy suggested to address nurses' job dissatisfaction (Stedman & Nolan, 2007). A coach helps the staff member focus on solving a specific problem or conflict that interferes with the employee's satisfaction at work. Coaches are often nurses or human resources staff within the organization prepared to help resolve conflicts. Conflicts could be between two nurses, between a nurse and a patient, or between a nurse and a physician. In a confidential environment, the coach helps the staff member explore the exact nature of the problem, consider various alternatives (e.g., transfer, quit, do nothing), delve into embedded issues (e.g., values conflict with organization, unmatched expectations), discover links (e.g., working with friends), and the disadvantages of leaving (e.g., start over with vacation time, benefits, leave friends). The goal is to reduce turnover from issues that can be resolved.

### Nurse Residency Programs

Residency programs, 12 or 18 months in length, are designed to acclimate new graduates to the work environment. One example is the Versant RN Residency Program™, an 18-month residency that includes both educational and emotional components. Novice nurses receive lectures and online access to best practices as well as a nurse partner who maintains an ongoing relationship and teaches professional accountability and critical thinking. In addition, residents participate in emotional support groups to share experiences and feelings. New-graduate turnover rates have gone from 35 percent to less than 6 percent, according to surveys of hospitals using the program (Mcpeck, 2006).

One-year residency programs for new graduates implemented at 12 sites have been shown to be effective in reducing turnover (Williams et al., 2007). Each residency involved a partnership between a school of nursing and a hospital. The program included a core curriculum, clinical guidance by a nurse preceptor, and a resident facilitator for professional role development assistance in addition to the usual orientation at the institution. The results showed that turnover of new graduates averaged 12 percent, more than half the national average.

Later reports of the residency program, implemented in 26 sites, found turnover rates declined to a low 5.7 percent (Lynn, 2008). The program continues to be refined with recent offerings including peer, preceptor, and manager participation and employee recognition components (Goode et al., 2009). It follows that programs that reduce turnover have been successful in motivating employees.

### Career Advancement

One example of a career advancement development strategy is the clinical ladder program. It uses a system of performance indicators to advance an employee within the organization. The three key components are:

1. Horizontal promotion
2. Clinical ladder
3. Clinical mentee

**Horizontal promotion** rewards the excellent clinical nurse without promoting the nurse to management. A clinical ladder, based on Benner's (2000) novice-to-expert concepts, includes:

1. Clinical apprentice—new nurse or nurse new to the area

2. Clinical colleague—a full partner in care

3. Clinical mentee—demonstrates preceptor ability

4. Clinical leader—demonstrates leadership in practice

5. Clinical expert—combines teaching and research with practice

The strength of the system is that superb, clinical nurses can remain at the bedside, clinical excellence can be rewarded, and nurses can move back and forth among the levels based on their personal and professional goals and needs.

Another example of clinical advancement program was used at a Magnet-certified institution, Cincinnati Children's Hospital Medical Center (Allen, Fiorini, & Dickey, 2010). The program's goal was to improve the quality of patient care, provide career opportunities for participating nurses, and to enhance job satisfaction and nurse retention. Evaluation of the program illustrated that goals were met. An additional finding revealed that the program had a substantial positive fiscal impact on the organization as well.

## Leadership Development

Developing internal staff is a cost-effective way to build leaders within the organization. The advantages include knowledge of the skills and strengths of the candidates, the cost saving in retaining high-performing staff, and the ability to design a program that fits the organization's specific needs. In fact, many nurse leaders fail not because they don't want to do the job, but because they don't have the leadership tools required.

Built around Benner's novice to expert concepts (Benner, 2000), one hospital designed a leadership curriculum that targeted the learning needs of staff at different developmental levels, e.g., 200 level for charge nurses, 300 level for assistant nurse managers, 400 level for nurse managers (Swearingen, 2009). As a result, the organization developed a pool of candidates available for promotion to higher-level positions. In addition, they found nurse retention rates improved.

# Succession Planning

Due to an aging nursing workforce, as well as the overall shortage of nurses, succession planning at all levels of nursing management is essential to ensure a smooth transition after a manager leaves or retires (Ponti, 2009). Succession planning is a strategic process that is a natural outgrowth of leadership development. It involves identifying core competencies required at each level of management, recognizing potential recruits, and providing opportunities for development and growth.

One institution developed a nurse management internship program to prepare first-line managers from an internal pool of interested nurses (Wendler, Olson-Sitki, & Prater, 2009). The one-year program successfully prepared several nurses for management positions in its first year. Those costs were recouped when a long term management opening was filled by one of the nurses who completed the internship.

There is no one single way to motivate people. The organization and the manager must use various tools to offer incentives and rewards that satisfy their staff. Increased productivity, patient care quality, job satisfaction, and retention are all outcomes that can result in appropriate motivational activities.

Case Study 17-1 illustrates how one nurse manager used her ingenuity to motivate staff.

## CASE STUDY 17-1

### MOTIVATING STAFF

Jamie Edgar is nurse manager of the mental health outpatient clinic for a large county health department. Her staff includes nurses, licensed clinical social workers, licensed mental health technicians, and clerical support staff. State funding for mental health services has been drastically cut. Jamie had a difficult decision to make regarding who on the staff would receive pay increases and who would not. Compounding her problem is the shortage of qualified psychiatric nurses and two vacant nursing positions that she has been unable to fill due to the low starting salary.

Jamie decides that the nursing staff will receive a four percent raise and the licensed clinical social workers will receive a three percent raise. The mental health technicians and clerical staff will not receive a wage increase this year. The mental health technicians and clerical staff members are upset when Jamie tells them there will not be any pay increases this year. Kevin Adams, a licensed mental health technician, and Charlotte DuBois, an administrative assistant, have both expressed frustration about the disparity in pay increases. Over the past two workweeks, Kevin has been clocking in 10 minutes late each work day and taking longer lunch periods than scheduled. The quality of Charlotte's work has decreased, and she is using more business time for personal telephone calls and personal business.

Jamie is concerned that Kevin's and Charlotte's negative attitudes will continue to affect their work as well as the morale of the staff. Initially, she tried more frequent praise of Kevin's and Charlotte's work, but after three weeks, noted no improvement in their attitude or performance. She counseled each employee individually about performance expectations; however, neither employee made an effort to improve his or her behavior. After receiving a final budget for her clinic, Jamie allocated $800 for training of clerical staff and mental health technicians. She met with Kevin, Charlotte, and two other staff members. Jamie asked the group to assist her in determining how to best spend the $800 training budget. The group agreed that time-management skills could be improved among many of the staff. After reviewing the cost associated with several time-management

training programs, the group was surprised at the expense. Jamie challenged her group to think of alternative ideas other than sending staff members to a seminar and offered a restaurant gift certificate for the most creative ideas.

At their next meeting, Kevin produced reviews of several interactive CD-ROM training programs. Kevin had searched the Internet for the best price for the programs and brought in several demonstration CDs of the top two time-management programs. Charlotte proposed purchasing planners for those staff members who didn't already have a planner or electronic calendar. Charlotte had spoken to the supplier who had the contract for county office supplies. They had agreed to a price of $12 per planner for a complete year of time-planning supplies. The group agreed that both Kevin and Charlotte's ideas were excellent, as well as coming in under the $800 limit.

Kevin and Charlotte were responsible for implementing their ideas with staff who requested training in time management. Although neither employee received a raise in base salary, Jamie was able to secure approval for both to work extra hours to complete training for the clinic staff. Jamie continued to praise both employees for their commitment to the clinic and their coworkers. Kevin began to arrive promptly for each work shift and kept his lunch periods to 30 minutes. Charlotte was eager to demonstrate to coworkers how her new planner helped her prioritize work and personal tasks. Her use of work time for personal business greatly decreased.

### Manager's Checklist

The nurse manager is responsible for:

- Understanding motivating factors for employees and how motivation affects job performance
- Using motivational techniques to enhance employee performance
- Utilizing creative techniques to motivate staff when traditional rewards such as pay or benefit increases are unavailable
- Empowering staff to use creativity to enhance job performance

## What You Know Now

- Job performance is determined by motivation and ability.
- Motivational theories (e.g., reinforcement, expectancy, equity, and goal-setting theories) describe the factors that initiate and direct behavior.
- The manager serves as a role model for staff.
- Staff development methods include orientation, preceptors, and on-the-job instruction.

- Nurse residencies, career advancement opportunities, and leadership development programs can help motivate staff members.
- Succession planning is a strategic process to develop future nurse leaders.

## Tools for Motivating and Developing Staff

1. Recognize that an employee's job performance includes both ability to do the job and motivation.
2. Become familiar with various theories of motivation and use the information to help you motivate others.
3. Be aware that you may be a role model to other staff regardless of your formal position.
4. Identify core competencies involved in specific positions and high performers with the potential to fill those positions.
5. Encourage staff development at all levels, including your own.

## Questions to Challenge You

1. What motivational theory appeals to your sense of how you learn? Why?
2. You are a new nurse manager:
   a. How would you discover what motivates the individuals on your staff?
   b. How could you utilize the organization's resources to motivate your staff?
   c. What staff development programs are available in your organization or community?
   d. How could you make those resources available to your staff?
3. What recommendations would you make to a new nurse manager regarding motivating staff? Have you seen any of these work? Explain.

### Pearson Nursing Student Resources

Find additional review materials at

**www.nursing.pearsonhighered.com**

Prepare for success with additional NCLEX®-style practice questions, interactive assignments and activities, Web links, animations and videos, and more!

## References

Adams, J. S. (1963). Toward an understanding of inequity. *Journal of Abnormal and Social Psychology, 67*, 422.

Adams, J. S. (1965). Injustice in social exchange. In L. Berkowitz (Ed.), *Advances in experimental social psychology* (Vol. 2). New York: Academic Press.

Allen, S. R., Fiorini, P., & Dickey, M. (2010). A streamlined clinical advancement program improves RN participation and retention. *Journal of Nursing Administration, 40*(7/8), 316–322.

Benner, P. (2000). *From novice to expert: Excellence and power in clinical nursing practice.* Upper Saddle River, NJ: Prentice Hall.

Butler, M. R. & Felts, J. (2007). Tool kit for the staff mentor: Strategies for improving retention. *Journal of Continuing Education in Nursing, 37*(5), 210–213.

Doucette, J. N. (2009). Create a great work culture. *American Nurse Today, 4*(6), 13–14.

Failla, K. R., & Stichler, J. F. (2008). Manager and staff perceptions of the manager's leadership style. *Journal of Nursing Administration, 38*(11), 480–487.

Goode, C. J., Lynn, M. R., Krsek, C., & Bednash, G. D. (2009). Nurse residency programs: An essential requirement for nursing. *Nursing Economics, 27*(3), 142–159.

Hersey, P., Blanchard, K. H., & Johnson, D. E. (2007). *Management of organizational behavior* (9th ed.). Upper Saddle River, NJ: Prentice Hall.

Locke, E. A. (1968). Toward a theory of task motives and incentives. *Organizational Behavior and Human Performance, 3*, 157.

Lynn, M. R. (2008). *UHC/AACN nurse residency programs.* Paper presented at the University Health-System Consortium Performance Excellence Forum, Dallas, TX.

McPeck, P. (2006). Residencies ease new grads into practice. *NurseWeek*, September 11, 2006. Retrieved January 2008 from http://www.versant.org/item.asp?id=70

Ponti, M. D. (2009). Transition from leadership development to succession management. *Nursing Administration Quarterly, 33*(2), 125–141.

Skinner, B. F. (1953). *Science and human behavior*. New York: Free Press.

Stedman, M. E., & Nolan, T. L. (2007). Coaching: A different approach to the nursing dilemma. *Nursing Administration Quarterly, 31*(1), 43–49.

Swearingen, S. (2009). A journey to leadership: Designing a nursing leadership development program. *Journal of Continuing Education in Nursing, 40*(3), 107–112.

Urquhart, C. (2009). How to motivate your staff. *American Nurse Today, 4*(7), 27–28.

Vroom, V. H. (1964). *Work and motivation*. New York: Wiley.

Wendler, M. C., Olson-Sitki, K., & Prater, M. (2009). Succession planning for RNs. *Journal of Nursing Administration, 39*(7/8), 326–333.

Williams, C. A., Goode, C. J., Krsek, C., Bednash, G. D., & Lynn, M. R. (2007). Postbaccalaureate nurse residency 1-year option. *Journal of Nursing Administration, 37*(7/8), 357–365.

# Evaluating Staff Performance

## The Performance Appraisal
EVALUATION SYSTEMS
EVIDENCE OF PERFORMANCE
EVALUATING SKILL COMPETENCY
DIAGNOSING PERFORMANCE PROBLEMS
THE PERFORMANCE APPRAISAL INTERVIEW

## Potential Appraisal Problems
LENIENCY ERROR

RECENCY ERROR
HALO ERROR
AMBIGUOUS EVALUATION STANDARDS
WRITTEN COMMENTS PROBLEM

## Improving Appraisal Accuracy
APPRAISER ABILITY
APPRAISER MOTIVATION

## Rules of Thumb

## Learning Outcomes

*After completing this chapter, you will be able to:*

1. Describe criteria that can be used to evaluate staff performance.
2. Discuss different methods used to evaluate performance.
3. Describe problems to expect when evaluating performance.
4. Explain how to use critical incidents to improve annual evaluations.
5. Explain how to conduct a performance appraisal interview.

## Key Terms

Ambiguous evaluation
   standards problem
Behavior-oriented rating
   scales

Critical incidents
Group evaluation
Halo error
Leniency error

Performance appraisal
Recency error
Written comments problem

The goal of a performance evaluation is to support nursing practice development (Schoessler et al., 2008). Evaluating past performance, compared to specified standards, enables the employee and the manager to identify developmental needs. Performance-related behaviors are directly associated with job tasks and need to be accomplished to achieve a job's objectives (Topjian, Buck, & Kozlowski, 2009).

## The Performance Appraisal

The primary purpose of performance evaluations is to give constructive feedback. A good appraisal system ensures that staff know what is expected and how well they meet those expectations. Performance appraisals serve as developmental tools as well as providing information for salary increases and promotions.

The **performance appraisal** process includes:

- Day-to-day manager–employee interactions (coaching, counseling, dealing with policy violations, and disciplining are discussed in Chapter 19)
- Making notes about an employee's behavior
- Encouraging the employee to complete a self evaluation
- Directing peer evaluation, if used
- Conducting the appraisal interview
- Following up with coaching and/or discipline when needed

In addition, performance appraisals and the decisions based on those appraisals, such as layoffs, are covered by several federal and state laws. In the past, employees have successfully sued their organizations over discriminatory employment decisions that were based on questionable performance appraisal results.

There are several steps to help ensure that an appraisal system is nondiscriminatory.

1. The appraisal is in writing and carried out at least once a year.

2. The performance appraisal information is shared with the employee.

3. The employee has the opportunity to respond in writing to the appraisal.

4. Employees have a mechanism to appeal the results of the performance appraisal.

5. The evaluator has adequate opportunity to observe the employee's job performance during the course of the evaluation period. If adequate contact is lacking (e.g., the appraiser and the appraisee work different shifts), then appraisal information should be gathered from other sources.

6. Anecdotal notes on the employee's performance are kept during the entire evaluation period (e.g., three months, one year). These notes, called critical incidents, and discussed later, are shared with the employee during the course of the evaluation period.

7. Evaluators are trained to carry out the performance appraisal process, including

   a. What is reasonable job performance;
   b. How to complete the form; and
   c. How to carry out the feedback interview.

8. The performance appraisal focuses on employee behavior and results rather than on personal traits or characteristics, such as initiative, attitude, or personality.

Regardless of how an organization uses performance appraisals, they must accurately reflect the employee's actual job performance. If performance ratings are inaccurate, an inferior employee may be promoted, another employee may not receive needed training, or there may not be a tie between performance and rewards (thus lessening employee motivation). For appraisals to be successful, the needs of the staff and requirements of the organization must be bridged.

## Evaluation Systems

Nurses engage in a variety of job-related activities. To reflect the multidimensional nature of the job, the performance appraisal form should cover different performance dimensions, such as pain management. In addition, the form should state specific criteria to be evaluated, such as "Evaluates pain levels and administers appropriate medications." Finally, the form should include the individual's goals for the year based on the previous year's evaluation.

### Results-Oriented System

All organizations need to be concerned with the bottom line. If a hospital has a 35 percent occupancy rate or a 20 percent employee absenteeism rate, its future is in jeopardy. In recent years, therefore, top management has turned to appraising some employees at least partly on results. With a results-oriented appraisal system, employees know in advance what is expected. Results are quantifiable, objective, and easily measured.

A focus on results requires setting objectives for what the employee is to accomplish. Although this technique has many variations, basically it involves two steps.

First, a set of work objectives is established at the start of the evaluation period for the employee to accomplish during some future time frame. These objectives can be developed by the employee's supervisor and given to the employee; however, it is better if the manager and employee work together to develop a set of objectives for the employee.

Each performance objective should be defined in concrete, quantifiable terms and have a specific time frame. For example, one objective may need to be accomplished in one month (e.g., "Revise the unit orientation manual to reflect the new Joint Commission standards"); another objective may not have to be met for 12 months (e.g., "Take and pass the CCRN examination within the next year"). In setting objectives, it is important that the employee perceive them as challenging yet attainable.

*Sylvia is an experienced critical care nurse. Her goals for the year include:*

- *Complete advanced cardiac life support (ACLS) recertification.*
- *Obtain CCRN credentialing.*
- *Precept one new graduate nurse.*
- *Serve on hospital shared governance committee.*

The second step involves the actual evaluation of the employee's performance. At this time, the supervisor and employee meet and focus on how well the employee has accomplished his or her objectives.

*At Sylvia's annual performance review, her manager noted that she had:*

- *Become ACLS recertified.*
- *Obtained CCRN credentialing.*
- *Precepted a new graduate nurse who was functioning above expectations.*
- *Chaired subcommittee of hospital shared governance committee.*

### Behavior-Oriented System

Behavior-oriented systems focus on what the employee actually does, as exemplified in Table 18-1.

Focusing on specific behaviors in appraising performance gives new employees specific information on how they are expected to behave and facilitates development of current staff members. Although there are several varieties of **behavior-oriented rating scales**, they all have a number of things in common:

1. Groups of workers who are very familiar with the target job (generally, individuals doing the job and their immediate supervisors) provide written examples (*critical incidents*) of superior and inferior job behaviors.

**TABLE 18-1** **Hill Top Healthcare System**

Employee Performance Evaluation Form

Employee Name: _____

Position: Registered Nurse

Department: _____

Hire Date: _____

Evaluation Review Period: _____

Manager Reviewer: _____

This appraisal contains a five-point scale that each performance expectation is rated on. The description of each number ranking on the five point scale is:

5 Significantly Exceeds Expectations—Staff member consistently goes above and beyond ordinary expectations. Staff member is the pillar role model of excellence 100% of the time.

4 Exceeds Expectations—Staff member frequently does things that are beyond their ordinary expectations. Peers and patients comment that staff member goes beyond others and routine expectations.

3 Meets Expectations—Staff member always meets expectation as expected.

2 Usually Meets Expectations—Staff member is able to demonstrate meeting performance expectations at times.

1 Does Not Consistently Meet Expectations—In this category, remediation work is necessary.

| Performance Expectations | 5–Significantly Exceeds Expectations | 4–Exceeds Expectations | 3–Meets Expectations | 2–Usually Meets Expectations | 1–Does Not Consistently Meet Expectation |
|---|---|---|---|---|---|
| 1. Models critical thinking and expert judgment in patient care. | | | | | |
| 2. Completes assessments, plans of care, and documentation as expected. | | | | | |
| 3. Has developed technical skills and seeks opportunity to enhance skills as appropriate. | | | | | |
| 4. Develops trusting, collaborative relationships with patients and peers. | | | | | |
| 5. Maintains confidentiality of information. | | | | | |
| 6. Demonstrates accountability for actions | | | | | |
| 7. Follows policies and protocols appropriately. | | | | | |
| 8. Completes annual education competencies and all education on new policies and procedures as expected. | | | | | |
| 9. Demonstrates care, respect, and compassion in all interactions. | | | | | |

| **TABLE 18-1** Continued |
| --- |

10. Ensures patients are safe and implements all safety protocols for patients that are appropriate.

11. Brainstorms ideas of needed improvement on the unit and offers ideas to the group along with solutions.

12. Is flexible with staffing and works with peers to meet the needs of patients when planning schedule.

13. Shows commitment to learning and expanding knowledge.

14. Serves as a preceptor and charge nurse as requested.

15. Demonstrates cost awareness and uses supplies and equipment appropriately.

16. Embraces personal responsibility to the organization, patient care, and unit team.

17. Works well with multidisciplinary team, recognizing many people must work together to make great patient care.

18. Participates in a hospital or unit committee.

19. Models direct, purposeful communication.

20. Works in harmony with coworkers, being a team player and settling conflicts professionally.

---

Employee's Goals for Next Year

What is the goal the employee will complete in the next 12 months? How can the manager support this goal?

_____

_____

_____

Signatures

This verifies that this review was completed and does not necessarily signify agreement or disagreement with the contents of the review.

_____

Employee's Signature

Date _____

Manager's Signature _____                                    Date _____

Human Resource's Signature _____                    Date _____

2. These critical incidents are stated as measurable/quantifiable behaviors. (Examples are given in Box 18-1.)

3. Critical incidents that are similar in theme are grouped together. These behavioral groupings (*performance dimensions*) are labeled, for example, patient safety.

Such behavior-oriented appraisal measures can be used only for one job or a cluster of similar jobs, so these scales are time-consuming and therefore expensive to develop. For these reasons, behavior-oriented systems are generally developed when a large number of individuals are doing the same job, such as critical care nurses.

### Evidence of Performance

Evidence of an individual's performance is collected in several ways, including peer review, self-evaluations, group evaluations, and the manager's notes and evaluation.

#### Peer Review

This is a process by which nurses assess and judge the performance of professional peers against predetermined standards (Davis, Capozzoli, & Parks, 2009). Peer review is designed to make performance appraisal more objective because multiple ratings give a more diverse appraisal. It is used frequently in clinical ladder programs, self-governance models, and evaluation of advanced practice nurses.

The steps for peer review are as follows:

1. The manager and/or employee select peers to conduct the evaluation. Usually, two to four peers are identified through a predetermined process.

2. The employee submits a self-evaluation portfolio. The portfolio might describe how he or she met objectives and/or predetermined standards during the past evaluation cycle. Supporting materials are included.

3. The peers evaluate the employee. This may be done individually or in a group. The individuals or group then submit a written evaluation to the manager.

---

## BOX 18-1 Example of a Critical Incident

1. Name of employee: Cindy Siegler
2. Date and Time of incident: March 22, 23, 24, at 0915
3. Description: Ms Siegler, patient care assistant, for the third time this week had nurses complain to manager that 0800 vital signs and finger sticks were not completed at 0900. Nurses use the vital signs and finger stick results as supporting facts in safely administering their medications that are scheduled for 0900. When the nurses go to find Ms. Siegler, each time she has been in the break room on her cell phone and eating. The nurses asked Ms. Siegler why she is in the break room for long periods of time. Ms. Siegler reported to them that she's not going to "push herself early in the day" and she likes to "ease into her shift." The nurses also asked Ms. Siegler why she must take a break when her work isn't done and it is a critical assessment and medication pass time for the unit. The nurses shared with Ms. Siegler that

they depend on her for vital sign and finger stick results. Ms. Siegler has told the nurses on three occasions now "I'll get there in a bit."

4. Comments: Ms. Siegler was counseled by manager. Manager told Ms. Siegler her one priority at work has to be meeting the needs of patients. Ms. Siegler was told that her role on the team is important and vital sign data and finger stick results must be completed and entered into the computer system for nurses before 0900. Ms. Siegler was instructed to not be in the breakroom unless the charge nurse had approved the break. She was also educated on proper break length being 15 minutes. Ms. Siegler was told that failing to meet any of the expectations discussed would result in written warning counseling. Ms. Siegler acknowledged understanding. She said, "I'll try harder." Manager stated she would talk with Ms. Siegler to touch base in two weeks.

4. The manager and employee meet to discuss the evaluation. The manager's evaluation is included, and objectives for the coming evaluation cycle are finalized.

Implementing a peer review involves several considerations. First, it is best to avoid selecting personal best friends for the review. Friends can provide poor ratings as well as inflated ratings, resulting in a negative experience. Second, consider how often to evaluate expert practitioners—for example, those nurses who have reached the top of a clinical ladder. Third, monitor the time needed for portfolio preparation. The object is to improve professionalism and quality of patient care, not to create more paperwork.

## Self-Evaluation

Self-evaluations help the employee examine performance over the year and consider improvements to be made. It is difficult for anyone to accurately rate one's own performance, so self-evaluations tend to be overly positive or, in some cases, excessively negative. Nonetheless, it is a valuable exercise to require employees to focus attention on how well they have met the requirements of the job regardless of whether the appraisal is behavioral-oriented ("Completes patient care plan within 24 hours of admission") or results-oriented ("Presented one in-service on the unit").

## Group Evaluation

Another technique is **group evaluation**. Here, several managers are asked to rank employee performance based on job descriptions and performance standards. Usually, one manager facilitates the process. In addition to evaluating individual performance, the performance of groups of nurses can also be evaluated in this way, and group variances can be benchmarked and evaluated. Using group evaluation reduces personal bias, is timely, and can be effective.

## Manager's Evaluation

Appraising an employee's performance can be a difficult job. A nurse manager is required to reflect on a staff member's performance over an extended period of time (usually 12 months) and then accurately evaluate it. Given that nurse managers have several employees to evaluate, it is not surprising that they frequently forget what an individual did several months ago or may actually confuse what one employee did with what another did.

A useful mechanism for fighting such memory problems is the use of **critical incidents**, which are reports of employee behaviors that are out of the ordinary, in either a positive or a negative direction. Critical incidents include four items: name of employee, date and time of incident, a brief description of what occurred, and the nurse manager's comments on what transpired (Box 18-1). Electronic devices, index cards, or a small notebook are best to use because they allow notes to be taken immediately. In addition, lag time increases the likelihood of errors and the possibility that the manager will neglect to share the incident with the employee (see next section).

Recording critical incidents as they occur is bound to increase the accuracy of year-end performance appraisal ratings. Although this type of note taking may sound simple and straightforward, a manager can still run into problems. For instance, some managers are uncomfortable about recording behaviors; they see themselves as spies lurking around the work area attempting to catch someone. What they need to remember is that this note taking will enable them to evaluate the employee more accurately and makes recency error (described later) much less likely.

The best time to write critical incidents is just after the behavior has occurred. The note should focus specifically on what took place, not on an interpretation of what happened. For example, instead of writing, "Ms. Hudson was rude," write, "Ms. Hudson referred to the patient as a slob."

Once a critical incident has been recorded, the manager should share it with the employee in private. If the behavior is positive, it is a good opportunity for the nurse manager to praise the employee; if the behavior is considered in some way undesirable, the manager may need to coach the employee (see Chapter 19).

Because most managers are extremely busy, they sometimes question whether note taking is a good use of their time. In fact, keeping notes is not a time-consuming process. The average note takes less than two minutes to write. If one writes notes during the gaps in the day (e.g., while waiting for a meeting to start), little, if any, productive time is used. In the long run, such note taking saves time. In addition, keeping and sharing notes forces a manager to deal with problems when they are small and thus are more quickly addressed. Then completing the appraisal form at the end of the evaluation period takes less time with notes for reference.

A key factor in effectively using this note-taking approach is how nurse managers introduce the technique to their staff. To get maximum value out of note taking, managers need to keep in mind two important facts:

1. The primary reason for taking notes is to improve the accuracy of the performance review.

2. When something new is introduced, people tend to react negatively to it.

Managers should be open and candid about the first fact, admitting that they cannot remember every event associated with every employee and telling employees that these notes will make more accurate evaluations possible. Even then, employees will still be suspicious about this procedure. One way to get the procedure off to a good start is for managers to make the first note they record on an employee a positive one, even if they have to stretch a bit to find one. By doing this, each employee's first contact with critical incidents is positive.

Three types of mistakes common with using notes are:

1. Some managers fail to make them specific and behavior oriented; rather, they record that a nurse was "careless" or "difficult to supervise."

2. Some managers record only undesirable behavior.

3. Some managers fail to give performance feedback to the employee at the time that a note was written.

Each of these errors can undermine the effectiveness of the note-taking process. If the notes are vague, the employee may not know specifically what he or she did wrong and therefore does not know how to improve. If only poor performance is documented, employees will resent the system and the manager. If the manager does not share notes as they are written, the employee will often react defensively when confronted with them at the end of the evaluation period. In sum, any manager who is considering using this powerful note-taking procedure needs to take the process seriously and to use it as it is designed.

By increasing the accuracy of the performance review, written notes also diminish the legal liability of lawsuits. If a lawsuit is brought, written notes are very persuasive evidence in court. Sharing the notes with employees throughout the evaluation period also improves the communication flow between the manager and the employee. Having written notes also gives the manager considerable confidence when it comes time to complete the evaluation form and to carry out the appraisal interview.

The manager will feel confident that the appraisal ratings are accurate. Not only does the manager feel professional, but the staff nurse also shares that perception. In fact, it is typically found that with the use of notes, the performance appraisal interview focuses mainly on how the employee can improve next year and what developmental activities are needed rather than on how he or she was rated last year. Thus, the tone of the interview is constructive rather than argumentative.

One final issue needs to be addressed. Different employees react differently to the use of notes. Good employees react positively. Although the manager records both what is done well and what is done poorly, good employees will have many more positive than negative notes and therefore will benefit from notes being taken. In contrast, poorer employees do not react well to notes being taken.

Whereas once they could rely on the poor memory of the nurse manager to produce inflated ratings, note taking is likely to result in more accurate (i.e., lower) ratings for poor employees. The negative reaction of poor employees, however, tends not to be a lasting one. Generally, the poor performers either leave the organization, or when they discover that they no longer can get away with mediocre performance, their performance actually improves.

In most organizations, an employee's immediate manager is in charge of evaluating her or his performance. If the immediate supervisor does not have enough information to evaluate an employee's performance accurately, alternatives are necessary. The manager can informally seek out performance-related information from other sources, such as the employee's coworkers, patients, or other managers who are familiar with the person being evaluated. The manager weighs this additional information, integrates it with his or her own judgment, and completes the evaluation.

## Evaluating Skill Competency

Health care organizations are required to assess their employees' abilities to perform the skills and tasks required for their positions (Joint Commission, 2011). Validation of competency is an ongoing process, initiated in orientation, followed up by development, and assessed on an annual basis and, possibly, remediation. Skill evaluation most commonly takes place in a skills lab, with simulation models, or by direct observation at the point of care. The manager plays a key role in determining the competences required on the job, especially for unit or department-specific competencies.

## Diagnosing Performance Problems

If the manager notes poor or inconsistent performance during the appraisal process, the manager must investigate and remedy the situation. Certain questions should be asked:

"Is the performance deficiency a problem?"
"Will it go away if ignored?"
"Is the deficiency due to a lack of skill or motivation? How do I know?"

The first step is to begin with accepted standards of performance and an accurate assessment of the current performance of the staff member. This means job descriptions must be current and performance appraisal tools must be written in behavioral terms. It also implies that employee evaluations are regularly carried out and implemented according to recognized guidelines. Also, the employee must know what behavior is expected.

Next decide whether the problem demands immediate attention and whether it is a skill-related or motivation-related problem. Skill-related problems can be solved through informal training, such as demonstration and coaching, whereas complex skills require formal training (e.g., in-service sessions or workshops). If there is a limit to the time an employee has to reach the desired level of skill, the manager must determine whether the job could be simplified or whether the better decision would be to terminate or transfer the employee.

If the performance problem is due to motivation rather than ability, the manager must address a different set of questions. Specifically, the manager must determine whether the employee believes that there are obstacles to the expected behavior or that the behavior leads to punishment, reward, or inaction. For example, if the reward for conscientiously coming to work on holidays (rather than calling in sick) leads to always being scheduled for holiday work, then good performance is associated with punishment.

Only when the employee sees a strong link between valued outcomes and meeting performance expectations will motivation strategies succeed. The manager plays a role in tailoring motivational efforts to meet the individual needs of the employee (see Chapter 17). Unfortunately, creating a performance–reward climate does not eliminate all problem behaviors. When

**Figure 18-1** ●
Decision tree
for evaluating
performance.

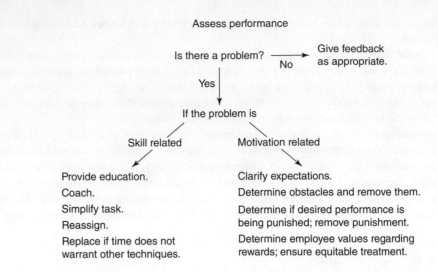

the use of rewards proves ineffective, other strategies, such as coaching and discipline, are warranted (see Chapter 19).

To differentiate between lack of ability and lack of motivation, the manager can analyze past performance. If past performance has been acceptable and little change in standards of performance has taken place, then the problem results from a lack of motivation. In contrast, if the nurse has never performed at an acceptable level, then the problem may be primarily skill related. Different intervention strategies should be used, depending on the source of the problem. The objective should be to enhance performance rather than to punish the employee. Figure 18-1 summarizes the steps to take.

## The Performance Appraisal Interview

Once the manager completes an accurate evaluation of performance, an appraisal interview can be scheduled. The appraisal interview is the first step in employee development.

### Preparing for the Interview

Keep in mind what needs to be accomplished during the interview. If the appraisal ratings are accurate, they are more likely to be perceived as such by the employee. This perception should, in turn, make the employee more likely to accept them as a basis for both rewards as well as developmental activities. More specifically, to motivate employees, rewards need to be seen as linked to performance.

The performance appraisal interview is the key to this linkage. In the interview, establish that performance has been carefully assessed and that, when merited, rewards will be forthcoming. Developmental activities also need to be derived from an accurate evaluation. If an employee is rated as "needs immediate improvement" on delegation skills, for example, any effort to remedy this deficiency must stem from the employee's acceptance of the need for improvement in delegation.

Even though managers try to fill out the appraisal form accurately, they should still anticipate disagreement with their ratings. Most employees tend to see themselves as above-average performers. This tendency to exaggerate our own performance results from the fact that we tend to forget our mistakes and recall our accomplishments; we often rationalize away those instances where our performance was substandard (e.g., "I forgot, but with this heavy workload, what do you expect?"). Given this tendency to over evaluate one's own performance and the fact that most staff previously have had poor experiences with the evaluation process, expect that staff will lack confidence in the whole appraisal process.

A key step for making the appraisal interview go well is to set up the performance appraisal interview in advance, preferably giving at least two days' notice. Schedule enough time: most interviews last 20 to 30 minutes, although the time needed will vary considerably depending on the degree to which the nurse manager and the staff nurse have talked regularly during the year.

In preparing for the appraisal interview, have specific examples of behavior to support the ratings. Such documentation is particularly important for performance areas in which an employee receives low ratings. In addition, try to anticipate how the staff member will react to the appraisal. For example, will the individual challenge the manager's ratings as being too low? Anticipating such a reaction, one can respond by saying, "Before I made my ratings, I talked with two other unit managers to make sure my standards were reasonable."

The setting should also be considered in planning the meeting. It is critical that the interview take place in a setting that is private and relatively free from interruptions. This allows a frank, in-depth conversation with the employee. Although it is difficult to limit interruptions in a health care setting, choosing the meeting time carefully will help. You may be able to schedule the meeting when another manager can cover, or at a time when interruptions are least likely to occur. The most important point to remember is that a poor setting limits the usefulness of the interview. No one wants weaknesses discussed in public. Similarly, interruptions destroy the flow of the feedback session.

## The Interview

The appraisal interview is most likely to go well if the nurse manager has written and shared critical incidents throughout the evaluation period. If such feedback has occurred, staff members go into the interview with a good idea of how they are likely to be rated, as well as what behaviors led to the rating. If the nurse manager has not kept notes throughout the year, it is important to recall numerous, specific examples of behavior, both positive and negative, to support the ratings given.

The major focus of the feedback interview should be on how the nurse manager and the staff member can work together to improve performance in the coming year. However, establishing such an improvement-oriented climate is easier said than done. In giving feedback, be aware that every employee has a tolerance level for criticism beyond which defensiveness sets in. Thus, in reviewing an employee's performance, emphasize only a few areas—preferably, no more than two—that need immediate improvement.

Unfortunately, evaluators often exceed an employee's tolerance level, particularly if performance has been mediocre. Typically, the manager will come up with an extensive list of areas needing improvement. Confronted with such a list, the staff member gradually moves from a constructive frame of mind ("I need to work on that") after one or two criticisms are raised to a destructive perspective ("She doesn't like me," "He's nitpicking," "How can I get even?") as the list of criticisms continues.

Following are recommendations for conducting an appraisal interview:

1. *Put the employee at ease.* Most individuals are nervous at the start of the appraisal interview, especially new employees who are facing their first evaluation or those who have not received frequent performance feedback from their manager over the course of the evaluation period. Begin the interview by giving an overview of the type of information that was used in making the performance ratings, such as, "In preparing for this review, I relied on the notes I have taken and shared with you throughout the year." Rather than trying to reduce the tension an employee may have at the start of the interview, it is better to ignore it.

2. *Clearly state the purpose of the appraisal interview.* An improvement-oriented theme should be conveyed at the beginning of the interview, can lead to identifying development activities, and will help the employee do the best possible job in the coming year.

3. *Go through the ratings one by one with the employee.* Provide a number of specific examples of behavior that led to each rating. Be careful not to rush. By systematically going through the ratings and providing behavioral examples, nurse managers project an image of being prepared and of being a professional. This is important for getting the staff nurse to accept the ratings and act on them.

4. *Draw out the employee's reactions to the ratings.* Ask for the employee's reaction to the ratings and then listen, accept, and respond to them. Of the seven key behaviors for doing performance reviews, nurse managers have the most difficulty with this one. To carry out this phase of the interview effectively, you must have confidence in the accuracy of the ratings.

   When asked to express their reactions, individuals who have received low ratings will frequently question the rater's judgment ("Don't you think your standards are a little high?"). Not surprisingly, the manager whose judgment has been questioned tends to get defensive, cutting off the employee's remarks and arguing for the rating in question. Being cut off sends a contradictory message to the employee. The individual was asked for reactions, but when given, the supervisor did not want to hear them. You should anticipate that the ratings will be challenged and must truly want to hear the staff nurse's reaction to them.

   After having listened to the employee's reactions, accept and respond to them in a manner that conveys that you have heard what the employee said (e.g., paraphrase some of the comments) and accept the individual's opinion ("I understand your view"). In addition, you may want to clarify what has been said ("I do not understand why you feel your initiative rating is too low. Could you cite specific behavior to justify a higher rating?"). Strive for a candid, two-way conversation to find out exactly how the employee feels.

5. *Decide on specific ways in which performance areas can be strengthened.* The focus of the interview should now shift to the future. If a thorough review of an employee's performance reveals deficiencies, you and the employee may jointly develop action plans to help the individual improve. An action plan describes mutually agreed-on activities for improving performance. Such developmental activities may include formal training, academic course work, or on-the-job coaching. Together, you and the staff nurse should write down the resulting plans.

   Because of the possibility of defensiveness, address only one or two performance areas needing improvement. Choose only the areas that are most troublesome and focus attention on these. In arriving at plans for improving performance, begin by asking the staff member for ideas on how to enhance personal performance. After the individual has offered suggestions, you can offer additional suggestions.

   It is critical that such performance plans refer to specific behavior. In some cases, not only will the staff member be expected to do things in a different manner ("I will refer to a patient as Mr., Mrs., or Ms. unless specifically told otherwise"), but you may also be expected to change your behavior ("I will post changes in hospital policy before enforcing them").

6. *Set a follow-up date.* After having agreed on specific ways to strengthen performance in problem areas, schedule a subsequent meeting, usually four to six weeks after the appraisal interview. At this later meeting, provide specific feedback on the nurse's recent performance.

   This meeting also gives you and the nurse an opportunity to discuss any problems they have encountered in attempting to carry out their agreed-on performance/improvement plans. In most cases, this follow-up session is quite positive. With only one or two areas to work on and a specific date on which feedback will be given, the nurse's performance usually improves dramatically. Thus, the follow-up meeting is one in which you have the opportunity to praise the employee.

7. *Express confidence in the employee.* The final key behavior is simple but often over-looked. It is nevertheless important that a manager indicate confidence that improvement will be forthcoming.

Since no more than two problem areas should be addressed in the appraisal interview, other problem areas may be considered later in the year. If the targeted performance areas continue to improve significantly, then meet again with the staff member one or two weeks after this follow-up session to raise another area that needs attention. As before, develop and write down specific ways to improve the performance deficiency and schedule another follow-up meeting. In short, performance deficiencies are not ignored, they are merely temporarily overlooked.

## Potential Appraisal Problems

No matter what type of appraisal system is used, problems that lessen the accuracy of the performance rating can arise, such as leniency, recency, and halo errors; ambiguous evaluation standards; and written comments problems. These, in turn, limit the usefulness of the performance review.

### Leniency Error

Managers tend to overrate their staff's performance. This is called **leniency error**. For example, a manager may rate everyone on her or his staff as "above average." Although numerous reasons are given for inflated ratings (e.g., "I want my nurses to like me," "It's difficult to justify giving someone a low rating"), these reasons do not lessen the problems that leniency error can create for both the manager and the organization. If you give a mediocre nurse lenient ratings, it is difficult to turn around and take corrective action, such as discipline.

Leniency error can also be demoralizing to the best performers, because they would have received high ratings without leniency. However, with leniency error, these outstanding nurses look less superior compared to their coworkers. Thus, leniency error tends to be welcomed by poorer performers and disliked by better ones.

### Recency Error

Another difficulty with most appraisal systems is the length of time over which behavior is evaluated. In most organizations, employees are formally evaluated every 12 months. Evaluating employee performance over such an extended period of time, particularly if one supervises more than two or three individuals, is a difficult task. Typically, the evaluator recalls recent performance and tends to forget more distant events. Thus, the performance rating reflects what the employee has contributed lately rather than over the entire evaluation period. This tendency is called **recency error**; it too can create both legal and motivational problems.

> *Shelby Miller, RN, transferred from a medical unit to the telemetry unit nine months ago. Overall, her performance has been good and she is an excellent team member. On two occasions, other nursing staff told the nurse manager, Lucinda Amos, about Shelby's quick and accurate assessment of critical changes in patient status. Last week, Shelby mis-read a physician's order and didn't administer pre-procedure medications as directed. The procedure had to be rescheduled, resulting in surgical delays as well. The physician was angry and complained to both Lucinda and the cardiology nursing director. On her annual performance appraisal, Lucinda rated Shelby "below average" on patient care delivery.*

Legally, if a disgruntled employee can demonstrate that an evaluation that supposedly reflects 12 months actually reflects performance over the last 2 or 3 months, an organization will have difficulty defending the validity of its appraisal system. In terms of motivation, recency error demonstrates to all employees that they only need to perform at a high level near the time of their performance review. In such situations, an employee is highly motivated (e.g., asking the supervisor for more work) just prior to appraisal but considerably less motivated as soon as it is completed.

As with leniency error, recency error benefits the poorly performing individual. Nurses who perform well year-round may receive ratings similar to those mediocre nurses who noticeably improve as their evaluation time approaches. Fortunately, recording critical incidents during the year lessens the impact of recency error.

### Halo Error

Sometimes an appraiser fails to differentiate among the various performance dimensions (e.g., nursing process, communication skills) when evaluating an employee and assigns ratings on the basis of an overall impression, positive or negative, of the employee. Thus, some employees are rated above average across dimensions, others are rated average, and a few are rated below average on all dimensions. This is referred to as **halo error**.

If a nurse is excellent, average, or poor on all performance dimensions, she or he deserves to be rated accordingly, but in most instances, employees have uneven strengths and weaknesses. Thus, it should be relatively uncommon for an employee to receive the same rating on all performance dimensions. Although halo error is less common and troublesome than leniency and recency error, it still is not an accurate assessment of performance.

### Ambiguous Evaluation Standards

Most appraisal forms use rating scales that include words such as "outstanding," "above average," "satisfactory," or "needs improvement." However, different managers attach different meanings to these words, giving rise to what has been labeled the **ambiguous evaluation standards problem**.

One organization dealt with the problem by identifying core competencies and skill level descriptors and tagging them with evaluation criteria, such as "exceeds expectation," "meets expectation," or "requires improvement" (Schoessler et al., 2008). Senior leadership validated that competency statements met accepted standards. Another approach is to develop rating forms that have each gradation along the performance continuum (e.g., excellent, satisfactory) anchored by examples of behavior that is representative of that level of performance.

### Written Comments Problem

Almost all performance appraisal forms provide space for written comments by the appraiser. The wise manager uses this space to justify in detail the basis for the ratings, to discuss developmental activities for the employee in the coming year, to put the ratings in context (e.g., although the evaluation period is 12 months, the appraiser notes on the form that he or she has only been the nurse's manager for the past 3 months), or to discuss the employee's promotion potential. Unfortunately, few nurse managers use this valuable space appropriately; in fact, the spaces for written comments are often left blank. When there are comments, they tend to be few and general (e.g., "Joan is conscientious"), focus totally on what the individual did wrong, or reflect only recent performance.

> *Dawn Stanley, RN, is director of nursing for an assisted living center. Two certified nurse aides transferred to her center from other facilities in the health care system. Both CNAs have struggled to meet performance expectations in the first 90 days of their new positions. In preparing performance appraisals for both employees, Dawn reviewed previous appraisals to see if other managers had indicated areas for improvement or performance trends. Both employees were rated as "marginal performers" but no written comments were provided, making the appraisal process more difficult for Dawn.*

The existence of the **written comments problem** should not be surprising. Most managers wait until the end of the evaluation period to make written comments; thus, the manager is faced with a difficult, time-consuming task. Small wonder, then, that the few comments tend to be vague, negative in tone, and reflect recent events. Fortunately, regular note taking can lessen the problems associated with written comments.

# Improving Appraisal Accuracy

For the manager and employee to get maximum benefit from an appraisal, it needs to encompass all facets of job performance and be free from rater error. Although attempting to get completely accurate evaluations is often impossible, there are ways to greatly improve the accuracy of appraisals.

## Appraiser Ability

Accurately evaluating an employee's performance involves using the job description, skill level descriptors, or core competency statements to identify behaviors required, then observing the employee's performance over the course of the evaluation period and recalling it, and knowing how to use the appraisal form accurately. To the extent that any of these things are lacking, a manager's ability to rate accurately is limited.

Fortunately, a manager's ability to rate employees can be improved. An organization can develop detailed job descriptions, skill level descriptors, and competency statements. The rater can be given more opportunities to directly or indirectly observe an employee's behavior. For example, other supervisors can provide information on an employee's performance when the immediate supervisor is not present. Managers can be taught to take notes on an employee's behavior to facilitate recall. In addition, managers can learn to use the appraisal form better through formal training.

Formal training programs help to increase appraiser ability by making raters aware of the various types of rating errors (the assumption being that awareness may reduce the error tendency), by improving raters' observational skills, and by improving raters' skill in carrying out the performance appraisal interview.

> *Simone Hurtado is team manager for the pediatric home services team. In previous years, Simone has struggled to adequately evaluate her employees. Since all of the patient care is delivered in client's homes, Simone relied on sporadic client feedback and review of patient care documentation to complete employee appraisals. Recently Simone attended an appraisal workshop. Using some of the suggested strategies, Simone and the other team managers have set up an observation schedule for their employees. Each employee will be randomly observed by a team manager in a client's home every six to eight weeks. Additionally, employees will be asked to complete self-evaluations as well as evaluations of other team members they work with on a regular basis. Simone has also established a system for compiling ongoing employee performance documentation.*

## Appraiser Motivation

Managers have a multitude of tasks to perform, often immediately. Not surprisingly, then, they often view performance appraisals as a task that can be done later. Furthermore, many managers do not see doing appraisals as particularly important, and some question the need for doing them at all. This is especially true if all employees receive the same percentage salary increase. Thus, if nurse managers are to be motivated to do appraisals well, they need to be rewarded for their efforts.

A nurse manager may spend little time on appraisals for several reasons:

- The organization does not reward the person for doing a good job.
- The manager's supervisor spends little time on the manager's own appraisal (thus sending the message that doing appraisals is not important).
- If a manager gives low ratings to a poor employee, a superior may overrule and raise the ratings.

In short, in many health care organizations, the environment may actually dampen appraiser motivation rather than stimulate it. Given these reasons for not spending time on appraisals, it is fairly obvious how an organization can enhance appraiser motivation:

- The manager needs to be rewarded for conscientiously doing performance reviews.
- The manager's supervisor needs to present a good model of how an appraisal should be carried out.
- As far as possible, the manager should be able to reward the highly rated staff.

This becomes more likely as outcomes are used as the basis for reimbursement to the organization and, subsequently, the organization bases rewards on productivity. For the organization and its employees to benefit from the performance appraisal system, pay increases should not be across the board, layoffs should not be based on seniority, and promotions should be tied to superior performance.

Learn how one manager used a performance evaluation to help a staff member and benefit the organization at the same time (see Case Study 18-1).

## CASE STUDY 18-1

### EVALUATING STAFF

Brenda Tice has been nurse manager for the medical intensive care unit (MICU) in a large urban hospital for six months. The MICU rarely has staff openings and the average nurse has 12 years of experience on the unit. Brenda herself was a nurse on the unit for 10 years prior to her promotion to nurse manager.

Lori Cook has been an RN on the MICU day shift for the past 18 months. Lori is pleasant and tries hard to please her patients and coworkers. However, she consistently stays late to complete her charting, relies heavily on coworkers to help her throughout the shift, and has little confidence in her own ability to handle complex patients. Often Lori will break down and cry during a patient code and is seemingly overwhelmed by the code process. Although the other nurses are supportive of Lori, they are aware of her limitations. Several nurses have complained when they have been assigned two high acuity patients and Lori is assigned one lower acuity patient.

Brenda discussed the issues with Lori. Brenda told Lori that she would help her attempt remediation as part of an action plan for performance improvement in order to meet minimum expectations for her position. Brenda arranged for Lori to attend several training programs designed specifically for ICU nurses, provided opportunities for experienced nurses to mentor Lori on more complex patients, and provided her with reference materials to reinforce Lori's skill set. Brenda also reviewed Lori's personnel records for the past 18 months. While Lori is rated high for attendance and her interpersonal skills, her clinical skills are rated as fair. Brenda notices three separate performance counseling documents dated within the past 12 months, with little improvement noted in her clinical performance.

Following another code incident in which Lori started crying and was asked to leave by a physician, Brenda determines that while Lori has many positive qualities, she does not have the clinical skills necessary to function independently in the MICU. Brenda had provided Lori with an action plan and fair warning and conversation about her not meeting expectation in the ICU and shared that Lori may not be a fit in the ICU environment. After contacting the human resources department to discuss the transfer process because of Lori's continued lack of ability to meet ICU performance expectations, she schedules a meeting with Lori to discuss her performance issues. Brenda reviews the performance concerns with Lori and informs her that due to her continued lack of ability to meet expectations she has 30 days to accept reassignment within the hospital to a unit that more closely matches her clinical abilities. Lori decides to interview for positions in the geriatric psychiatric unit and the psychiatric day treatment program.

### Manager's Checklist

The nurse manager is responsible for:

- Understanding the performance appraisal process and appraisal tools used by the organization
- Providing honest and timely feedback to all employees
- Communicating as needed with the human resources department when performance issues arise
- Accurately and thoroughly documenting all performance-related issues
- Identifying the impact of poor performers on the morale and productivity of staff
- Making staffing decisions in a timely manner

# Rules of Thumb

For approximately five percent of employees, the prescriptions given in this chapter will not work, for reasons yet unknown. Additional suggestions or "rules of thumb" derived from practical experience include the following:

- *Go beyond the form.* Too often, people doing evaluations cite an inadequate form as an excuse for doing a poor job of evaluating their employees. No matter how inadequate an appraisal form is, managers can go beyond it. They can focus on behavior even if the form does not require it. They can set goals even if other supervisors do not. They can use critical incidents. In short, managers should do the best job of managing they can and not let the form handicap them.

- *Postpone the appraisal interview if necessary.* Once the appraisal interview begins, there is often the belief that the session must be completed in the time allotted, whether the session is going well or not. Managers forget the goal of the appraisal interview is not merely to get an employee's signature on the form but also to get the employee to improve performance in the coming year. Therefore, if the interview is not going well, a manager should discontinue it until a later time. Such a postponement allows both the manager and the employee some time to reflect on what has transpired as well as some time to calm down.

    In postponing the meeting, the manager should not assign blame ("If you're going to act like a child, let's postpone the meeting"), but should adopt a more positive approach ("This meeting isn't going as I hoped it would; I'd like to postpone it to give us some time to collect our thoughts"). Most managers who have used this technique find that the second session, which generally takes place one to two days later, goes much better.

- *Don't be afraid to change an inaccurate rating.* New managers often ask whether they should change a rating if an employee challenges it. They fear that by changing a rating, they will be admitting an error. They also fear that changing a rating will lead to other ratings being challenged. A practical rule of thumb for this situation is if the rating is inaccurate, change it, but never change it during the appraisal interview. Rather, if an employee challenges a rating and the manager believes the employee has a case, the manager should tell the person that some time is needed to think about the rating before getting back to the employee.

    The logic behind this rule of thumb is as follows: If a manager does a careful job of evaluating performance, few inaccurate ratings will be made. But no one is perfect, and on occasion, managers will err. When such an error occurs, the manager should correct it. Most employees respect a manager who admits a mistake and corrects it. By allowing for time to reflect on the ratings, a manager eliminates the pressure to make a snap judgment.

An effective performance evaluation contributes to the employee's development, improves job satisfaction, and enhances employee morale. Learning how to evaluate employees is one of the nurse manager's useful activities.

## What You Know Now

- Doing performance appraisals is one of the most difficult and most important management activities.
- Accurate appraisals provide a sound basis for both administrative decisions (e.g., salary increases, promotions) and employee development.
- The evaluations system may be results oriented or based on behavioral criteria.
- Evaluation standards must be based on identified criteria, such as job descriptions, skill level descriptors, or core competencies, and based on performance as evaluated over the course of a year.
- To enhance the accuracy of the performance appraisal, the manager should record critical incidents throughout the evaluation period.
- Self-evaluation, peer review, group evaluations, and the manager's evaluation are examples of ways to collect evidence of performance.

- To improve the value of the appraisal interview, the manager should follow the key behaviors for conducting an appraisal interview.
- Problems with employee appraisal include leniency error, recency error, halo error, ambiguous standards, and the inadequate use of written comments.
- The manager's ability to accurately evaluate staff can be improved through formal training and a positive example from the manager's supervisor.

## Tools for Evaluating Staff Performance

1. Become familiar with the evaluation process adopted by your organization.
2. Familiarize yourself with the appraisal instrument used for staff evaluation.
3. Learn to use critical incidents and include positive behaviors as well as those needing improvement.
4. Be alert to the chances for error in the appraisal process.
5. Prepare for an appraisal interview using the strategies suggested in the chapter.
6. Follow the key behaviors for conducting an appraisal interview.

## Questions to Challenge You

1. What evaluation method is used at your workplace or clinical site? If you do not know, find out and share it with a colleague or class.
2. If you have been evaluated in the skills lab, on a simulator, or at the point of care, which assessment best evaluated your skills?
3. What components of your job (or clinical placement) are evaluated? Are they the appropriate ones?
4. What types of assessment methods have been used to evaluate you? Were they the best ones to evaluate your performance? What would you suggest?
5. If you have been evaluated as an employee, did your evaluator follow the key behaviors in this chapter? What improvements would you suggest?
6. Have you ever evaluated someone else's performance at work? How closely did your actions follow the suggestions in the chapter?

**Pearson Nursing Student Resources**

Find additional review materials at

**www.nursing.pearsonhighered.com**

Prepare for success with additional NCLEX®-style practice questions, interactive assignments and activities, Web links, animations and videos, and more!

## References

Davis, K. K., Capozzoli, J., & Parks, J. (2009). Implementing peer review: Guidelines for managers and staff. *Nursing Administration Quarterly, 33*(3), 251–257.

Joint Commission. (2011). Comprehensive accreditation manual for hospitals: The official handbook. Retrieved July 28, 2011 from http://www.jcrinc.com/Accreditation-Manuals/PCAH11/2130/

Schoessler, M. T., Aneshansley, P., Baffaro, C., Castellan, T., Goins, L., Largaespada, E., Payne, R., & Stinson, D. (2008). The performance appraisal as a developmental tool. *Journal for Nurses in Staff Development, 24*(3), E12–E18.

Topjian, D. F., Buck, T., & Kozlowski, R. (2009). Employee performance? For the good of all. *Nursing Management, 40*(4), 24–29.

# Coaching, Disciplining, and Terminating Staff

Day-to-Day Coaching

Positive Coaching

Dealing with a Policy Violation

Disciplining Staff

Terminating Employees

## Learning Outcomes

*After completing this chapter, you will be able to:*

1. Describe how to coach an employee.
2. Discuss positive coaching.
3. Explain how to confront an employee about a policy violation.

4. Discuss how to discipline an employee.
5. Describe how to terminate an employee.

## Key Terms

Coaching
Discipline

Progressive discipline
Terminate

One of the most challenging problems for managers is knowing what to do when employees fail to perform to expectations. Managers often want to ignore the problems, hoping they'll disappear, but that seldom happens. Instead, the manager can learn how to handle these problems.

## Day-to-Day Coaching

**Coaching**, the day-to-day process of helping employees improve their performance, is an important tool for effective nurse managers. Yet coaching is probably the most difficult task in management and is often neglected. In one short interaction, it encompasses needs analysis, staff development, interviewing, decision making, problem solving, analytical thinking, active listening, motivation, mentoring, and communication skills. Intervening immediately in performance problems on a day-to-day basis usually eliminates small problems before they become larger ones and the subject of discussion in performance appraisal interviews or disciplinary actions. Coaching should also be used when performance meets the standard but improvement can still be obtained.

The goal of coaching is to eliminate or improve performance problems, but few nurses are prepared to coach and are often hesitant to confront employee problems. Coaching employees when the problem initially surfaces can potentially save time, prevent poor morale from occurring, and avoid more difficult action later, such as discipline or termination (Palermo, 2007). Additionally, appropriate and timely coaching can help retain employees and reduce turnover (Stedman & Nolan, 2007). (See Chapter 20 for more on reducing turnover and retaining staff.)

Examples of problems that coaching can improve or eliminate are incorrect flow sheet documentation, excessive absenteeism, or frequent personal phone calls or excessive texting. Before entering into a coaching session, the nurse manager (coach) should prepare for the interaction and try to anticipate how the employee will react ("Everybody gets personal phone calls") in order to formulate an appropriate response ("I am here to talk about the number of personal phone calls you receive"). In general, coaching sessions should last no more than 5 to 10 minutes. The steps in successful coaching are:

1. *State the targeted performance in behavioral terms.* "For the past two days, the physical assessment portions of your flow sheets have not been filled out."

2. *Tie the problem to consequences for patient care, the functioning of the organization, or the person's self-interest.* "It's difficult for other nurses and physicians to know whether the patient's status is changing, and therefore it's hard to know how to treat the patient. Physical assessments are a standard of practice in our unit. Failure to document assessments could lead to legal problems should the patient's record go before a court of law." This is an important but often overlooked step because it cannot be taken for granted that the employee knows why the behavior is a problem. If employees are expected to act in a certain way, they need to understand why the behavior is important and be rewarded when it has improved. Avoid threatening language, such as "If you want to stay in this unit, you had better complete your documentation." This puts the employee on the defensive and makes the person less receptive to change.

3. *Having stated the problem behavior, avoid jumping to conclusions but instead explore reasons for the problem with the employee.* Listen openly as the employee describes the problem and the reasons for it. If the problem was caused by ignorance—for instance, lack of familiarity with the standard of care on performing and documenting assessments—simply inform the nurse of the appropriate behavior and end the coaching session.

4. *Ask the employee for his or her suggestions and discuss ideas for how to solve the problem.* In many cases, the employee knows best how to solve the problem and is more likely to be committed to the solution if it is his or her own. It is better to encourage employees to solve their own problems; however, this does not mean that managers cannot add suggestions for improvement. It is essential to listen openly to understand the employee's perspectives.

5. *How formal should the coaching session be?* If the problem is minor and a first-time occurrence, you may simply state what actions will be taken to solve the problem and end the meeting. In most cases, however, you and the employee should agree on specific behavioral steps each will take to solve the problem; write down these steps for later reference.

6. *Arrange for a follow-up meeting, at which time the employee will receive performance feedback.* It is possible that an employee may bring up personal problems as a cause for the work problems. The coaching session then verges on becoming a counseling session. When the employee brings up personal problems, nurse managers should convey their concern and willingness to work with the employee to get help for the problems. In most cases, nurse managers will not be the direct source of the help but rather will help the employee seek out other, more appropriate, sources, such as the organization's employee assistance program. Do not delve into potential personal problems ("Are there problems at home that I should know about?") unless staff raise them. The employee's personal life is not the manager's business.

## Positive Coaching

Coaching as a strategy to improve problem performance has been discussed, but coaching can also be used as tool to reinforce positive behaviors (Karsten et al., 2010). In fact, negativity is a far more common experience than a positive experience (Huseman, 2009). Coaching can be a leadership development tool as well.

Coaching has been shown to help leaders become more confident and competent and to improve their team's functioning as well (McDermott & Levenson, 2007; McNally & Lukens, 2007). Coaching leaders is especially useful during times of transition, but historically, asking a leader to use a coach has been seen as punitive (Karsten et al., 2010). Often a senior executive uses a coach to model the importance to administrative staff. Coaching administrators is also a strategy for succession planning (McNally & Lukens, 2006).

Leadership coaching can be undertaken as one-on-one interactions with a coach, a group with similar needs participating in coaching sessions together, or individual and group sessions. Such coaching is results oriented, and its purpose is to help the participant become more self-aware, ensure accountability, and attain professional goals (McNally & Lukens, 2006).

## Dealing with a Policy Violation

As with day-to-day coaching, the manager must prepare to confront an employee about a policy violation. The leadership style of the manager is important in determining whether the employee perceives that he or she is being told what to do versus being sold on the idea that she or he is an important contributor to the staff. The steps involved in confrontation are similar to coaching. These steps are outlined in Box 19-1.

The first key behavior is to determine whether the employee is aware of the policy. The employee should have received policy information at orientation, and an updated policy manual should be readily accessible to all employees. It is also important to know whether the policy has been enforced consistently. If policies regarding tardiness are not applied to everyone on a daily basis, efforts to change this behavior in one individual predictably will be unsuccessful. It is better to identify policies and procedures that the majority of staff accept and to determine which employees need direction in compliance.

Second, describe the behavior that violated the policy in a manner that conveys concern to the employee regarding the outcome. By focusing on the employee's behavior, you avoid making the interaction a personal issue.

After stating that the policy has been violated, obtain a document that states the policy so that interpretation issues can be clarified. For example, if the policy being violated is the requirement that nurses report to a peer about their patients when leaving the unit, have a copy of the policy in hand.

## BOX 19-1 Steps in Confrontation

1. Prepare before the meeting.

Is the employee aware of the policy and procedure? Desired behavior?

Has the policy/procedure been consistently enforced?

How will the employee react?

2. Without attacking the person, describe the undesired behavior. Tie that behavior to its consequences for the patients, organization, or employee.

Jane, were you aware that it is clinic policy to notify *both* the clinic manager and the hospital supervisor when you will be absent from work? Not only were we worried about you, but we had to reschedule patient procedures because we did not have the staff to attend to both clinic appointments and special procedures.

3. Solicit and openly listen with empathy to the employee's reasons for the behavior.

Why didn't you notify someone about your absence?

4. Explain why the behavior cannot continue, and ask for suggestions in solving the problem. If none are offered, suggest solutions. Agree on steps each will take to solve the problem.

In the future, you will need to notify both the clinic manager and the hospital supervisor if you cannot come in. How do you suppose you might do this, since you do not have a phone?

5. Set and record a specific follow-up date.

Can we meet again in one month to review this plan?

The next step is to solicit the employee's reason for the behavior (e.g., what is preventing the person from informing a peer about patients when leaving the unit). Allow sufficient time for the employee to respond while at the same time guarding against the pursuit of extraneous, unrelated issues. In the latter event, redirect the employee's attention to the policy violation and suggest dealing with other issues at another time.

Convey to the employee that she or he cannot continue breaking an established policy. In the previous example, you could discuss the effects of the behavior, such as medications not given, IVs running dry, and patients being left unattended, as reasons for having the policy.

Next, explore alternative solutions so that negative outcomes will be avoided. Ask the employee for suggestions for solving the problem, and discuss each of the suggestions. Offer help if it is appropriate. Decide and agree on a course of action. The last step in the process is to set up a reasonable date to follow up with the employee on adherence to the established policy.

Although dealing with policy violations in a distinct step-by-step sequence is not always possible, proceed in an orderly manner. Many policy violations require early and decisive interventions, and these must be handled in an immediate, forthright manner.

## Disciplining Staff

Most managers dread having to **discipline** an employee. Nevertheless, there will be occasions where discipline is necessary (e.g., when a regulation has been violated that jeopardizes patient safety). Managers may hesitate to discipline for many reasons, including:

- Lack of management support or training
- Letting past inappropriate behavior go by without mention
- Rationalizing to avoid disciplining
- Previous poor experience with attempting to discipline employees
- Fear that the employee will respond negatively (White, 2006)

Learning how to discipline effectively can reduce your concerns and improve morale for all employees. Keep in mind, though, that the primary function of discipline is not to punish the guilty party, but to teach new skills and encourage that person and others to behave appropriately in the future.

## BOX 19-2  Guidelines for Effective Discipline

1. Get the facts before acting.
2. Do not act while you are angry.
3. Do not suddenly tighten your enforcement of rules.
4. Do not apply penalties inconsistently.
5. Discipline in private.
6. Make the offense clear. Specify what is appropriate behavior.
7. Get the other side of the story.
8. Do not let the disciplining become personal.
9. Do not back down when you are right.
10. Inform the human resources department and administration of the outcome and other pertinent details.

When faced with a disciplinary situation, maintain close contact with the organization's human resources department and administration. Before taking any disciplinary action, discuss the action you intend to take and seek approval for it. This close coordination with administration is essential to guarantee that any disciplinary action is administered in a fair and legally defensible manner.

To further ensure fairness, rules and regulations must be clearly communicated, a system of progressive penalties must be established, and an appeals process must be available. To enforce rules or regulations, managers must inform employees of them ahead of time, preferably in writing. Guidelines for effective discipline can be found in Box 19-2.

Penalties should be progressive. **Progressive discipline** is the process of increasingly severe warnings for repeated violations that can result in termination. Questions to ask include:

- How many different offenses are involved?
- What is the seriousness of the offense?
- What were the time interval and employee responses to prior disciplinary action?
- What is the previous work history of the employee?

Penalties are also progressive, beginning with a verbal warning (Box 19-3), and followed by a written warning (Box 19-4), suspension, and discharge.

For minor violations (e.g., smoking outside in an unauthorized area), penalties may progress from an oral warning, to a written warning placed in the employee's personnel folder, to a suspension, and ultimately to discharge. For major rule violations (e.g., theft of property), however, initial penalties should be more severe (e.g., immediate suspension).

## BOX 19-3  Verbal Warning Form

Employee's name:
Date of verbal warning:
Specific offense or rule violation:
Specific statement of the expected performance:



Any explanation given by the employee or other significant information:




_____
Supervisor

Date _____

| BOX 19-4 | Written Warning Form |
|---|---|

Employee's name:
Date of conversation:
Specific rule violation or performance problem:


Previous conversations about the rule violation or performance problem:


Specific change in the employee's performance or behavior expected:


Employee's comments:


Supervisor's comments:


Employee's signature:
-or-
Employee was asked to sign this written warning on _____ but declined to sign.

_____
Supervisor

Date _____

At each stage of the disciplinary process, documentation is essential. In addition, an appeals process should be built into an organization's disciplinary procedures to ensure that discipline is carried out in a fair, consistent manner.

Case Study 19-1 shows how one nurse manager handled a disciplinary problem.

## Terminating Employees

Unfortunately, some employees do not respond to either coaching or discipline, and nurse managers will face the day when they must **terminate**, or fire, an employee (Bing, 2007). The steps in terminating an employee are similar to those for disciplining, except there are no plans to correct the behavior and no follow-up. As with a disciplinary action, nurse managers must maintain close contact with the organization's human resource department and nursing administration. They must discuss the termination and seek approval for it.

Preparation before terminating an employee is essential (Cohen, 2006). To prepare, answer the following questions:

1. Did you set your expectations clearly from the beginning? Did you review the job description, performance appraisal criteria, and pertinent policies and procedures with the employee? These expectations should have been in writing.

2. Did you document the employee's performance on a continuing basis, using the critical incident or a similar method?

## CASE STUDY 19-1

### PROGRESSIVE DISCIPLINE

Katie Connors is nurse manager of the birthing center in a metropolitan hospital. The hospital has several different nursing programs that utilize various patient care units for clinical instruction. A student nurse, Amber Schroeder, was assigned to work with Natalie Cole, RN, for the day shift. Natalie and Amber's patient arrives at the birthing center for induction of labor. During the admission process, the patient confides to Natalie and Amber that she is terrified that she might need a caesarean section. Amber tells the patient that a young woman and her baby recently died at the hospital during an emergency C-section. The patient begins to hyperventilate, refuses to let Natalie continue with the admission, and threatens to leave the birthing center. Natalie is so angry at Amber for scaring the patient that she grabs her by the arm and pulls her out of the room. Natalie loudly berates Amber in the hallway to the point that Amber is crying.

Katie hears the commotion in the hallway and instructs Amber to sit in the staff lounge until her instructor can return to the unit. Katie and Natalie reassure the patient, who allows Natalie to complete the admission process. Throughout the shift, Natalie tells every staff member and physician about Amber's "stupid comment." Katie speaks with the nursing instructor and Amber about the incident. She also checks back with the patient and gently gathers facts about the incident.

Katie is concerned about Natalie's response to the situation. While Natalie has excellent nursing skills, she has often been abrupt or rude to other staff members. Katie has coached Natalie on her communication skills in three other specific incidents and verbally warned Natalie about her lack of professional communication. After discussing the incident with the human resources manager, Katie agrees that a written warning will be placed in Natalie's personnel file.

At the end of the shift, Katie requests that Natalie come to her office to discuss what happened with the student nurse. Katie informs Natalie she is disappointed in how she reacted to the inappropriate comment made by the student nurse. Specifically, physically grabbing the student and verbally attacking her in front of patients and staff was unacceptable and violates hospital policy. Further, Natalie continued to disparage the student to other staff and physicians, which is also unacceptable. Natalie expresses her frustration at the thoughtlessness of Amber's comment. Katie tells Natalie that while Amber's comment was inappropriate, Natalie's response was also inappropriate. Katie reinforces to Natalie the importance of professional communication at all times and reviews the communication points she had provided to Natalie in the past. She also informs Natalie that she will have a written warning placed in her personnel file. Natalie apologizes for her actions and assures Katie she will work on her communication skills. Katie documents the incident and follow-up action in Natalie's personnel file.

### Manager's Checklist

The nurse manager is responsible for:

- Collecting all necessary facts related to the disciplinary situation
- Communicating with the human resources department and nursing administration about the offense and appropriate penalty
- Disciplining the employee in a timely manner
- Providing strategies to the disciplined employee to improve his or her behavior
- Clearly and firmly communicating expectations for appropriate behavior
- Documenting the outcome of the discipline as appropriate
- Following up with the human resources department and nursing administration regarding the outcome of the discipline

3. Did you keep the employee informed about his or her performance on a regular basis?

4. Did you conduct coaching sessions or deal with policy or procedure violations in a timely manner? Were the sessions and the agreed-on actions in these meetings documented?

5. Were you honest with the employee about the poor performance or the policy that was violated? Were you specific about behaviors that failed to meet expected standards? Was the expected performance stated in behavioral terms?

6. Were you consistent among employees in how you dealt with performance issues and policy or procedure violations?

7. Did you follow up? Did you deliver the actions you agreed to in the coaching sessions?

8. Did you document everything in writing? The importance of this cannot be overstated.

9. Have you notified security so that the terminated employee may be escorted out?

This checklist applies to almost every instance of termination. The few exceptions might be theft or physical abuse of a patient or assault on others. Even in the latter instances, observation and documentation are crucial to avoid legal challenges.

A sample script for a termination conversation is shown in Box 19-5.

See how one manager handled terminating an employee in Case Study 19-2.

Terminating an employee affects the morale of the entire unit. Coworkers may take sides, and the manager may need to share pertinent facts if they relate to patient safety or acceptable behavioral standards. Not terminating poor performing staff, conversely, can hurt the manager's credibility and decrease performance on the unit (Hader, 2006).

Employees cannot be fired simply for being a member of a protected class, including their race, sex, national origin, or religion, or their disability as long as their disability does not prevent them from doing their job. In addition, a nurse, for example, cannot be fired for refusing to follow medical orders that he or she believes might harm a patient.

Even with careful documentation and the most conscientious adherence to organizational policies regarding termination, firing an employee may be followed by legal action, grievance procedures, and stressful and time-consuming hearings. A preferable alternative is that the employee voluntarily resign. Careful documentation may allow the manager to suggest that the employee voluntarily leave the organization. This allows the employee to leave without a record of termination.

Being a nurse manager is a challenging, ever-changing job and seldom more difficult than when employees must be disciplined or terminated. Even coaching employees can be a stressful experience. Developing the skills to intervene early with employee problems and follow-up as necessary should the problem continue or escalate will help reduce incidents and improve performance and morale.

---

## BOX 19-5   Script for a Termination Conversation

Manager: Lucy, we are here today to have the conversation I told you we would be having about your attendance. On March 13, you received a written warning counseling for your attendance. Since then, you have accumulated the following unscheduled absences:

On March 17, you missed work because of car problems. Then on May 2, you didn't report to work because you said you forgot you were working, and then refused to come in. You have now accumulated eight incidents of unscheduled absence this year. Our hospital attendance policy states that the hospital relies on employees being dependable to take excellent care of patients and that when employee attendance interrupts the ability to provide excellent care, we must advance the corrective action process. At our hospital, eight absences in a 12-month period is considered an unacceptable, very serious violation of our hospital's policy.

Prior to today, you received a verbal counseling and a written warning for your attendance. At the time of your verbal counseling, you had accumulated the following unscheduled absences:

August 23, last year, you missed your shift at work, stating you had a family issue.

September 8, you missed work, stating you were ill.

September 24, you called in reporting GI illness and did not come to work.

November 20, you called in to work reporting you had overslept and wouldn't be reporting to work.

On November 25, you were given verbal counseling concerning your attendance. A copy of the policy was given to you at that time, your absences were reviewed, and you acknowledged that you understood you should not miss more work unplanned.

You continued to accumulate unscheduled absences and were given a written warning on February 1. These absences included the following:

On December, 16 you called in to work reporting a scheduling conflict.

On January 27, you called in and said you had a cold and weren't coming to work.

In addition to your verbal and written warnings, I, as your manager, spoke with you on other occasions as well to remind you about the attendance policy and the seriousness of your current attendance situation. You have continued to accumulate absences and have seriously violated the attendance policy despite multiple attempts at coaching. Therefore today, May 3, your employment is terminated. Human Resources is here with us to provide you all information on your benefits, retirement fund, and to answer any questions you have.

## CASE STUDY 19-2

### TERMINATING STAFF

Carrie Lyle is nurse manager of a 20-bed medical–surgical unit in a suburban hospital. Six months ago, Margaret Johnson, LPN, transferred to the unit from the skilled nursing unit. Carrie noted that although Margaret had been an employee of the hospital for 12 years, her personnel record included several entries regarding substandard performance. Carrie also found gaps in her performance appraisals from other units. Carrie discussed these issues with Margaret prior to her transfer and clearly indicated performance expectations. However, Margaret often arrives late to work and leaves before report is finished for the day shift.

Claire Kindred, RN and night shift charge nurse, has worked with Margaret for the past six months. Claire requested a meeting with Carrie to discuss patient care concerns. Claire indicated that during most shifts, Margaret takes extended meal and break times. She has been found sleeping during her shift in empty patient rooms. Recently, Claire helped one of Margaret's patients to the bathroom. When recording the patient's output, she noted that Margaret had charted the patient's IV intake for the entire shift even though it was only three hours into the night shift. When confronted, Margaret laughed and told Claire she was "just saving time." Claire had documented the dates of the incidents and provided them to Carrie.

Carrie met that evening with Margaret to discuss her performance and informed her that she will be on probation for the next 30 days. During the probation time, Margaret's performance would be reviewed each shift to ensure she is completely meeting all expectations for patient care and performance. The next morning, Robert Adams, RN, brought one of his patient's charts to Carrie's office. The patient had been assigned to Margaret on the night shift. In addition to diabetes, the patient has bilateral below-the-knee amputations. On the patient's physical assessment, Margaret had charted

positive pedal pulses. She also charted she had changed the patient's IV tubing and IV dressing. On closer inspection, Robert found that the date stickers had been covered over by new stickers and no IV tubing changes were noted on the patient's chart. Carrie immediately contacted the human resources department. She tells them that Margaret has falsified patient documentation in direct violation of her probation and hospital policy. The human resources department reviews Margaret's file and concurs that immediate termination is appropriate. Exit paperwork is initiated by the human resources department and forwarded to Carrie.

Carrie meets Margaret as she arrives for her scheduled shift. She asks Margaret to come into her office to discuss her immediate termination of employment. Margaret is visibly shaken and says "I'll do better," then "You can't do this to me." Carrie calmly outlines the performance problems and compliance issues that support Margaret's termination. She has a security officer escort Margaret to her locker to gather her personal items. Carrie documents the meeting outcome in Margaret's personnel file.

### Manager's Checklist

The nurse manager is responsible for:

- Understanding the organization's discipline and termination policies and procedures
- Reviewing personnel files and identifying past performance problems that may affect current or future performance
- Addressing employee performance issues in a timely manner
- Verifying performance problems rather than personality problems
- Working with the human resources department when employee termination is indicated

## What You Know Now

- Coaching is the day-to-day process of helping employees improve their performance or eliminate a performance problem.
- Coaching can reinforce positive behaviors, serve as a leadership development tool, and assist with succession planning.
- To confront an employee, make the employee aware of the policy violation and its consequences, elicit reasons for the behavior, and agree on steps to prevent future recurrence.
- When rule violations occur, disciplinary action is needed. Penalties should be progressive.
- When staff members do not respond to discipline, managers must terminate their employment.
- If an employee must be terminated, the manager must stay in close contact with the human resources department and administration when planning and carrying out the termination.

## Tools for Coaching, Disciplining, and Terminating Staff

1. To prepare and conduct a coaching session
   a. Note the behavior and why it is unacceptable
   b. Explore reasons for the behavior with the employee
   c. Ask the employee for suggestions to solve the problem
   d. Arrange for follow-up
2. To conduct a discipline session
   a. Be certain you are calm before beginning
   b. Assure privacy before beginning
   c. Apply rules consistently
   d. Get both sides of a story
   e. Keep the focus on the problem, not the person
   f. Arrange for follow-up
   g. Inform the human resources department and administration
3. To prepare to terminate a staff member
   a. Inform the human resources department and administration beforehand
   b. State the offending behavior and the reason for termination
   c. Explain the termination process
   d. Remain calm
   e. Arrange for employee to be escorted out
   f. Report back to the human resources department and administration

## Questions to Challenge You

1. Have you ever been coached, confronted, or disciplined in your workplace or clinical site? How well did the intervenor handle the situation? How well did you handle it? Did you learn from it?
2. Have you ever had to coach, confront, or discipline someone? How did the person respond? How well did you do? What did you learn?
3. Do you think you could terminate a staff member? If not, how would you prepare yourself?
4. Select a colleague or classmate and role-play four situations:
   a. A coaching session
   b. A confrontation
   c. A discipline session
   d. A termination
   After you have completed these sessions, reverse positions and play the opposite role.
5. Critique each other's performance.

**Pearson Nursing Student Resources**

Find additional review materials at

**www.nursing.pearsonhighered.com**

Prepare for success with additional NCLEX®-style practice questions, interactive assignments and activities, Web links, animations and videos, and more!

# References

Bing, S. (2007). A tale of three firings. *Fortune, 156*(2), 210.

Cohen, S. (2006). How to terminate a staff nurse. *Nursing Management, 37*(10), 16.

Hader, R. (2006). Put employee termination etiquette to practice. *Nursing Management, 37*(12), 6.

Huseman, R. C. (2009). The importance of positive culture in hospitals. *Journal of Nursing Administration, 39*(2), 60–63.

Karsten, M., Baggon, D., Brown, A., & Cahill, M. (2010). Professional coaching as an effective strategy to retaining frontline managers. *Journal of Nursing Administration, 40*(3), 140–144.

McDermott, M., & Levenson, A. (2007). What coaching can and cannot do for your organization. *Human Resources Planning, 30*(2), 30–37.

McNally, K., & Lukens, R. (2006). Leadership development: An external-internal coaching partnership. *Journal of Nursing Administration, 36*(3), 155–161.

Palermo, J. C. (2007). Well-crafted worker discipline program diminishes risk. *Business Insurance, 41*(8), 9.

Stedman, M. E., & Nolan, T. L. (2007). Coaching: A different approach to the nursing dilemma. *Nursing Administration Quarterly, 31*(1), 43–49.

White, K. M. (2006). Better manage your human capital. *Nursing Management, 37*(1), 16–19.

# CHAPTER 20

# Managing Absenteeism, Reducing Turnover, Retaining Staff

## Absenteeism

A MODEL OF EMPLOYEE ATTENDANCE

MANAGING EMPLOYEE ABSENTEEISM

ABSENTEEISM POLICIES

SELECTING EMPLOYEES AND MONITORING ABSENTEEISM

FAMILY AND MEDICAL LEAVE

## Reducing Turnover

COST OF NURSING TURNOVER

CAUSES OF TURNOVER

UNDERSTANDING VOLUNTARY TURNOVER

## Retaining Staff

EMPLOYEE ENGAGEMENT

HEALTHY WORK ENVIRONMENT

IMPROVING SALARIES

RECOGNIZING STAFF PERFORMANCE

ADDITIONAL RETENTION STRATEGIES

## Learning Outcomes

*After completing this chapter, you will be able to:*

1. Explain absenteeism.
2. Discuss ways to manage absenteeism.
3. Describe how nursing turnover affects the organization.
4. Explain voluntary turnover.

5. Discuss what organizations can do to improve retention of nurses.
6. Discuss what managers can do to help retain nurses.

## Key Terms

Absence culture
Absence frequency
Attendance barriers
Engagement
Family and Medical Leave Act

Involuntary absenteeism
Involuntary turnover
Presenteeism
Salary compression
Total time lost

Turnover
Voluntary absenteeism
Voluntary turnover

Keeping higher-performing nurses is a priority in health care. Appropriate hiring decisions begin the process, but once employment begins organizations can do much to ensure that they retain their best performers. It is appropriate to mention several suggestions here from Chapter 17, Motivating and Developing Staff. Mentoring, coaching, nurse residency programs, and clinical ladder advancement programs all help retain nurses. In order to understand why nurses are absent or leave the organization and develop ways to retain them, it is necessary to consider absenteeism, turnover, and retention.

# Absenteeism

Although the extent or the cost of nurse absenteeism is difficult to determine, it is well established that absenteeism in health care organizations is both pervasive and expensive. The costs of absenteeism, however, can also have a detrimental effect on the work lives of the other staff. Working shorthanded, especially for an extended period of time, can create both physical and mental strain. Even if temporary replacements are called in, the work flow of the unit will still be disrupted as hurried staff must take time to explain standard organizational procedures to replacement nurses.

## A Model of Employee Attendance

To understand employee absenteeism, it is important to distinguish voluntary from involuntary absenteeism. For example, not coming to work in order to finish one's income taxes would be seen as **voluntary absenteeism** (i.e., absenteeism under the employee's control). In contrast, taking a sick day because of food poisoning would be considered **involuntary absenteeism** (i.e., largely outside of the employee's control). Although this distinction seems reasonable in theory, in practice it is often difficult to distinguish these two categories because of a lack of accurate information (few employees will admit to abusing sick leave). In fact, 65 percent of employees call in sick for reasons other than illness (CCH Survey, 2007).

Some organizations try to distinguish voluntary from involuntary absenteeism by the way they measure absenteeism. Traditionally, health care organizations have measured absenteeism in terms of **total time lost** (i.e., the number of scheduled days an employee misses). Given that one long illness can drastically affect this absenteeism index, total time lost is clearly not a perfect measure of voluntary absenteeism. In contrast, **absence frequency** (i.e., the total number of distinct absence periods, regardless of their duration) is somewhat insensitive to one long illness.

This distinction between absence frequency and total time lost should make sense to managers. For example, an employee who missed nine Mondays in a row would have nine absence frequency periods as well as nine total days absent. In contrast, a person who missed nine consecutive days of work would have nine total days lost but only one absence frequency period. Intuitively, it seems likely that the first individual was much more prone to being absent voluntarily than the second.

An employee's attendance at work is largely a function of two variables: the individual's ability to attend and motivation to attend as shown in Figure 20-1.

As seen in Figure 20-1, an employee's ability to attend can be affected by such **attendance barriers** as:

- Personal illness or injury
- Family responsibilities (e.g., a sick child)
- Transportation problems (e.g., an unreliable automobile)

Although it is natural to view such barriers as resulting in involuntary absenteeism, sometimes this is too simplistic a judgment. For example, an employee whose car was not running may consciously have not made alternative arrangements to get to work the next day because he or she was not motivated to attend. This example illustrates that some of the distinctions

**Figure 20-1** ●
A diagnostic model of
employee attendance.

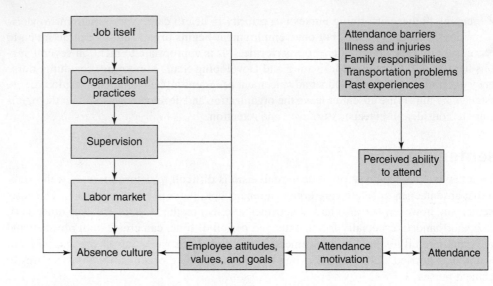

portrayed in Figure 20-1 are not always clear-cut. In trying to understand employee absenteeism, a manager will have to make assumptions about why the behavior is occurring (e.g., a manager cannot be certain that a person was actually ill).

According to the attendance model, an employee's motivation to attend is affected by several factors: the job itself, organizational practices, the absence culture, generational differences, management, the labor market, and the employee's personal characteristics.

### The Job Itself

In assessing the job itself, employees holding more enriched jobs are less likely to be absent than those with more mundane jobs. Enriched jobs may increase attendance motivation because employees believe that what they are doing is important and because they know that other employees are depending on the job holder (i.e., if the job holder doesn't do his or her job, other employees can't do theirs).

The nature of a job influences attendance through its effect on attendance motivation as well as on illness and injuries (i.e., attendance barriers). For example, a job that requires heavy lifting (e.g., moving patients from beds to stretchers) may increase the likelihood that a staff nurse will be injured. Similarly, a job that exposes a nurse to patients with highly contagious conditions, such as in an outpatient clinic, may increase the likelihood of illness.

### Organizational Practices

As portrayed in Figure 20-1, organizational practices can also influence attendance motivation. Some health care organizations have absence control policies that reward employees for good attendance and/or punish them for excessive absenteeism. An organization may also be able to increase attendance motivation by carefully recruiting and selecting employees (see Chapter 15). In addition to affecting attendance motivation, organizational practices may influence an employee's ability to attend. Organizational activities, such as offering wellness programs, employee assistance programs, van pools, on-site child care, or coordinating car pools could influence an employee's ability to attend work.

### Absence Culture

The **absence culture** of a work unit (or an organization) can also influence employee attendance motivation. Some work units have an absence culture that reflects a tolerance for absenteeism. Other units have a culture in which being absent is frowned upon. Although an organization's absence culture can be affected by organizational practices (e.g., attendance policies) and the nature of the jobs involved (e.g., people in higher-level jobs tend to be less accepting of coworkers calling in sick), it is also affected by informal norms that develop among work-group members. For example, people in a cohesive work group may develop an understanding that missing work, except for an emergency or a serious illness, is unacceptable. Such an attendance culture is likely to emerge if the employees work in jobs that they see as important (e.g., providing direct patient care) and if an employee being absent causes a hardship for coworkers (e.g., forced overtime, being called in on a day off).

## Generational Differences

Today's workforce includes nurses from four generations, and each cohort (traditionals, baby boomers, Generation X, and Generation Y) has different expectations in the workplace (Dols, Landrum, & Wieck, 2010). Younger nurses expect to have flexible scheduling and may use absenteeism to achieve it.

Older nurses may resent the younger ones, especially their technology skills and their lower need for social interaction. Here is an example:

> *Kirsten McNamara is 24 years old. She spends her lunch break relaxing and returning text and e-mail messages on her phone while she eats; she uses the quiet time to rejuvenate. Her coworkers, traditionals and baby boomers, are offended, and complain that she was "on her phone and rude" the whole lunch hour.*

Generational differences affect retention as well. Generation X and Y nurses want challenging careers that offer opportunities for growth and advancement as well as time for lives outside of work. Flexible schedules and time off are valued by these cohorts, and organizations can expect high turnover if these expectations are not met.

Expectations of the younger generational cohorts affect supervision as well. They expect independence and to be involved in decision making (Farag, Tullai-McGuinness, & Anthony, 2009). Thus, shared governance is an appropriate structure, and consultation is an effective management strategy.

## Management

Management influences attendance motivation of all staff as well. A nurse manager can influence the nature of a staff nurse's job (e.g., the degree of responsibility given and participation in decision making), decisions about personnel, the consistency with which organizational practices are applied (e.g., whether sanctions are enforced for abuse of sick leave), and a work unit's absence culture by stressing the importance of good attendance.

A shared governance organizational model encourages attendance because of the emphasis on cooperative decision making. The manager who consults frequently with staff supports this model. Knowing that their input is valuable to the unit's functioning promotes participation and, thus, attendance.

Cost-cutting is here to stay (Ferenc, 2009), and managers must be flexible in the work environment. Recognize staff performance, make any enhancement or flexibility necessary in order to keep staff. Evaluate work flow and consider creative ways to use staff to get all the work done. Be open to potentially having to work in a different way or change a work flow.

## Labor Market

Another factor that influences attendance is the labor market. If the nurse believes that plenty of equivalent jobs are available locally, he or she might be less motivated to attend than if fewer jobs were available.

To the extent that the local employment market for nurses leads an employee to perceive it would be easy to find an equivalent job if she or he lost or disliked the current one, one would expect a lower level of attendance motivation than if market conditions were less favorable. This might happen during a nursing shortage.

### Personal Characteristics

Although features of the job itself, organizational practices, absence culture, generational differences, supervision, and the labor market can all have a direct effect on employee attendance motivation, these factors can also interact with an employee's attitudes (e.g., job satisfaction), values (e.g., personal work ethic), or goals (e.g., desire to get promoted). If a person who seeks variety works in a job that does not provide it, the employee may become dissatisfied and thus more likely to abuse sick leave.

The reverse is also true. Employees' attitudes, values, and goals can also have a direct effect on attendance motivation. For example, a staff nurse with a high personal work ethic or a goal of getting promoted should be more highly motivated to attend work than a nurse who lacks such a work ethic.

An employee's attendance behavior is also influenced by past experiences. For example, if an employee's perfect attendance in the previous year was not recognized, we might expect the employee's attendance motivation to decrease in the coming year. Conversely, if a coworker with an outstanding attendance record received a promotion, peers who value a promotion and who witnessed this link between performance and reward would be more motivated to attend work in the upcoming year.

## Managing Employee Absenteeism

The attendance model in Figure 20-1 is useful not only for understanding why absenteeism occurs, but also for developing strategies to control it. Some causes of absenteeism, such as transportation difficulties or child care problems, may be beyond the direct control of nurse managers. A manager, however, should try to do what is possible, either in interactions with staff or by attempting to influence the organization to change policies that may be interfering with a nurse's ability or motivation to attend work. On the other hand, the manager must be careful that the steps taken do not go so far as to discourage the legitimate use of sick leave. Clearly, one does not want sick nurses coming to work and exposing patients and coworkers to their illnesses.

To diagnose the key factors leading to absenteeism, the manager needs information from several sources, including staff, the human resources department, other nurse managers, and administration. Absence patterns can answer such questions as:

- Is absenteeism equally distributed across all nurses?
- In comparison to other units, does your area of responsibility have a high absenteeism rate?
- Are most absences of short or long duration?
- Does the absenteeism have a consistent pattern (e.g., occur predominantly on weekends or shortly before a person quits)?

Although a manager may not be able to do much to affect the staff's ability to attend, the organization can take several actions. For example, to lessen child care problems, the organization could set up or sponsor a child care center. To reduce transportation problems, an organization could provide shuttle buses or coordinate car pools. Health fairs, exercise programs, and stress-reduction classes could be offered to promote health. Given that alcoholism and drug abuse are widely recognized as important causes of absenteeism, an employee assistance program may be cost-effective. In addition to these organizational actions, a nurse manager, through coaching, may be able to influence a staff nurse's attendance. (See Chapter 19 for information on how to coach staff.)

Clearly, the best way for nurse managers to control absenteeism is by encouraging their staff's motivation to attend. Other absenteeism management strategies that a nurse manager might consider include:

- Enriching the staff nurse's job by increasing its responsibility, variety, or challenge
- Reducing job stress (e.g., by providing timely and more concrete information)
- Creating a norm of excellent attendance (e.g., by emphasizing the negative impact of a nurse not coming to work)
- Enhancing advancement opportunities (e.g., by providing developmental experiences so that the best employees are promotable)
- Improving coworker relations (e.g., by considering coworker compatibility when scheduling work and/or creating work teams)
- Trying to select employees who will be satisfied with and committed to their jobs
- Being a good role model by rarely taking sick days
- Discussing the employee's attendance during the performance appraisal interview
- Rewarding good attendance with salary increases and other rewards
- Enforcing absenteeism control policies (e.g., carrying through on employee discipline when there is an attendance problem)

## Absenteeism Policies

Most organizational policies allow employees to accrue paid sick days—typically, one sick day for every month employed. Unused sick days accrue across time to some maximum number (e.g., 60 days). Typically, if an employee leaves the organization with accumulated sick leave or days above the maximum, the person simply loses it.

Although such a policy may seem reasonable, it may actually encourage unwanted behavior. For example, once a nurse has reached the maximum limit for accrued sick days, the person may see no reason for not using sick days that would otherwise be lost. Such a policy also encourages employees who know they will be leaving the organization (e.g., those about to retire or change jobs) to use accumulated sick leave.

An innovative approach for managing absenteeism is substituting personal days for unused sick days. Two problems arise if personal days are not given: Employees are forced to lie (i.e., say they are sick when they are not) to carry out what they see as legitimate activities (e.g., attending a conference with their child's teacher), and their manager has no warning and therefore may have difficulty covering for the absent employee.

By substituting personal days for sick days, the employee no longer has to lie, and the nurse manager may have time to plan for a replacement. In moving to a policy that incorporates the use of personal days, an organization typically allocates fewer paid sick days but adds personal days. For example, instead of 12 sick days, an employee may annually receive nine sick days and three personal days. With the availability of personal days, a staff nurse can inform the manager in advance of the need for a personal day off. In many cases, the two of them can arrive at a day off that is optimal for both of them.

Realizing that they have not been motivating good attendance, some progressive organizations have allowed sick days to accumulate without an upper limit. Then, when an employee leaves the organization, she or he is paid for unused sick days (e.g., one-half day's pay for each unused sick day). Other organizations allow retiring employees to add unused sick days to days worked. Still other organizations have paid employees for their sick days, or allowed the conversion of sick days to vacation days or additional pay.

Obviously, changing an organization's paid sick leave policy is beyond the control of the nurse manager. However, a concerted effort by an organized group of managers may be effective in encouraging the human resources department and administration to initiate such changes. Considering the high costs of absenteeism, these changes can be quite cost-effective.

Most health care organizations have formal policies concerning how much absenteeism is allowed. Once this limit is reached, disciplinary steps are prescribed. In disciplining an employee, the manager must follow the discipline policy carefully. The effectiveness of discipline as a strategy for reducing absenteeism is limited. Most discipline policies only take effect after excessive absenteeism. Not surprisingly, most employees know what this is and are careful not to exceed it. In effect, the nurse manager is left with an absenteeism problem but not one that she or he is able to address through the use of discipline.

## Selecting Employees and Monitoring Absenteeism

Many of the managerial actions addressed in other chapters of this book are relevant to the control of absenteeism. For example, in recruiting employees, the use of a realistic job preview should increase the congruence between job characteristics and employee values and expectations. Similarly, basing merit pay and advancement opportunities on an employee's overall performance appraisal rating (which is partly based on attendance) will motivate better attendance. Also, leadership skills are important in getting the organization to change policy to lessen absenteeism (e.g., providing payment for unused sick days).

Strategies for dealing with employees with excessive absences include:

- Set expectations with each new employee. Give her or him the attendance policy in writing, and clarify any questions.
- Monitor each individual's attendance, and document it.
- Intervene early and consistently, coaching and dealing with policy or procedure violations as appropriate.
- If discipline is called for, use the key behaviors for disciplining in Chapter 19.
- Be sure to reward staff who have good attendance. Ensure that any organizational rewards are delivered, and give your personal reward through feedback in performance appraisals.
- Be a role model for good attendance yourself.

These steps will set a tone of intolerance for poor attendance. The opposite of absenteeism is **presenteeism** when the employee is at work although disabled by physical or mental illness. Those employees who were sick more often, who had heavier workloads, were highly skilled, enjoyed positive relationships with coworkers, or whose job status was precarious were more likely to be present at work even though ill (Biron, Brun, Ivers, & Cooper, 2006). Additionally, high psychological distress and psychosomatic illness were predictors of presenteeism.

## Family and Medical Leave

The federal **Family and Medical Leave Act (FMLA)** took effect in 1993 and has been amended by federal statute as well as court decisions (U.S. Department of Labor, 2011). Under this act, all public employers (federal, state, and local) and all private employers employing 50 or more individuals must provide their eligible employees with leave of up to 12 weeks during any 12-month period for the employee's own serious illness, the birth or adoption of a child, the placement of a foster child into the household, or the care of a seriously ill child, spouse, or parent.

The FMLA also allows eligible employees to maintain health insurance coverage while on leave and allows them to return to the same or equivalent position at the end of the leave period. The leave may be taken all at once, intermittently, or by working a reduced work schedule, if available. The employee must be allowed to take leave for qualified purposes without pressure or discouragement by the employer or manager. More generous collective bargaining agreements or state laws supersede the FMLA, but the FMLA supersedes any inconsistent or less generous provisions. FMLA may run concurrently with other leaves, including state workers' compensation leave.

Employees are eligible to take leave if they:

- Have worked for the employer for at least 12 months
- Have worked at least 1,250 hours during the previous 12 months
- Are at a work site with 50 or more employees, or at a site where 50 workers are employed within 75 miles of the work site (50 employees/75 miles rule)

The FMLA is quite complex. (See U.S. Department of Labor Web site for updated information at http://www.dol.gov/compliance/laws/comp-fmla.htm.)

State law and collective bargaining agreements may make the organization's leave policy unique. Furthermore, the overlap and interaction between the Americans with Disabilities Act and the FMLA is complicated. The organization is responsible for assuring that the employee can perform the job while at the same time ensuring that the employee's legal rights are not violated (Lester, 2011). The human resources department at each organization is the best source of information about FMLA and ADA requirements.

# Reducing Turnover

Closely related to absenteeism is employee **turnover**, the number of staff members who vacate a position. Reducing turnover begins with recruitment and selection (see Chapter 15) and continues with motivation and development of staff. Retaining both experienced nurses and new graduates is essential (Hill et al., 2010; Hirschkorn et al., 2010; Salt, Cummings, & Profetto-McGrath, 2008).

## Cost of Nursing Turnover

Two interrelated factors affect the nurse turnover rate: market opportunities and the economy. When the economy is robust, health care organizations tend to hire more staff; during a recession, the hospital may cut staff or leave positions vacant. At the same time, nurses are more apt to stay in a position if the economy is poor or if there are few other opportunities (Healthcare Association of New York State, 2010).

Data from a national survey in 2009 found that turnover rates that year (7.1 percent) had declined from the 10.1 percent of the previous year (Healthcare Association of New York State, 2010). The surveyors attributed the change to the poor economy and the lack of opportunities.

Given the expense in hiring a new nurse (e.g., recruiting, selection, orientation, on-the-job training) and temporarily replacing a nurse who quits or is fired (e.g., paying other nurses to work overtime or filling the vacancy with a temporary replacement), the costs are certainly sizable. Thus, nursing turnover needs to be understood better and controlled more effectively.

Turnover has been thought of in simplistic terms and seen as universally negative. Such a primitive view of turnover is not helpful to managers as they attempt to deal with this costly problem. Rather, varieties of turnover need to be differentiated:

- Did the employee leave of her or his own accord, or was the person asked to leave?
- Was the departed individual's performance exceptional or mediocre?
- Did the employee leave for career development (e.g., return to school) or because of dissatisfaction with the organization?
- Will the departed nurse be easy or difficult to replace?

Turnover has consequences that go far beyond direct dollar costs. Turnover can have a number of repercussions among other nurses who worked with the departed nurse (Jones, 2008). They may have to work longer hours (overtime) or simply work harder to cover for a departed nurse; this can cause both physical and mental strain and may result in additional departures. Thus, departed nurses may begin a cycle of nurses leaving, resulting in a turnover spiral. If temporary replacements are used, problems still can result as the work flow of the unit is disturbed and communication patterns within the unit are disrupted.

Turnover is not always undesirable. Anyone with work experience can remember some individual (e.g., coworker, administrator) whose departure would have improved the organization's functioning significantly. Furthermore, what may be seen as a desirable departure by some (e.g., the nurse manager) may be viewed as a loss by others (e.g., a subset of coworkers). If the departed nurse was a poor performer, performance may improve. Recently hired staff may be more enthusiastic, long-running conflicts between people may be reduced or eliminated, or administration may be challenged to improve the work environment (see the Healthy Work Environment section later in the chapter).

## Causes of Turnover

Before turnover can be managed, its causes must be understood. Traditionally, organizations have attempted to determine the reasons for voluntary turnover through two sources: the exiting employee's supervisor is asked why the employee is leaving, and an exit interview with the departing employee is conducted by someone in the human resources department.

Such an approach for determining the cause of voluntary turnover is certainly straightforward, but departing employees may not give honest answers in their exit interviews because they know that future employers will ask for references. Thus, exiting employees may provide safe responses (e.g., "a better opportunity came along") during an exit interview.

Although this tendency for departing employees to make safe responses is understandable, it makes it difficult to determine why turnover is occurring. Surveys sent to former employees several weeks after they have resigned may be more useful. Former employees need to be assured that their responses will not influence any future reference information furnished about them, but rather will be used only to help the organization identify the reasons why nurses are leaving. Another way to attempt to discover the cause of nurse turnover is to conduct interviews with the former employee's coworkers, who often know why an employee left.

## Understanding Voluntary Turnover

The discussion in this chapter focuses on **voluntary turnover** (i.e., employees choose to leave). If an organization finds a significant amount of **involuntary turnover** (i.e., employees being terminated), then it needs to carefully examine the way it recruits, selects, motivates, and develops employees. (See Chapters 15 and 17.)

The goal should be to reduce voluntary turnover. The manager's first opportunity to reduce turnover is when the decision to hire is made. An individual's length of stay at past employers is an indication of how long the person could be expected to stay on a new job.

Turnover is a direct function of a nurse's perceptions of both the ease and the desirability of leaving the organization. Perceived ease of movement depends on the nurse's personal characteristics, such as:

- Education
- Area of specialization
- Age
- Geographic mobility
- Contacts at other hospitals
- Transportation

As well as external forces, such as:

- Job openings at other organizations
- Non–health care organizations hiring nurses for nursing or nonnursing positions
- Economy

As with ease of movement, perceptions of the desirability of movement can be affected by several factors. One is the opportunity for movement within the organization. If other positions exist within the organization, the less turnover there should be; that is, a nurse may be able to leave the current position by means of a lateral transfer, promotion, or demotion. For example, a nurse who is having problems with a coworker may be able to transfer to a new unit rather than leave the organization.

Turnover and employee absenteeism have been referred to as withdrawal behaviors because they allow an employee to leave the workplace, in one case temporarily and, in the other, permanently. In many cases, these withdrawal behaviors share a common cause: job dissatisfaction discussed next.

# Retaining Staff

Job satisfaction is a key component to retaining staff (Wisotzkey, 2011). Job satisfaction is affected by various facets of the work environment, including:

- Relationships with the nurse manager, other staff nurses and unit employees, patients, and physicians
- Shift worked (e.g., day versus evening, rotating versus fixed)
- Fit between nurse values and institutional culture
- Expectations of practice setting
- Compensation level
- Equal and fair distribution of rewards and punishments

## Employee Engagement

Employee engagement is tied to employee retention as well as customer satisfaction, but employees engaged in their workplace are in the minority across industries (Advisory Board Company, 2007). Additionally, in a survey of more than 4,000 nurses, researchers found uneven levels of engagement among them (Advisory Board Company, 2007). **Engagement** is defined as being inspired by the organization, willing to invest effort, likely to recommend the organization, and planning to remain in the organization.

Rivers, Fitzpatrick, and Boyle (2011) studied factors that affect employee engagement. Key factors of engagement were control over practice, professional development and growth, teamwork, and nurse–physician collaboration. The least important factors related to engagement were salary and benefits. The implications for managers and administration suggest that an organizational structure that encourages staff input, frequent communication and attention to problems as soon as they occur, and development opportunities are some of the ways to encourage employee engagement.

## Healthy Work Environment

A healthy work environment increases nurse job satisfaction, a necessary condition for retaining nurses (Paris & Terhaar, 2011; Weston, 2010). Environmental factors can improve job satisfaction and reduce the intention to leave, according to Applebaum, Fowler, and Fiedler (2010). Miracle (2008) posits that both nurse satisfaction and excellent nursing care is the product of a healthy work environment.

The American Association of Critical Care Nurses (AACN, 2005) established six criteria for a healthy work environment to "foster excellence in patient care" (p. 1). These criteria are:

- Skilled communication—as important as clinical skills
- True collaboration—between and among nurses and other health care professionals
- Effective decision making—involved as partners in making policy and leading organizations
- Appropriate staffing—effective match between patient needs and nurse competencies
- Meaningful recognition—for value of work
- Authentic leadership—leaders embrace, live, and engage others in it

## Improving Salaries

As the largest group of health care professionals, nurses' wages account for the majority of an organization's salary budget. It is reasonable (although not cost-effective) that organizations imagine they can reduce expenses by constraining nurses' salaries or allowing open positions to go unfilled. Thus, nurses employed for many years find their salaries only slightly greater than (or even less than) nurses with only a few years of experience. This effect is known as **salary compression**. Paying new nurses a higher starting salary or rewarding those with fewer years of experience with higher increases results in the salaries of long-term employees being at or below those of less-experienced nurses.

Sign-on bonuses and loan-forgiveness programs, for example, are strategies used to attract new graduates. They are, however, only quick fixes that serve to disadvantage already-employed nurses whose salary ceilings remain fixed. Pay scales, however, can be reconfigured to reflect achievement and accomplishment.

### Recognizing Staff Performance

Recognizing the contributions of staff is not necessarily expensive or time-consuming. The manager can integrate some strategies into the everyday managing of staff. Here are some examples:

- Provide personalized immediate feedback of a job well done.
- Write a personal note acknowledging an employee's good performance. Leave in the employee's mailbox or mail to a home address.
- Publicly recognize an employee's good performance—at staff meeting, in an e-mail to all, with kudos on the unit bulletin board.
- Encourage staff to post notes on the bulletin board to thank a coworker for a great job or recognize a peer for impressive observed work with a patient.
- Design a bulletin board to highlight one employee. Change it every two weeks or once per month. The employee can bring in personal and family photos as well as post facts about them. This facilitates employee recognition and a sense of camaraderie as employees get to know each other better.

Examples of low-cost and formal rewards for staff are shown in Box 20-1.

---

### BOX 20-1    Rewarding Employees

**Low-Cost Rewards for Employees**

- Allow staff to have a half day, whole day, or Friday off for excellent performance by flexing hours and completing hours for week in fewer days. For example, allow an employee to choose four 10-hour shifts one week as a treat instead of five 8-hour days.
- Give magazine subscriptions.
- Have a monthly birthday celebration potluck to recognize all employees with a birthday that month—rotate the theme for different kinds of food/activities.
- Initiate an employee of the month program— reward the employee with a gift card, certificate of recognition, or some other small gift.
- Start a newsletter and devote a section to describing excellent employee performance and including staff kudos to one another.

**Formal Rewards for Employees**

- Give awards for perfect attendance, patient advocate, clinical leader, expert nurse, most cost–effective, etc. Present the awards at a hosted annual awards banquet, with food and formal recognition.
- Start a reward points system in which employees earn points for great customer service/teamwork. Make a "treat box" that has small gift items such as snacks, pens, notepads, etc. Assign a point value to each gift item and let staff accumulate points. Staff can then "buy" items with their points.
- Provide continuing education opportunities presented by physician sponsors or nurses from the community. Start a program that gives staff the opportunity to take time off to attend an educational offering once per year or a set number of times as determined by the group.
- Help with tuition reimbursement for continuing education.
- Give customer service awards based on years of service.

## Additional Retention Strategies

In addition to the work environment, salary adjustments, and staff recognition, managers can use several other strategies to help retain a valued employee in the organization. These include:

- Providing a realistic job preview to new hires
- Facilitating movement within the organization
- Coordinating with other managers to influence organizational policy
- Adapting to turnover rate

### Provide Realistic Job Preview and Follow-up

Retaining nurses begins with the interview when the manager has an opportunity to present the job realistically. Retention continues with orientation and socialization of the new nurse to the unit (Hatler et al., 2011). Both clinical advancement programs and preceptorships, discussed in Chapter 17, have been found to improve retention (Allen, Fiorini, & Dickey, 2010; Salt, Cummings, & Profetto-McGrath, 2008).

### Facilitate Intraorganizational Movement

If a staff nurse is "burned out" from working on an oncology floor, one option is to allow a transfer to another service area in the organization (e.g., home care). Unfortunately, some managers hinder or even prohibit such a transfer (particularly if the potential transferee is an excellent performer), not wanting to lose a good nurse. However, this perspective is shortsighted. If the staff nurse cannot transfer to another area (intraorganizational mobility), she or he may leave the organization entirely (interorganizational mobility).

One nurse manager decreased voluntary turnover on her unit without incurring additional costs (see Case Study 20-1).

---

## CASE STUDY 20-1

### RETENTION

Mona Karnes is nurse manager of labor and delivery at a suburban hospital. Over the past 12 months, the voluntary turnover rate among full-time RNs has been 15 percent for her unit and 25 percent for the hospital as a whole. Despite increasing starting salary rates and offering signing bonuses, turnover rates have remained high. Administration is in the process of conducting an annual salary review as well as a benefits review.

Mona has collected information from exit interviews conducted by the human resources department. From these data, Mona has developed three strategies to aid in retention for her unit:

1. Rotate leadership responsibilities on the unit to offer all nurses the opportunity to develop leadership and management skills. These responsibilities currently include a weekly charge nurse role for each shift, education committee chair, physician relations liaison, women's health service line representative, and information technology representative. Other leadership roles will be added as appropriate.

2. Survey staff to determine interests and strengths and connect staff members with a mentor. For example, Debbie Edwards, RN, enjoys developing patient education modules. Debbie will work with Heather Adams, new nurse graduate, to develop Heather's patient education skills.

3. Schedule free monthly CEU offerings during staff meetings that are presented by staff members, physicians, or pharmaceutical company representatives. By attending monthly staff meetings, most RNs will complete 90 percent of state-required CEUs for license renewal.

All three strategies are at no cost to the unit or hospital. After six months, the voluntary turnover rate on Mona's unit has decreased to 8 percent.

### Manager's Checklist

The nurse manager is responsible for:

- Understanding the financial impact of voluntary turnover on the unit and the organization
- Gathering and analyzing data that provide insight into the reasons for voluntary turnover
- Utilizing creative solutions to increase staff retention
- Establishing open and effective communication with staff members
- Evaluating retention strategies in a timely manner and adjusting processes as appropriate
- Communicating successful strategies to colleagues and administration

### Adapt to Turnover Rate

Sometimes the organization may simply need to adapt to a high turnover rate. Even if this is the case, the manager may be able to lessen potential problems by doing two things:

1. Manage beliefs about why a nurse left. Sometimes, the reason is unclear, and the grapevine will often provide an inaccurate and less attractive reason from the organization's perspective (e.g., "He left for $1.05 more an hour at a competitor institution").

2. Provide human resources with a preferred list of replacement workers. Some organizations keep an up-to-date list of former nurses who will fill in on an occasional basis. Such former employees are familiar with organizational procedures and can handle the work more efficiently.

The strategies outlined in this chapter have been shown to be effective in addressing absenteeism and reducing turnover. However, not all are equally applicable to all situations. Situational factors determine what is appropriate. For example, flexible work hours may be suitable for a clinic but not for an around-the-clock operation. By being creative, nurse managers not only can reduce absenteeism and turnover, but can also have an influence on nurses' attendance and on which nurses leave by providing incentives for the exceptional nurse to stay and by doing less to retain mediocre nurses.

## What You Know Now

- Employee attendance is affected by the job, organizational practices, absence culture, generational differences, labor market, management, and the employee's characteristics.
- An organization can improve employee attendance by addressing specific barriers, such as adding a child care center, coordinating car pools, or offering health promotion and employee assistance programs.
- Innovative solutions to absenteeism problems include substituting personal days for sick days, allowing sick days to accrue and unused days to be paid to the employee, or converting unused sick days to paid days at retirement.
- Turnover may be voluntary or involuntary, but it is always costly to the organization.
- Many factors cause voluntary turnover, including job dissatisfaction, undesirable work environment, and ease of movement.
- Organizations can help retain nurses by providing healthy work environments, improving salaries, and recognizing performance.
- Managers can help reduce turnover by providing realistic job previews and follow-up, facilitating intraorganizational movement, but may have to adapt to turnover rate.

## Tools for Reducing Turnover, Retaining Staff

1. Become familiar with your organization's policies on employee attendance.
2. Identify attendance problems and monitor them, if necessary.
3. Monitor turnover and evaluate the causes.
4. Provide realistic job previews to new hires, especially new graduates.
5. Monitor new graduates' performance and offer additional support and training as needed.
6. Consider ways to improve the work environment.

## Questions to Challenge You

1. As a nurse manager, what would you do to reduce absenteeism?
2. Can you recall instances where an employee's leaving has benefited the organization? Describe what happened.
3. Have you voluntarily left a job?
   a. What was the reason? Was there more than one reason?
   b. What reason did you give your supervisor?
   c. Was it the same rationale that you answered in part *a* of this question?

4. In addition to ideas presented in the chapter, can you think of other ways to reduce voluntary turnover?
5. Have you seen managers be effective in retaining staff? What did they do that worked especially well?
6. If you were a manager, what specific actions would you take to retain staff?

**Pearson Nursing Student Resources**
Find additional review materials at
**www.nursing.pearsonhighered.com**

Prepare for success with additional NCLEX®-style practice questions, interactive assignments and activities, Web links, animations and videos, and more!

# References

Advisory Board Company (2007). *Engaging the nurse workforce: Best practices for promoting exceptional staff performance.* Washington, DC: Advisory Board Company.

American Association of Critical Care Nurses. (2005). *AACN's healthy work environments initiative.* Retrieved August 22, 2011 from http://www.aacn.org/wd/hwe/content/hwehome.pcms?menu=practice

Allen, S. R., Fiorini, P., & Dickey, M. (2010). A streamlined clinical advancement program improves RN participation and retention. *Journal of Nursing Administration, 40*(7/8), 316–322.

Applebaum, D., Fowler, S., & Fiedler, N. (2010). The impact of environmental factors on nursing stress, job satisfaction and turnover intention. *Journal of Nursing Administration, 40*(7/8), 323–328.

Biron, C., Brun, J., Ivers, H., & Cooper, C. L. (2006). At work but ill: Psychosocial work environment and well-being determinants of presenteeism propensity.

*Journal of Public Mental Health, 5*(4), 26–37.

CCH survey finds most employees call in "sick" for reasons other than illness. (2007). Wolters Kluwer Press Release (October 10, 2007). Retrieved August 22, 2011 from http://www.wolterskluwer.com/Press/Latest-News/2007/Pages/pr_11oct07_2.aspx

Dols, J., Landrum, P., & Wieck, K. L. (2010). Leading and managing an intergenerational workforce. *Creative Nursing, 16*(2), 68–74.

Farag, A. A., Tullai-McGuinnes, S., & Anthony, M. K. (2009). Nurses' perception of their manager's leadership style and unit climate: Are there generational differences? *Journal of Nursing Management, 17*(1), 26–34.

Ferenc, J. (2009). Cost cuts to stay. *Material Management in Health Care, 18*(12), 4–12.

Hatler, C., Stoffers, P., Kelly, L., Redding, K., & Carr, L. L. (2011). Work unit transformation to welcome new graduate nurses. *Nursing Economics, 29*(2), 88–93.

Healthcare Association of New York State (2010). *Nurses*

*needed: Short-term relief, ongoing shortage. Results from the 2010 nursing workforce survey.* Retrieved August 22, 2011 from http://www.hanys.org/workforce/reports/2010-06-07_nurse_survey_results_2010.pdf

Hill, K. S., Cleary, B. L., Hewlett, P. O., Bleich, M. R., Davis, K., & Hatcher, B. J. (2010). Commentary: Experienced RN retention strategies. *Journal of Nursing Administration, 40*(11), 468–470.

Hirschkorn, C. A., West, T. B., Hill, K. S., Cleary, B. L., & Hewlett, P. O. (2010). Experienced nurse retention strategies. *Journal of Nursing Administration, 40*(11), 463–467.

Jones, C. B. (2008). Revisiting nurse turnover costs. *Journal of Nursing Administration, 38*(1), 11–18.

Lester, R. L. (2011). Ensuring the health care worker can perform the essential functions of their position in the increasingly restricted legal environment governing hiring and disability accommodation. *Kentucky Bar Association Bench & Bar, 75*(3), 10–16.

Miracle, V. A. (2008). A healthy work environment. (Editorial). *Dimensions of Critical Care Nursing, 27*(1), 41–42.

Paris, L. G., & Terhaar, M. (2011). Using Maslow's pyramid and the national database of nursing quality indicators to attain a healthier work environment. *The Online Journal of Issues in Nursing, 16*(1). Retrieved August 22, 2011 from http://www.nursingworld.org/MainMenuCategories/ANAMarketplace/ANAPeriodicals/OJIN/TableofContents/Vol-16-2011/No1-Jan-2011/Articles-Previous-Topics/Maslow-and-NDNQI-to-Assess-and-Improve-Work-Environment.aspx

Rivera, R. R., Fitzpatrick, J. J., & Boyle, S. M. (2011). Closing the RN engagement gap: Which drivers of engagement matter. *Journal of Nursing Administration, 41*(6), 265–272.

Salt, J., Cummings, G. G, & Profetto-McGrath, J. (2008). Increasing retention of new graduate nurses. *Journal of Nursing Administration, 38*(6), 287–296.

U. S. Department of Labor. (2011). *The Family and Medical Leave Act (FMLA).* Retrieved August 22, 2011 from http://www.dol.gov/compliance/laws/comp-fmla.htm

Weston, M. J. (2010). Strategies for enhancing autonomy and control over nursing practice. *The Online Journal of Issues in Nursing, 15*(1). Retrieved August 22, 2011 from http://www.nursingworld.org/MainMenuCategories/ANAMarketplace/ANAPeriodicals/OJIN/TableofContents/Vol152010/No1Jan2010/Enhancing-Autonomy-and-Control-and-Practice.aspx

Wisotzkey, S. (2011). Will they stay or will they go? Insight into nursing turnover. *Nursing Management, 42*(2), 15–17.

# Dealing with Disruptive Staff Problems

**Harassing Behaviors**
- BULLYING
- LACK OF CIVILITY
- LATERAL VIOLENCE

**How to Handle Problem Behaviors**
- MARGINAL EMPLOYEES
- DISGRUNTLED EMPLOYEES

**The Employee with a Substance Abuse Problem**
- STATE BOARD OF NURSING
- STRATEGIES FOR INTERVENTION
- REENTRY
- THE AMERICANS WITH DISABILITIES ACT AND SUBSTANCE ABUSE

## Learning Outcomes

*After completing this chapter, you will be able to:*

1. Identify harassing behaviors, including bullying, incivility, and lateral violence.
2. Describe strategies to deal with bullying behaviors.
3. Explain how to manage staff with problem behaviors.

4. Discuss how to handle marginal and disgruntled employees.
5. Explain how to handle staff with a substance abuse problem.

## Key Terms

Lateral violence                          Marginal employees

A major challenge confronting managers today is not only improving individual performance and productivity, but also enhancing the efforts of the entire work group. Some of the general techniques for enhancing performance described in Chapter 17 are ineffective because individual problems affect group functioning.

Harassing behaviors—including bullying, incivility, and lateral violence—marginal staff, disgruntled employees, and employees abusing alcohol or drugs are addressed in this chapter. There are no proven methods for managing these problems; the strategies presented here are a starting point. Assistance from administration and the human resources department often is needed.

## Harassing Behaviors

### Bullying

Bullying in the workplace increases staff dissatisfaction, turnover, and litigation, and can damage the organization's reputation as well (Dempster, 2006). In a health care setting, bullying threatens not only the victim (the "target"), but poses a danger to patients too (Stokowski, 2010). Called incivility, verbal abuse, or vertical or horizontal violence, all such behaviors are examples of bullying (Broome, 2008). Nurses report verbal abuse as the most frequent form of bullying (Christmas, 2007) with senior nurses, managers, and physicians the most likely perpetrators (Vessey, DeMarco, Gaffney, & Budin, 2009).

Bullying can occur online, via text messages, or in person. Bullies use words, nonverbal behaviors, or involve other people, such as with gossiping. Bullying behaviors can range from mildly irritating to dangerously violent (Stowoski, 2010). Examples include:

- Being ignored or given the "silent treatment"
- Treated in a condescending or patronizing manner
- Derogatory remarks made within hearing
- Dismissive body language, such as eye rolling
- Ridicule, sarcasm
- Verbal abuse
- Scapegoating
- Isolating
- Failure to assist
- Sexual harassment
- Physical attack

Policy efforts to combat bullying in health care settings have been launched by the Joint Commission and the American Nurses Association. Joint Commission recommends zero tolerance of disruptive or abusive behavior (Joint Commission, 2008). The American Nurses Association recommends strategies to combat hostility, abuse, and bullying in the workplace (ANA, 2010).

Several states are considering healthy workplace bills that would allow workers to sue for harm from abusive treatment (Stowoski, 2010). As widespread reports of abuse surface, it is hoped that swift legal action will offer redress for victims (Sullivan, 2013).

### Lack of Civility

At times, an instance of bullying is not so obvious. Lack of civility is an example. Uncivil behavior creates an environment that also endangers patients (Covell, 2010). Lack of civility includes any behavior that is:

- Rude
- Disrespectful
- Impolite
- Ill-mannered

Examples are aggressive behaviors, such as:

- Yelling
- Swearing
- Spreading rumors
- Destroying or taking another's property

Here's an example:

*Reid Martin, nurse manger, has encouraged new graduate nurse Joy Gabriel, to develop an informational presentation for a staff meeting as a strategy to improve her self-confidence. At the next monthly staff meeting, Joy presents information about a new occlusive dressing. Joy is shy, and public speaking is difficult for her. Her voice shakes, and she drops the box of new dressings she brought to demonstrate. Kristi Sanderson, RN, has been rolling her eyes and sighing loudly throughout Joy's presentation. At the end of the meeting, Kristi makes a point of telling several other staff members that it was "painful" to sit through Joy's presentation. Joy overhears Kristi's comments.*

This example is a situation that does not quite rise to the level of bullying. Nonetheless, the manager must confront Kristi and explain why nonverbal signals are inappropriate. (Remember you learned in Chapter 9 that nonverbal communication is more powerful than verbal communication.) Kristi must be also told that *sotto voce* criticisms will not be tolerated. Following the suggestions on coaching and progressive discipline, the manager must explain the consequences for repeated instances of discourtesy to her fellow staff members and insist that Kristi conduct herself in a civil manner. The manager also followed up with Joy and shared that her presentation was excellent and apologized for the inappropriate comments. The manager told Joy that the issue was being handled so that another staff member would not face such uncivil behavior in the future.

## Lateral Violence

Another example of the complexity of bullying is **lateral violence**, harassment between employees of equal rank. See the following example:

*Jeana Rossi, RN, is a staff nurse on a medical unit. At 0700, she took over care for five patients from Greg Robeson, RN, an agency nurse who had worked the 7p–7a shift. During her review of patient medication administration records, Jeana noted that an IV antibiotic scheduled to be administered at 2300 had not been charted. Checking the IV bin, Jeana found the 2300 dose. Greg had already left the unit. Per hospital policy, Jeana completed a missing dose report and turned it in to her manager. Two days later, Greg corners Jeana in the staff lounge and loudly berates her in front of other staff members for completing a missing dose report. "You're so stupid!" Greg shouts. "You just wanted to make me look bad, didn't you?"*

This example shows how difficult some staff problems can be to manage. If you were the manager on this unit, how would you handle the situation? Here are some alternatives. The manager could report Greg to the agency and request that he no longer be assigned to the unit, but then a replacement must be found and the manager may have concerns about the competency of other nurses this agency might send. Remember, Greg was the only nurse on the night shift. The manager could also discuss the event with Greg and counsel him on violating hospital policy. In the end, the manager reported the situation to her supervisor and called the director of the agency, who assured the manager that the agency would provide a competent nurse for the next shift.

The manager has a special duty to protect staff from bullying by others, to each other, or to students. Take every report of verbal aggression seriously, document events, and use the appropriate conflict strategy to resolve it. Left on its own, bullying is likely to continue and escalate.

One caveat regarding bullying: if the situation becomes threatening, seek help immediately, preferably from security. Also see the section in the next chapter, Preventing Workplace Violence, for specific strategies.

# How to Handle Problem Behaviors

Here is another example of a complex staff problem.

*The staff at the outpatient imaging center all share a common break room. Over the past several months, several staff members have complained to their nurse manager, Julie Fredrickson, that their lunches are missing from the break room refrigerator or particular items such as desserts or cans of soda are missing. One afternoon, Julie enters the break room to get a cup a coffee and sees one of the radiologists, Dr. Gibson, eating a brownie and looking through several lunch bags. "I never get a chance to get out for lunch," Dr. Gibson said. "I'm sure your staff doesn't mind sharing with a hungry physician."*

If you were the nurse manager at this outpatient center, how would you handle this situation? Dr. Gibson was committing theft, even if the items he stole were inexpensive. Nonetheless, his behavior caused nurses to go without some of their own food, and, more importantly, it was disrespectful to them. It implied that he thought his needs were more important than any of theirs. When informed, the manager alerted his supervisor and then confronted Dr. Gibson who, after threatening to report the manager to administration, calmed down, said he would donate pizza for the staff the next day, and agreed to stop stealing (yes, the manager used the word "stealing").

Managers and nurses are faced with any number of other problems presented by employees, including staff who are marginally competent, perpetually complaining, verbally abusive, or who lack civility in the workplace. Still others may have a substance-abuse problem.

## Marginal Employees

Some staff, no matter how many times they are coached or disciplined, never seem to reach the level of competence expected of an experienced nurse (Arnold, Pulich, & Wang, 2008). These are **marginal employees**. Work habits may be sloppy, communication skills poor, or decision making inadequate. Discipline does not help either in spite of the employee's attempts to improve.

Marginal employees present the manager with a unique challenge. The manager can ignore the problem and hope that the employee will improve, a largely ineffective strategy. This also leaves the unit vulnerable to complaints from other staff who must cover for the marginal employee, and affects the unit's morale.

The manager could, in contrast, follow the organization's procedures for progressive discipline and termination (see Chapter 19), which may leave the unit understaffed. Furthermore, the nurse may move on to another institution, perpetuating the poor performance.

In some organizations (e.g., government institutions and those with union contracts), the manager must follow strict guidelines for discipline and, especially, for dismissal. Because of the time and effort involved, managers in these organizations may allow the behavior to persist (Abbassi, Hollman, & Hayes, 2008).

It is crucial, then, for the manager to address the poor performance of a marginal employee. By not having crucial conversations with a marginal employee, action planning to improve performance, and following through with formal corrective action if behavior does not improve after coaching, the manager is failing the high-performing employees (Weston, 2009). If the manager is persistent, fair, and consistent, employees are more likely to perceive the policies are just (Henle, Kohut, & Booth, 2009).

## Disgruntled Employees

Disgruntled employees are those who are always complaining; their behavior affects morale on the unit. They complain about anything and everything, but they direct most of their complaints against the organization. They may air them in public, which can affect how others view the organization. Although the temptation is to label this as an attitude problem, complaining is a behavior and as such can be addressed by the following:

- Remember to set standards of performance and communicate them to the employee.
- Keep notes about incidents of complaining in behavioral terms.
- Take action early, and be consistent among employees.
- Use key behaviors for coaching found in Chapter 19.
- Follow up as scheduled.

Case Study 21-1 describes one manager's experience with an employee with another problematic behavior.

---

### CASE STUDY 21-1

#### PROBLEM STAFF

Gene Marshall is the nurse manager for a general medical–surgical unit in a veteran's hospital. His busy unit primarily serves elderly male patients. Felicia Ralston, RN, has worked on the medical–surgical unit for three years. Since her hiring, Felicia has obtained several body piercings, including her nose, eyebrow, and tongue. She usually wears large hoops or bars in her facial piercings. Not long ago, Felicia added a visible tattoo to the back of her neck and upper shoulder. The tattoo on her lower back can often be seen despite her uniform. Recently, she came to work after adding purple highlights to her hair.

As the number and prominence of Felicia's piercings and body art have increased, several patients and their family members have told Gene that they were "uncomfortable" having Felicia as their nurse. Some patients feel intimidated by her unusual appearance. Gene speaks with Felicia about the patient and family member concerns and reviews the hospital's dress code with her. Felicia becomes angry and tells Gene that hair color, body piercings, and tattoos are a form of individual expression and have nothing to do with her performance as a nurse.

Later, Felicia tells everyone on the unit about her discussion with Gene, speaking loudly and inappropriately in patient care areas. She asks the unit clerk if she knows which patients or family members complained to Gene about her appearance. The following day, Felicia asks each of her assigned patients if they "have a problem" with her. Felicia reports back to Gene that none of her patients said they had any problems with her or her appearance. After discussing the situation with the human resources department, Gene meets with Felicia and provides her with a written warning regarding her body piercings, tattoos, and hair color as well as her unprofessional behavior following their initial meeting. Gene tells Felicia that she must remove jewelry from her nose and eyebrows prior to reporting for work and that her hair color must be a natural color. He also tells her that her tongue jewelry must be small and unnoticeable. Felicia's uniforms are to cover her tattoos completely.

Gene also provides Felicia with a copy of the federal court ruling in which the court ruled that body piercings and tattoos are not considered protected as free speech and that employers have the right to set standards of dress and appearance for their employees. Gene tells Felicia that not only has her behavior been inappropriate and unprofessional but, because it made staff and patients uncomfortable, it could be considered harassment or workplace violence. Finally, Gene emphasizes to Felicia that she should directly speak with him regarding any performance issues or problems and not involve staff or patients in the situation. If Felicia does not comply with these standards within 10 working days, she will be terminated from her position.

#### Manager's Checklist

The nurse manager is responsible for:
- Understanding the human resources policies for their organization
- Consistently applying policies to all employees
- Providing timely and appropriate feedback when an employee is in violation of policies
- Remaining professional at all times when dealing with an irate or angry employee
- Maintaining accurate and thorough documentation of performance issues
- Following up with the human resources department as necessary

## The Employee with a Substance Abuse Problem

As substance abuse has become increasingly prevalent in society, nursing has not remained immune. Substance abuse not only is detrimental to the impaired nurse, but also jeopardizes patients' care, thereby also exposing the employing agency to greater liability.

Early recognition of alcohol or drug dependency and prompt referral for treatment is essential. Some general signs and symptoms may become evident as a nurse's dependency progresses (Boxes 21-1 and 21-2).

In addition to the signs and symptoms listed in Boxes 21-1 and 21-2, the nurse manager should be alert for workplace indications of drug abuse as shown in Box 21-3.

If the manager discovers signs or symptoms in an employee or becomes aware of the unit changes described, further investigation is warranted, and administration should be informed.

---

**BOX 21-1   Signs of Alcohol or Drug Dependency**

- Family history of alcoholism or drug abuse
- Frequent change of work site (same or other institution)
- Prior medical history requiring pain control
- Conscientious worker with recent decrease in performance
- Decreased attention to personal appearance
- Frequent complaints of marital and family problems
- Reports of illness, minor accidents, and emergencies
- Complaints from coworkers
- Mood swings/depression/suicide attempts
- Strong interest in patients' pain control
- Frequent trips to the bathroom
- Increasing isolation (night shift request; eating alone)
- Elaborate excuses for tardiness
- Difficulty in meeting schedules/deadlines
- Inadequate explanation for missing work

---

**BOX 21-2   Physical Symptoms of Alcohol or Drug Dependency**

- Shakiness, tremors of hands, jitteriness
- Slurred speech
- Watery eyes, dilated or constricted pupils
- Diaphoresis
- Unsteady gait
- Runny nose
- Nausea, vomiting, diarrhea
- Weight loss or gain
- Blackouts (memory losses while conscious)
- Wears long-sleeved clothing continuously

---

**BOX 21-3   Workplace Indications of Drug Abuse**

- Incorrect narcotics counts
- Alterations of narcotics containers
- Discrepancies on medication records or frequent corrections on them
- High wastage of narcotics
- Marked shift variations in the quantity of narcotics required on the unit
- Excessive patient reports that their pain medication was ineffective

## State Board of Nursing

State boards of nursing are charged with protecting the public, including the practice by nurses impaired by substance abuse. Reporting laws vary from state to state, as do consequences, but most state boards require the nurse manager to report an impaired colleague (Collins & Mikos, 2008).

Diversion programs offering referral, assistance, and monitoring may be offered in lieu of disciplinary action in some states. For example, the Kansas Nurse Assistance Program (KNAP) is offered to nurses whose practice is impaired by substance abuse (Sidlinger & Hornberger, 2008). Nurses who successfully complete the program are not reported to the Kansas State Board of Nursing (Kansas State Board of Nursing, 2008).

## Strategies for Intervention

Once the manager has identified a nurse with a substance abuse problem, intervention with that nurse must be planned. With the assistance of the human resources department and administration, the manager should examine the organization's policies and procedures and licensure laws as well as determine if a diversion program exists (see above).

Before intervening, the manager should collect all documentation or information about the nurse's behavior that would suggest an abuse problem. Documentation includes records of absenteeism and tardiness (especially recent changes), records of patient complaints about ineffective medications or poor care, staff complaints about job performance, records of controlled substances, and physical signs and symptoms noticed at different times. Dates, times, and behaviors should be carefully noted. Any one behavior means very little; it is the composite pattern that identifies the problem.

Next, the manager should identify appropriate resources to help the nurse. Internal resources include an employee assistance program (EAP) counselor, if the organization has one, or other nurses recovering from alcohol or drug dependency who have offered to help. External resources include the names and phone numbers of treatment center staff, other recovering nurses (if known), and Alcoholics Anonymous or Narcotics Anonymous. It is absolutely essential that several sources be provided so that the nurse knows that help from someone who knows how he or she feels is available, and also knows how to get it. This support cannot be emphasized enough. Failing to offer this assistance is like telling a diabetic he has diabetes and failing to tell him where he can get insulin.

In addition to assistance for the nurse, the manager should check on health insurance provisions for substance abuse treatment. Many insurance carriers have recognized that successful treatment reduces the use of other health care services and, thus, reduces the cost of health care. Accordingly, they offer coverage for treatment to encourage participants to enter recovery programs. Others, unfortunately, do not. Because many of an organization's employees may be covered under the same health care plan, the manager should be able to check these provisions. Few policies cover anything but brief inpatient care, usually only for detoxification, but they may cover outpatient treatment, which is considerably less expensive. Even when there is little or no insurance coverage, the nurse may be able to afford outpatient care. Alcoholics Anonymous and Narcotics Anonymous are effective alternatives, and both are free.

The goal of the intervention is to get the nurse to an appropriate place for an evaluation of the possible problem. Treatment centers or therapists who specialize in substance abuse are recommended to conduct the evaluation. They have the necessary experience for diagnosing and, if indicated, treating the disease.

The manager, human resources, and administration must also decide beforehand what action on the part of the nurse will be acceptable. If the nurse refuses to go for an evaluation, what will the consequences be? The organization's policies and the state board of nursing regulations must be met, and the manager must be clear about the consequences (e.g., discipline, termination) and willing to carry them out. Most experts in treating addictions in nurses recommend that the nurse be offered the option of substance abuse evaluation and, if needed, treatment. If she or he does not agree to that, then the manager should follow the usual disciplinary process and make a report to the state board of nursing, if indicated.

Once preparations have been made, the intervention should be scheduled as soon as possible. Others may be asked to join the manager, but the group should be small and restricted to only those involved in past problems, a substance abuse or human resource staff person, or the manager's supervisor. In some organizations, the top nursing administrator conducts all substance abuse interventions and, in that case, the nurse manager must fully inform the administrator of all circumstances leading to the intervention and provide all the documentation needed. Also, the manager should participate in the intervention so that all relevant information is presented and denial is kept to a minimum.

The intervention should be scheduled at a time and place when and where interruptions can be avoided. It is best to surprise the nurse with a request to come to the office. Denial can build, rationalizations can be developed, and defensiveness can increase if the nurse is given time to consider the problem.

The manager should present the nurse with the collected evidence showing a pattern of behaviors that suggests an abuse problem might be occurring and that an evaluation must be undertaken to know for sure. It is important to focus on the problem behaviors, not on the inadequacy of the person. The individual has already experienced shame and guilt about the use. The manager has an opportunity to help the nurse recognize that substance abuse is an illness that needs treatment; then the nurse will be better able to accept that a problem exists.

In the best-case scenario, the nurse admits the problem, is grateful to be getting help, and goes willingly to treatment. It is best to go directly to treatment from the work site if this can be arranged beforehand. It is important to move quickly before denial resurfaces.

Some nurses, of course, will continue to deny the obvious, in which case the manager must continue to confront the nurse with the reality of the circumstances. If the nurse refuses to go for an evaluation, the manager must follow the organization's disciplinary process. If the nurse is using alcohol or drugs at the time, immediate removal from patient care is necessary. The manager should arrange to have someone (either a family member or another staff member) drive the nurse home, whether the nurse is going to treatment or not. Not only do alcohol or drugs make the nurse an unsafe driver, but the stress of the intervention may distract the nurse even more.

If the nurse agrees to go for an evaluation and/or treatment, specific plans must be made. It should be clear to all parties when the nurse will contact the treatment center (the sooner the better, even if mood-altering chemicals are not being used at the time) and when the nurse will report back to the manager with the recommended course of action. It is possible to arrange with a treatment facility for reports to be made directly to the manager, but federal regulations regarding confidentiality prohibit treatment staff from reporting a patient's status to anyone without that person's written consent. Because the goal of treatment is recovery, which includes returning to work, most facilities request that the nurse give this consent.

The decision to allow an employee to return to work or even to require the employee to avoid returning for any period of time will be based on the recommended treatment. Withdrawal from narcotics very likely will require inpatient detoxification; partial hospitalization also may be recommended. If the employee needs time off for these treatments, sick leave can be used, or the employee may be given an unpaid leave of absence (see the section on the Americans with Disabilities Act and substance abuse).

### Reentry

Reentry to the workplace must be carefully planned, whether the employee has been absent for any length of time or not. It is especially important for the manager and administration to recognize the threat that access to the category of drugs the nurse was addicted to (e.g., narcotics) poses to recovery. Return to work is usually recommended, but not all treatment staff are familiar enough with nursing to be aware of the danger of putting the nurse in constant, daily contact with the drugs that may have been abused in the past. However, it is vitally important to the nurse's recovery that he or she return to work, preferably in the same setting.

This dilemma has often been dealt with in two ways. One method is to reassign the nurse for a period of time (possibly as long as two years) to a job or a unit where few mood-altering drugs are given, such as the nursery, department of education, rehabilitation, home care, dialysis, or patient care audits. Although reassignment presents a problem for the organization and may be disappointing to the nurse, it is far better to make this accommodation than to jeopardize the nurse's recovery by providing access to drugs too soon. This is less a concern with nurses who abused only alcohol.

Another method is to retain the nurse on the unit but not allow administration of mood-altering medications. In fact, state law or organizational policy may require that recovering nurses in the early posttreatment period be restricted from handling controlled substances, carrying narcotic keys, being in charge, or working overtime. This method requires that other staff not only know about the nurse's problem but also be willing to give pain and sleep medications to that nurse's patients. Because this involves disclosing the nurse's addiction, management and staff must decide whether this is reasonable, and the nurse must agree.

Recovering nurses may be discouraged from working evening or night shifts. A reentry contract may be used to specify these restrictions. The contract also may require documentation of participation in recovery groups and random urine drug tests. Ideally, the reentering nurse should have an identified support person available at work.

These restrictions are usually necessary only for the nurse who was addicted to narcotics, but each case should be individually decided based on the amount of stress in the job, the need for rotating shifts, and other factors that may inhibit recovery.

## The Americans with Disabilities Act and Substance Abuse

The Americans with Disabilities Act (ADA) went into effect in 1990 and was amended in 2009 (U.S. Department of Justice). The Act applies to employers of 15 or more people. This law prohibits discrimination in personnel policies (such as hiring and firing) and other employment-related issues if an individual has a qualifying disability. Because alcohol or drug dependency limits one or more of a nurse's activities, it is considered a disability under the ADA. Only those who have been identified with substance abuse disorders, either diagnosed or self-reported, are protected under the law. A person using drugs or who is under the influence of alcohol in the workplace is not protected from the job-related consequences of that use.

The same consideration must be given to the nurse addict as to a nurse with a hearing impairment. This means providing sick leave and treatment opportunity, as well as making reasonable job accommodations. Several reasonable job accommodations have been mentioned previously: assignment to a unit where narcotics and sedatives are not given or are given infrequently, exemption from shift rotation, exemption from charge duties, and the like. Furthermore, the employee's drug abuse history must be kept private. The ADA confidentiality provisions require the employer to keep records on employee substance abuse (i.e., disability) in separate, locked files with access limited to a need-to-know basis.

As with other chronic diseases, alcohol and drug dependency is a disorder prone to relapse. How relapses will be treated under this law is not clear. As with many other personnel issues, it is wise for the nurse manager to consult with human resources and administration about ADA requirements.

Health care today requires that every employee function at peak efficiency and effectiveness. Health care organizations cannot afford to protect an employee whose professional functioning is impaired by substance abuse. Discharging the employee and allowing the person to go to another institution to continue practicing and endangering patients, as well as himself or herself, cannot be allowed. The nurse manager is the frontline contact with staff and can be alert to the signs and symptoms of substance abuse problems, learn intervention techniques and skills, and help recovering nurses return to the workplace. Concern for patients' safety requires intervention, and humane concern for nurse colleagues mandates that such assistance be made available.

Dealing with employee problems present ongoing challenges for the nurse manager, but the steps are similar to those described in Chapter 19. That is, identify the problem, intervene appropriately, and follow up as necessary. In addition, the manager must be persistent, fair, and consistent when intervening with problem employees.

## What You Know Now

- Bullying increases staff dissatisfaction and turnover and can pose a danger to patients as well.
- Incivility and lateral violence are examples of bullying.
- The behaviors of employees who harass others, are marginal performers, are disgruntled, or abuse substances affect coworkers as well as patient care.
- Nurse managers need to identify staff problems early and intervene if necessary.
- Identifying, intervening, and returning nurses with substance abuse problems to the workplace help the organization, the manager, and the affected nurse.
- Substance abuse not only is detrimental to the impaired nurse but also jeopardizes patient care and places the organization at increased liability.
- The manager must be persistent, fair, and consistent when intervening with problem employees.

## Tools for Managing Staff Problems

1. Identify bullying behavior promptly and intervene as appropriate.
2. Document all instances of problem behavior.
3. Try to resolve conflicts and deal with problems as they appear.
4. Consult administration and human resources before intervening in serious problems, such as substance abuse.
5. Follow up problem behaviors with coaching, disciplining, or terminating if needed, using the guide in Chapter 19.

## Questions to Challenge You

1. Have you ever worked or shared a class with a person who caused problems? (Most of us have.) How did the problem manifest itself? How was it handled? How do you wish the problem had been handled?
2. Have you ever experienced bullying or seen others bullied? How did you or they handle it?
3. Are you familiar with the signs and symptoms of substance abuse? Have you seen someone exhibit these characteristics? What signs or symptoms did they exhibit? What happened?
4. Using the examples in the chapter, consider how you would respond to the problem behaviors.

**Pearson Nursing Student Resources**

Find additional review materials at

**www.nursing.pearsonhighered.com**

Prepare for success with additional NCLEX®-style practice questions, interactive assignments and activities, Web links, animations and videos, and more!

## References

Abbassi, S. M., Hollman, K. W., & Hayes, R. D. (2008). Bad bosses and how not to be one. *The Information Management Journal, 42*(1), 52–56.

American Nurses Association. (2010). House of Delegates Resolution. Hostility, abuse and bullying in the workplace. *The Kansas Nurse, 85*(6), 17.

Arnold, E., Pulich, M., & Wang, H. (2008). Managing immature, irresponsible, or irritating employees. *The Health Care Manager, 27*(4), 350–356.

Baird, C. (2010). Spotting alcohol and substance abuse.

*American Nurse Today, 4*(7), 29–31.

Broome, B. A. (2008, Winter). Dealing with sharks and bullies in the workplace. *ABNF Journal,* 28–30.

Christmas, K. (2007). Workplace abuse: Finding solutions. *Nursing Economics, 25*(6), 365–367.

Collins, S. E., & Mikos, C. A. (2008). Evolving taxonomy of nurse practice act violations. *Journal of Nursing Law, 12*(2), 85–91.

Covell, C. L. (2010). Can civility in nursing work environments improve medication safety? *Journal of Nursing Administration, 40*(7/8), 300–301.

Dempster, M. (2006). Turning blind eye to bullies hurts business. *Business Edge.* Retrieved December 2007 from http://www.businessedge.ca/article.cfm/newsID/9505.cfm

Henle, C. A., Kohut, G., & Booth, R. (2009). Designing electronic use policies to enhance employee perceptions of fairness and to reduce cyberloafing: An empirical test of justice theory. *Computers in Human Behavior, 25*(4), 902–910.

Joint Commission. (2008, July 9). Behaviors that undermine a culture of safety. Retrieved October 15, 2010 from http://www.jointcommission.org/SentinelEvents/SentinelEventAlert/sea_40.htm

Kansas State Board of Nursing. (2008). The Kansas nurses assistance program. Retrieved August 23, 2011 from http://www.ksbn.org/knap.htm

Sidlinger, L., & Hornberger, C. (2008). Current characteristics of the investigated impaired nurse in Kansas. *The Kansas Nurse, 83*(1), 3–5.

Stokowski, L. A. (2010). A matter of respect and dignity: Bullying in the nursing profession. Retrieved October 15, 2010 from http://www.medscape.com/viewarticle/729474

Sullivan, E. J. (2013). *Becoming influential: A guide for nurses* (2nd ed.). Upper Saddle River, NJ: Prentice Hall.

U. S. Department of Justice. (2009). Americans with disabilities act of 1990, as amended. Retrieved July 25, 2011 from http://www.ada.gov/pubs/ada.htm

Vessey, J. A., DeMarco, R. F., Gaffney, D. A., & Budin, W. C. (2009). Bullying of staff registered nurses in the workplace. *Journal of Professional Nursing, 25*(5), 299–306.

Weston, M. J. (2009). Managing and facilitating innovation and nurse satisfaction. *Nursing Administration Quarterly, 33*(4), 329–334.

# Preparing for Emergencies

## Learning Outcomes

*After completing this chapter, you will be able to:*

1. Identify examples of disasters that require preparation.
2. Describe potential emergency situations.
3. Explain triage in disaster situations.
4. Discuss the core competencies nurses must have to be prepared for emergencies.
5. Discuss how services can be continued during an emergency.
6. Identify the impact disasters may have on employees

## Key Terms

Emergency operations plan (EOP)

# Preparing for Emergencies

In the decade since September 2001, emergency preparedness has been the focus of national and local efforts. Emergencies can be natural disasters (e.g., tornadoes, hurricanes, earthquakes, or floods), or they may be man-made accidents (e.g., hazardous material spill) or intentionally created (e.g., acts of terrorism). Regardless of the cause, health care organizations must be prepared to deal with the mass casualties that may occur due to any type of emergency (see Box 22-1).

# Types of Emergencies

## Natural Disasters

Natural disasters include any disaster that is not man-made. Floods, hurricanes, tornadoes, volcanos, heat waves, and blizzards are examples of natural disasters. Location is a key element in preparing for natural disasters. Coastal areas must prepare for hurricanes, Mississippi River towns should prepare for flooding, and plains areas should plan for tornado disasters.

Health disasters are also natural disasters. Epidemics of diseases that spread rapidly through the population and pandemics that spread disease around the globe are health disasters. Severe acute respiratory syndrome (SARS), AIDS, antibiotic resistant bacteria, the Ebola virus, and the H1N1 influenza virus are examples of epidemics and pandemics.

## Man-Made Disasters

Sadly, man-made disasters are much more common today than just a few decades ago, when even a bomb threat would be unlikely and possibly thought a hoax. Now, any such threat would be deemed critical, and personnel would respond accordingly.

Man-made disasters can be accidental or intentional. Industrial hazards, structural collapses of buildings or bridges, and power outages are examples of accidental hazards. Subways, sports stadiums, and airplanes may be attacked. Chemical, physical, biological, radiological, or nuclear toxins may spread to the population causing illness and death. Anthrax, a bacterial toxin, and asbestos, a physical toxin, are examples of poisonous substances that can cause environmental disasters.

## Levels of Disasters

Disasters are further categorized by level as follows:

- Level I: Local level response and containment suffices
- Level II: Regional level response is necessary
- Level III: Statewide or national assistance is needed (Smeltzer et al., 2010)

---

**BOX 22-1** **Examples of Disasters**

**Natural Disasters**

Floods
Hurricanes
Earthquakes
Landslides and mudslides
Wildfires
Epidemics and pandemics (influenza, SARS, H1N1)

**Man-Made Disasters**

Accidental
   Structural collapse of buildings or bridges
   Industrial spills
   Power outages
Intentional
   Explosive or incendiary devices
   Sniper or mass casualty shootings
   Release of toxins (chemical, physical, biological, radiological, nuclear)
   Arson fires

Every health care organization must prepare for both natural and man-made disasters and the resulting mass casualty incidents (MCI). Unfortunately, efforts sometimes fall short of the goal.

The National Center for Health Statistics (NCHS) (Niska & Shimizu, 2011) found that only half of U.S. hospitals had plans for alternate care areas with beds, staffing, and equipment. Only half had arranged for advanced registration of health care professionals. More than half, however, had staged practice drills. NCHS has concluded that emergency response preparedness nationwide has not met the goal of full preparedness. Thus, national efforts are being directed toward improving disaster management.

## National Responses to Emergency Preparedness

At the national level, the Joint Commission and the federal government have created initiatives to help prepare first responders and health care organizations to handle emergencies (Sauer et al., 2009). The Joint Commission expanded its emergency management standards to include mitigation, preparedness, response, and recovery (The Joint Commission, 2009). The executive branch of the U.S. government issued executive orders establishing, among other initiatives, the Office of Homeland Security. The U.S. Congress passed legislation addressing bioterrorism and pandemics. Congress also directed the Federal Emergency Management Agency (FEMA) to coordinate disaster relief efforts.

## Hospital Preparedness for Emergencies

Plans for emergency management are required of all hospitals (The Joint Commission, 2009). Key to successful emergency management is a hospital **emergency operations plan (EOP)**. The EOP includes preparation, education and training, and implementation of the hospital's response to emergency situations.

### Emergency Operations Plan

The hospital's EOP includes the following components:

- Activation response
- Communication plan
- Patient care coordination plan
- Security plan
- Traffic flow plan
- Data management strategy
- Resources availability (Smeltzer et al., 2010)

Finally, the EOP must include plans to deactivate the response, follow-up with post-incident review, and a schedule for practice drills.

Implementation of the EOP includes three components: planning, preparing, and practicing (Smeltzer et al., 2010).

### Planning

Planning involves determining the hospitals' top three to five vulnerabilities based on its geographic location. For example, if the hospital is near a factory, the EOP would include plans for possible industrial accidents. If the hospital is located in a city near the Atlantic Ocean, they would prepare for hurricane victims. On the other hand, if the hospital sits on the Kansas plains, tornadoes are more likely. Once vulnerabilities have been determined, planning can proceed based on the possible patient injuries.

Preparing

Preparation includes staff education and training. Both knowledge and skills training are needed, and lectures and computer simulations may be used. Participants' knowledge and skills must be evaluated and, if deficient, retraining conducted.

Practicing

Hospitals are required to test their EOP twice a year (The Joint Commission, 2009). One practice can be a tabletop event, but one must involve realistic situations and simulated patients (Sauer, 2011). The timing of exercises should include occasions when the hospital is at low capacity to test its readiness in the most adverse situations. Evaluation of the hospital's EOP and performance should be evaluated annually.

## Disaster Triage

Similar to the triage system used by the military in war situations, hospitals must reverse their usual triage method of treating the most-seriously injured person first. Instead, they must prioritize scarce resources to those who can benefit the most (Kirwan, 2011). The Simple Triage and Rapid Treatment (START) system is an example (www.start-triage.com). The goal is to treat as many injured people as possible in the shortest time possible. Inundated with mass casualties, precious time must be directed to the least seriously injured first, then the more seriously injured, and so on.

## Core Competencies for Nurses

The National Emergency Preparedness Education Coalition (2003) established core competencies for nurses to prepare for mass casualties. These include:

- *Critical thinking.* Critical thinking in disasters is different than in normal health care situations. Mass casualties may inundate the facility, the triage system is reversed, and the nurse may be concerned about family at home. Nurses' abilities to prioritize, demonstrate clinical judgment, and make decisions are key to successful emergency responses (Coyle, Sapnas, & Ward-Presson, 2007).
- *Assessment.* Assessment includes self-assessment and situational assessment (Coyle, Sapnas, & Ward-Presson, 2007). Patient assessment includes physical injuries, as expected, but also emotional injuries and family assessments. During a disaster such as SARS, the hospital may be inundated with "psychological" casualties—people who think they have the symptoms. Triage must address how to treat these casualties as well.
- *Technical skills.* In addition to therapeutic interventions skills, nurses must be able to implement appropriate therapies, arrange transport, and maintain patient safety during an incident. The nurse must also be aware of hazardous substances, the isolation techniques necessary and use personal protective equipment as needed.
- *Communication.* When dealing with mass casualties, communication within the hospital and with local officials is essential. A system to track patients throughout their stay is necessary for staff follow-up so that families can be kept informed (Kirwan, 2011).

## Continuation of Services

Complicating emergency preparedness is the need to provide for continuation of services in the event of an emergency. Routine services may be disrupted. Loss of electrical power may be countered by the backup generators, but if computer capabilities close down, how will the electronic medical record and the medication system work? How will documentation continue? Resupply of medications, food, water, and supplies may be interrupted. What if resupply lines are impacted by a disaster (e.g., trucks delivering meds cannot get through due to flooded or washed out roads)? Furthermore, how will the facility handle a large influx of patients and/or casualties? If needed, how will the evacuation of the facility be handled? The EOP must address all of these issues.

Risk assessment is necessary to identify the hospital's vulnerability (Edwards et al., 2007). Hospitals are often the frontline responders to mass casualty events, but maintaining services in the face of overwhelming numbers of casualties can be challenging. Capabilities, resources, and education and training needs must be assessed.

Surge capacity describes an institution's ability to mobilize when suddenly confronted with a vast increase in patient demand (Hick et al., 2008). By planning ahead of time for an influx of patients, strategies can be put in place to mobilize emergency procedures. A surge system includes:

- Supplies
- Personnel
- Physical space
- Management infrastructure

These components are known as "stuff, staff, and structure" (Barbisch & Koenig, 2006). At the onset of a disaster and the impending arrival of mass casualties, a hospital incident command structure can be implemented, a rapid needs assessment conducted, and appropriate activities mobilized. Preparation and drills ensure that all components are in place. Post-incident follow-up is essential to continually evaluate performance and initiate improvements.

## Impact on Employees

Depending upon the nature of the emergency, staff will be affected. They may become ill themselves, their homes may be flooded, or they may have children left at home that they have to go to, for example. With the loss of staff, how will the agency continue to accept and care for new patients?

Employee fatigue and exhaustion, including mental fatigue, must be addressed. Personal protective equipment must be available and staff must be trained to use the equipment and know how to access it in an emergency. Protective equipment includes respiratory protection, eye and face protection, and hand, arm, and body protection, if needed.

Education, training, and practice drills help staff prepare for sudden MCI (Williams, Nocera, & Casteel, 2008). Key to maintaining operational readiness is the staff's willingness to come to work during a disaster (Davidson et al., 2009). The hospital's surge capacity includes a callback system to request that staff return to work during an emergency but doesn't address the staff member's willingness to come to work (Cone & Cummings, 2006).

Several factors determine staff members' decisions to come to work, including vulnerability of family, personal safety concerns, professional accountability, past experience with disasters, caring connection with the organization, and the desire to help (Davidson et al., 2009).

These factors suggest appropriate management responses. Developing a caring relationship with staff members and a compassionate response during and after a disaster may slightly help mitigate staff concerns about family vulnerability and personal safety. Worry about pets, children, dependent adults, and their own security will, of course, still affect employees' decisions to return to work (Davidson et al., 2009).

In addition to the complications of preparing for emergencies, the hospital also may not be reimbursed for care provided, standards of care may not be established or able to be maintained, and the hospital may incur liability for volunteers' safety or their performance (Hodge et al., 2009). Emergency preparedness, however, has improved in the past decade and promises to improve in the future.

See how one hospital prepared for an impending emergency in Case Study 22-1.

## CASE STUDY 22-1

### PREPARING FOR AN IMPENDING EMERGENCY

Weather forecasters were predicting 15 inches of snow to fall in the next 24 hours. It was likely to be the biggest snow storm the town had seen in as many years as anyone could remember. Everyone was in an uproar over the impending severe storm that threatened to shut the city down. Mt. Bethel Hospital administration wanted to make sure they were prepared for this blizzard ahead of time and had an effective emergency plan in place to get the patients good, uninterrupted care.

The snow was expected to start at four o'clock in the afternoon. Hospital managers and administrators met early that morning at seven o'clock to get a plan in place. It was decided that a message would go out to all staff who were scheduled to work that night, advising them to come into the hospital for their night shift early. The hospital would serve dinner in the cafeteria to those waiting for their shift to start. Getting night staff to the hospital before the blizzard was projected to be at its worst would allow the hospital to run in routine fashion overnight. The hospital also encouraged night shifters to bring a bag to stay over the next day at the hospital and asked them to consider working the following night shift too.

The administration team increased its linen and grocery orders with vendors so the hospital would be well stocked in case deliveries couldn't be made for a few days. The grocery order was delivered and included all items requested. The linen order was delivered that day; it was only double the routine delivery, because many other facilities had also requested excess linens to be delivered. The administration made a note in its plan to notify staff to conserve linen resources if a normal linen delivery couldn't occur the next day.

The administration announced to the day-time staff that all staff had been invited to spend the night at the hospital after their shift and asked to work the next day as well. Each staff member was provided with a cot to sleep on, blankets, meals, and scrubs. In addition, the hospital made shower facilities within the building available for staff, and even put up sign-up sheets for each shower so staff could schedule their time. Most day staff agreed to stay at the hospital to avoid driving home and so they would be available the next day when people at home were likely not going to be able to drive in for their shift.

Mt. Bethel was well prepared for the impending blizzard. With proper advance preparation, the hospital was able to operate under normal patient care standards. The staff had been so gracious to stay at the hospital and meet the staffing needs for patient care. Within 36 hours, the streets were cleared and the city was back to its usual operations. Staff was able to commute to work, deliveries of groceries and linens were back on schedule, and the hospital was operating under normal conditions again. Mt. Bethel administration was pleased it had been able to successfully plan and work through the weather emergency.

## What You Know Now

- Emergencies include natural disasters, man-made accidents, and acts of terrorism.
- Emergency preparedness is the focus of national efforts and promises to increase in the coming decade.
- Every hospital is required to have an emergency operations plan (EOP).
- Triage in a mass casualty incident is the reverse of normal standards: the goal is to treat the most people in the shortest time with the resources available.
- Planning, preparing, and practicing are the steps necessary to manage potential emergencies.
- Core competencies for nurses include critical thinking, assessment, technical skills, and communication.
- Surge capacity describes an institution's ability to mobilize when confronted with an influx of patients.
- Education, training, and practice drills help staff prepare for sudden MCI.
- Employees' caring connection with the institution may help mitigate their concerns about family vulnerabilities and personal safety.

## Tools for Preparing for Emergencies and Preventing Violence

1. Become familiar with your organization's emergency operations plan (EOP).
2. Participate in education and training sessions to prepare for emergencies.
3. Refresh your training regarding reverse triage.
4. Recognize that an actual disaster will challenge your ability to handle family situations, concerns about your personal safety, and effect your decision to come to work.
5. When an emergency occurs (practice or actual), recall your training and participate as required.

## Questions to Challenge You

1. Do you know what to do in an emergency? List the steps you would take. Then locate a copy of your organization's policies and procedures for emergencies and evaluate yourself.
2. Create a fictitious emergency situation with a classmate or colleague. Challenge each other on how each of you would handle the situation. Share your experience with others.
3. Have you participated in disaster drills? How well did you follow your training? How well did the organization handle the drill? Did you see areas for improvement?
4. Have you been involved in an actual disaster experience? If so, share your experience with classmates or colleagues. Nothing makes a situation real better than a factual account.

**Pearson Nursing Student Resources**
Find additional review materials at
**www.nursing.pearsonhighered.com**
Prepare for success with additional NCLEX®-style practice questions, interactive assignments and activities, Web links, animations and videos, and more!

## Web Resource

START Triage: http://www.start-triage.com

## References

Barbisch, D., & Koenig, K. L. (2006). Understanding surge capacity: Essential elements. *Academic Emergency Medicine, 13*(11), 1098–1102.

Cone, D. C., & Cummings, B. A. (2006). Hospital disaster staffing: If you call, will they come? *American Journal of Disaster Medicine, 1*(1), 28–36.

Coyle, G. A., Sapnas, K. G., & Ward-Presson, K. (2007). Dealing with disaster. *Nursing Management, 38*(7), 24–29.

Davidson, J. E., Sekayan, A., Agan, D., Good, L., Shaw, D., & Smilde, R. (2009). Disaster dilemma: Factors affecting decision to come to work during a natural disaster. *Advanced Emergency Nursing Journal, 31*(3), 248–257.

Edwards, D., Williams, L. H., Scott, M. A., & Beatty, J. (2007). When disaster strikes: Maintaining operational readiness. *Nursing Management, 38*(9), 64–66.

Hick, J. L., Koenig, K. L., Barbisch, D., & Bey, T. A. (2008). Surge capacity concepts for health care facilities: The CO-S-TR model for initial incident assessment. *Disaster Medicine and Public Health Preparedness, 2*(Supplement 1), 551–557.

Hodge, J. G., Garcia, A. M., Anderson, E. D., & Kaufman, T. (2009). Emergency legal preparedness for hospitals and health care personnel. *Disaster Medicine and Public Health Preparedness, 3*(Supplement 1), S37–S44.

Howard, P. K., & Gilboy, N. (2009). Workplace violence. *Advanced Emergency Nursing Journal, 31*(2), 94–100.

Kirwan, M. M. (2011). Disaster planning: Are you ready? *Nursing Made Incredibly Easy, 9*(3), 18–24.

Niska, R. W., & Shimizu, I. M. (2011, March 24). Hospital preparedness for emergency response: United States, 2008. *National Health Statistics Reports, 37*, 1–15.

Nursing Emergency Preparedness Education Coalition. (2003). *Educational competencies for registered nurses responding to mass casualty incidents.* Retrieved August 23, 2011 from http://www.nursing.vanderbilt.edu/incmce/competencies.html

Sauer, L. M., McCarthy, M. L., Knebel, A., & Brewster, P.

(2009). Major influences on hospital emergency management and disaster preparedness. *Disaster Medicine and Public Health Preparedness, 3*(Supplement 1), S68–S73.

Smeltzer, S., Bare, B., Hinkel, J., & Cheever, K. (2010). *Brunner and Suddarth's textbook of medical–surgical nursing* (12th ed.). Philadelphia, PA: Lippincott Williams & Wilkins.

The Joint Commission. (2009). Emergency management in *The Joint Commission Hospital Accreditation Program.* Oakbook Terrace, IL: The Joint Commission.

Williams, J., Nocera, M., & Casteel, C. (2008). The effectiveness of disaster training for health care workers: A systematic review. *Annals of Emergency Medicine, 52*(3), 211–222.

# Preventing Workplace Violence

## Violence in Heath Care
### INCIDENCE OF WORKPLACE VIOLENCE
### CONSEQUENCES OF WORKPLACE VIOLENCE
### FACTORS CONTRIBUTING TO VIOLENCE IN HEALTH CARE

## Preventing Violence
### ZERO-TOLERANCE POLICIES
### REPORTING AND EDUCATION
### ENVIRONMENTAL CONTROLS

## Dealing with Violence
### VERBAL INTERVENTION
### A VIOLENT INCIDENT
### OTHER DANGEROUS INCIDENTS
### POST-INCIDENT FOLLOW-UP

## Learning Outcomes

*After completing this chapter, you will be able to:*

1. Discuss what health care organizations can do to prevent violence.
2. Identify threats and threatening behaviors.
3. Describe how to recognize escalating violence.
4. Discuss how to respond to a violent incident.
5. Describe how to handle the follow-up to a violent incident.

## Key Term

Workplace violence

# Violence in Health Care

**Workplace violence** is any violent act, including physical assaults and threats of assault, directed toward persons at work or on duty. Those working in health care are among the most vulnerable to attack (Howard & Gilboy, 2009). Most assaults in health care are by patients, but attacks are also made by disgruntled family members, coworkers, vendors, employers, or even colleagues (Gates, Gillespie, & Succop, 2011). Some assaults are episodes of domestic violence that occur at work (Pollack et al., 2010).

Violence includes:

- Threatening actions, such as waving fists, throwing objects, or threatening body language
- Verbal or written threats
- Physical attacks, including slapping, hitting, biting, shoving, kicking, pushing, beating
- Violent assaults, including rape, homicide, and attacks with weapons, such as knives, firearms, or bombs

## Incidence of Workplace Violence

Violence in health care occurs more often than in other workplace settings (U.S. Department of Health and Human Services, 2008). Public focus, however, has been on other occupational settings with violence in health care receiving little attention (Gates, Gillespie, & Succop, 2011). This is in spite of an increase in assaults in health care (U.S. Department of Labor, Bureau of Labor Statistics, 2009).

## Consequences of Workplace Violence

Violence can range in intensity and cause physical injuries, temporary or permanent disability, psychological trauma, or death (Howard & Gilboy, 2009). In health care, violence is more likely to occur in psychiatric settings, emergency rooms, waiting rooms, and geriatric units, while clinics are reported to be less likely sites of violence (Nachreiner et al., 2007).

In addition to harming employees, violence in the workplace can affect worker morale, increase staff stress, cause a mistrust of administration, and exacerbate a hostile work environment (Gates et al., 2011). Furthermore, absenteeism and turnover are expensive, and the organization may incur additional health costs for care of injured workers.

## Factors Contributing to Violence in Health Care

Working with the public carries with it inherent risks, and the added stress by staff, patients, and families in health care settings increases that risk (Gates et al., 2011). Furthermore, hospitals have an "open door" policy for visitors. Visiting hours are not restricted, and visitors are often not required to check in when they enter.

Patients with head trauma, seizure disorders, dementia, alcohol or drug withdrawal, or who are homeless may lash out in violence. Crime victims and the perpetrators might be admitted to the same hospital, and gang violence could spill over into the hospital. In addition, family members' stress and fear as well as long waits can contribute to the possibility of violent actions. Finally, the absence of visible, armed, and adequately trained security personnel may make the setting less secure.

Although no workplace can be certain to be free from violence, especially random violence, some additional risk factors for potential violence in health care organizations include:

- Working understaffed, especially at meal times and visiting hours
- Long waiting times
- Overcrowded waiting rooms
- Working alone

- Inadequate security
- Unlimited public access
- Poorly lit corridors, rooms, and parking lots

Injuries to nurses from violence are likely underreported for several reasons (Gacki-Smith et al., 2009). The definition of workplace violence may not be clear, reporting policies may not be in place, and employees may simply believe that assaults are part of the job (Ray, 2007). Staff also may fear that reporting an assault will be construed as poor job performance (Gacki-Smith, 2009).

## Preventing Violence

### Zero-Tolerance Policies

The health care organization should cultivate a culture of intolerance to violence and set its violence prevention policies to reflect that position (Gates, Gillespie, & Succop, 2011). Appropriate personnel policies must state clearly what will happen if violence or the threat of violence occurs. Policies regarding patients and visitors must do the same. Specifically, anyone who becomes violent or who exhibits threatening behavior must be removed from the setting and the authorities contacted.

Questions to ask when developing policies regarding violence prevention are shown in Box 23-1.

### Reporting and Education

Employees must be educated to recognize the warning signs of violence and potential assailants or agitators, and be taught conflict resolution skills and de-escalation tactics. They should also be alerted to use care when storing health instruments (stethoscopes, hemostats, scissors) that could be used as weapons.

Once adequate policies are in place, employees must be informed about them so that they are prepared in case of an event or crisis. In addition, they need to know how to report and to whom to report as well as how to document problem situations. Employees should be reassured that reporting threatening behavior will not result in reprisals.

### Environmental Controls

The organization should institute environmental controls to ensure patient, visitor, and employee safety. These include:

- Adequate lighting
- Security devices
- Bullet-resistant barriers in the emergency department
- Curved mirrors in hallways

---

**BOX 23-1    Preventing Violence: Questions to Ask**

- Does your facility have a clear reporting procedure in the event that there's a workplace aggression incident?
- Whom does the staff inform of its concerns?
- What are the repercussions should individuals report an incident that makes them uneasy?

- Does your facility offer a mental health support program for staff? Is it effective in helping to reduce employee stress?
- When someone voices a concern to supervisory staff, is action taken to address the problem quickly?

*From:* DelBel, J. C. (2003). De-escalating workplace aggression. *Nursing Management, 34*(9), 30–34.

In addition, safe work practices should be implemented, such as:

- Escort services
- Adequate staffing
- Judicious use of restraints or seclusion
- Alerting staff about patients with histories of violent behavior, dementia, or intoxication

# Dealing with Violence

### Verbal Intervention

Verbal threats often precede a physically violent event; thus, all employees need to know techniques for reducing aggression in people who are making verbal threats. (See Box 23-2.)

When faced with a potentially violent situation, try to keep calm even when another person is screaming threats or abuse. Try to get the person away from others. A crowd might encourage the abuser, or the person might be afraid to "lose face" in the presence of others.

As you learned in Chapter 9, nonverbal communication is more powerful than your words, so watch your body language and keep a distance from the person. Use clear and direct words; anxiety could make it difficult for the person to comprehend. Reflect the person's words back; this lets the person know that you hear him or her. Silence is often effective because it forces the person to think about what is being said and may be calming in itself. Finally, keep your tone of voice calm, keep your volume normal, and slow your rate of speech. Together, these strategies may reduce the person's anxiety and aggression (Gates, Gillespie, & Succop, 2011).

### A Violent Incident

In spite of all that an organization and individuals do to try to prevent violence, the person's aggression may escalate. In the event that such a situation occurs, the organization should make certain that all employees are prepared. Each employee should:

- Recognize the signs of escalating violence
- Know the organization's violence policies
- Be prepared to protect their patients, their visitors, and themselves

Every employee should learn how to watch for threatening behaviors to evaluate when a person is likely to become violent. Law enforcement personnel recommend watching for these behaviors:

- Clenched fists
- Blank stare
- Fighting stance (one foot back with arm pulled back ready to strike)
- Arms raised in a fighting position
- Standing too close or advancing toward you
- Holding anything that might be used as a weapon, such as a pen, letter opener, heavy object, or an actual weapon—a gun or knife
- Overt intent (saying that they intend to "kick your —," or similar statements)
- Movement toward the exit to prevent you from leaving (Sullivan, 2013)

---

**BOX 23-2**    **Verbal Intervention Strategies**

1. Remain calm.
2. Isolate the individual.
3. Watch your body language.
4. Keep it simple.

5. Use reflective questioning.
6. Embrace silence.
7. Maintain moderation in speech.

*From:* DelBel, J. C. (2003). De-escalating workplace aggression. *Nursing Management, 34*(9), 30–34.

When these threatening behaviors are present, or if the person becomes physically violent, you must protect your patients, visitors, other staff, and yourself. Contact security immediately and follow the steps in Box 23-3.

### Other Dangerous Incidents

An infant abduction, a bomb threat, or a gun on the unit are some examples of other dangerous incidents that could occur. Most organizations now have a specific code to alert staff to a potential or real infant abduction, such as Code Pink, and many hospitals now also place security bands on babies and parents to prevent a baby being abducted from the nursing unit.

Policies are in place in most hospitals to address bomb threats or a gun on the unit and the procedures to follow, and the staff are trained to call the hospital's 911 number. Other threats also use specific codes for alerting security and obtaining assistance. In addition, drills for infant abductions, bomb threats, and firearms on the unit are practiced on a routine basis and included in yearly competency testing for employees. Keeping patients safe is always the focus.

### Post-Incident Follow-Up

After a violent incident, everyone involved will suffer some degree of emotional, if not physical, trauma. Gates, Gillespie, and Succop (2011) found that 94 percent of emergency department nurses experienced at least one symptom of posttraumatic stress disorder (PTSD) following an incident of violence, with 17 percent diagnosed with probable PTSD.

Post-incident follow-up is essential for the well-being of patients, visitors, and staff members. The steps to take are shown in Box 23-4.

A nurse manager used the steps in handling a violent incident and its follow-up in Case Study 23-1.

Violence in the workplace is a reality of life today, but organizations and individuals can take steps to reduce potential threats. Because the nursing shortage is continuing, and because nurses and women are more likely to be attacked, organizations must take all the necessary steps to ensure that their nurses are kept safe from harm. Additionally, nurses themselves must be informed about how to recognize potential threats and how to prevent violence from escalating. In this way violence may be prevented or, at the least, reduced.

---

**BOX 23-3**   How to Handle a Violent Incident

1. Notify security immediately.
2. Never try to disarm someone with a weapon.
3. If not armed, enlist staff help in restraining a violent person.
4. Put a barrier between you and the violent person.

---

**BOX 23-4**   How to Handle Post-Incident Follow-Up

1. Be certain that everyone is safe following a violent event.
2. Arrange immediate treatment for the injured.
3. Complete injury and incident reports.
4. Follow up with human resources regarding the worker's compensation process for the injured employees.
5. Contact security to determine if a police report should be filed.
6. Contact the injured employee at home to express concern for the person's well-being and follow up with any questions the person may have.

## CASE STUDY 23-1

### WORKPLACE VIOLENCE

Melanie Sanchez is nurse manager of a 30-bed skilled nursing unit (SNU) in an urban hospital. Patient confusion and aggression are not uncommon occurrences for her staff. Nursing and assistive staff have been trained on conflict resolution and methods for dealing with aggressive patients.

Sandra Porter, RN, has worked in the SNU for the past six years. Today, while administering medication to patients before lunch in the common dining room, Sandra noticed a newly admitted patient, Mr. B, yelling obscenities at another staff member. Sandra secured her medication cart and came to the aid of the nursing assistant. Sandra attempted to verbally de-escalate the situation, but Mr. B became increasingly aggressive. When Sandra turned to instruct the nursing assistant to clear patients from the dining room, Mr. B. picked up a chair and struck Sandra in the arm and shoulder. The nursing assistant alerted Melanie and several nurses to the problem. Melanie immediately called the hospital operator to request that security respond to a violent patient on the SNU. Upon entering the dining room, nursing staff were able to restrain Mr. B while Melanie accompanied Sandra to the emergency department for treatment of her injuries. Sandra sustained a broken arm, a laceration to her shoulder, and several contusions.

As soon as Sandra's injuries were treated and she was released from the emergency department, Melanie contacted the medical/surgical nursing division director and the human resources department about the assault and filled out an incident report. She also completed an injury report for Sandra's worker's compensation claim. Melanie contacted the security department and requested a meeting with the security director to determine if a police report should be filed regarding Mr. B's assault of Sandra. The next day, Melanie contacted Sandra at home and informed her that a case manager from human resources would call her within the week regarding her worker's compensation claim. Melanie also checked to see how Sandra was doing and encouraged her to call Melanie directly if she had questions or concerns.

### Manager's Checklist

The nurse manager is responsible for:

- Ensuring that appropriate action is taken to secure the safety and well-being of the injured employee, patients, and other staff immediately following a workplace violence incident
- Securing immediate and appropriate treatment for the injured employee
- Informing administration and human resources departments of the incident
- Completing required injury and incident reports in a timely manner
- Following up with human resources regarding the worker's compensation process for the injured employee
- Contacting security to determine if a police report should be filed regarding the incident.
- Contacting the injured employee at home to express concern for their well-being and follow up with any questions they may have
- Ensuring any scheduling problems due to the injured employee's absence are resolved

## What You Know Now

- Health care organizations are vulnerable to violence in the workplace, but incidents of violence may be underreported.
- Risk factors for violence in health care organizations include understaffing, patient conditions, family members' anxiety, unlimited public access, inadequate security, and an unsafe physical environment.
- The organization should establish a zero-tolerance for violence policy and make certain that all employees know it.
- All employees should be able to recognize potential threats and the warning signs of violence.
- All employees should know how to report threats and threatening behavior, to whom to report such episodes, and how to document the incidents.
- Employees should be assured that reporting potential threats will not result in reprisals.
- All employees should know the steps to take if a violent incident occurs.

## Tools for Preparing for Emergencies and Preventing Violence

1. Recognize potential threats and threatening behavior and how to report them.
2. Alert staff and administration to these threats.
3. Know how to respond to a person who becomes violent.
4. Know what to do following a violent incident.
5. Monitor the environment for dangerous areas and report your observations to administration.
6. Remain alert for potential violence and instruct staff to stay vigilant.

## Questions to Challenge You

1. Evaluate your current workplace or clinical site. See if you can find potential opportunities that would allow violence to occur. Describe them.
2. Ask to see the workplace violence policies at your school, clinical site, and/or workplace. Evaluate them. Are they adequate? Can you suggest changes?
3. Have you ever been the victim of violence or threats of violence? How did you handle the event and its aftermath? Would you do something differently now? How did the authorities respond? Could you suggest changes for them?
4. Are you aware of specific action that your school, workplace, or clinical site has done to protect people from violence? What more could you suggest?

**Pearson Nursing Student Resources**

Find additional review materials at
**www.nursing.pearsonhighered.com**

Prepare for success with additional NCLEX®-style practice questions, interactive assignments and activities, Web links, animations and videos, and more!

## References

DelBel, J. C. (2003). De-escalating workplace aggression. *Nursing Management, 34*(9), 30–34.

Gacki-Smith, Juarez, A. M., Boyett, L., Homeyer, C., Robinson, L., & MacLean, S. L. (2009). Violence against nurses working in U.S. emergency departments. *Journal of Nursing Administration, 39*(7/8), 340–349.

Gates, D., Gillespie, G., Smith, C., Rode, J., Kowalenko, T., & Smith, B. (2011). Using action research to plan a violence prevention program for emergency departments. *Journal of Emergency Nursing, 37*(1), 32–39.

Gates, D. M., Gillespie, G. L., & Succop, P. (2011). Violence against nurses and its impact on stress and productivity. *Nursing Economics, 29*(2), 59–66.

Howard, P. K., & Gilboy, N. (2009). Workplace violence. *Advanced Emergency Nursing Journal, 31*(2), 94–100.

Nachreiner, N. M., Hansen, H. E., Okano, A., Gerberich, S. G., Ryan, A. D., McGovern, P. M., Church, T. R., & Watt, G. D. (2007). Difference in work-related violence by nurse license type. *Journal of Professional Nursing, 23*(5), 290–300.

Pollack, K. M., McKay, T., Cumminskey, C., Clinton-Sherrod, A. M., Lindquist, C. H., Lasater, B. M., Hardison Walters, J. L., Krotki, K., & Grisso, J. A. (2010). Employee assistance program services of intimate partner violence and client satisfaction with these services. *Journal of Occupational and Environmental Medicine, 52*(8), 819–826.

Ray, M. M. (2007). The dark side of the job: Violence in the emergency department.

*Journal of Emergency Nursing, 33*(3), 257–261.

Sullivan, E. J. (2013). *Becoming influential: A guide for nurses* (2nd ed.). Upper Saddle River, NJ: Prentice Hall.

U.S. Department of Labor, Bureau of Labor Statistics.

(2009). Nonfatal occupational injuries and illnesses requiring days away from work, 2009. Retrieved August 24, 2011 from http://www.bls.gov/news.release/osh2.nr0.htm

U.S. Department of Health and Human Services.

(2008). *Understanding and responding to workplace violence.* Washington, DC: U.S. Department of Health and Human Services.

# Handling Collective Bargaining Issues

Laws Governing Unions

Process of Unionization

    THE GRIEVANCE PROCESS

    THE NURSE MANAGER'S ROLE

Status of Collective Bargaining for Nurses

    LEGAL STATUS OF NURSING UNIONS

    THE FUTURE OF COLLECTIVE BARGAINING
    FOR NURSES

## Learning Outcomes

*After completing this chapter, you will be able to:*

1. Discuss the laws that govern collective bargaining.
2. Describe the nurse manager's role in collective bargaining.
3. Explain what is involved in the grievance process.
4. Describe the legal issues involved for nurses.
5. Discuss the future of nursing unions.

## Key Terms

Collective bargaining        Grievances        Strike

# Laws Governing Unions

Before federal laws governing labor relations in this country were enacted, disputes between the owners or managers of a company and the company's labor force were settled by the judiciary branch of government. During this period of American history, the courts often ruled that **collective bargaining**, collective action taken by workers to secure better wages or working conditions, was illegal. Today, however, labor laws enacted by Congress, decisions by the U.S. Supreme Court, and the National Labor Relations Board (NLRB) guide labor relations between employers and employees.

Since enactment of the National Labor Relations Act in 1935, nurses and other employees of private, for-profit health care institutions have been protected in their right to organize for collective bargaining purposes. Under the provisions of the act, as amended in 1974, employees of voluntary, not-for-profit health care institutions also were granted the same rights and protections.

In the United States, a *closed shop* is a business in which union membership (often of a specific union and no other) is a precondition to employment. An *open shop* is a business in which union membership is not a component in hiring decisions and union members don't receive any preference in hiring.

A *right-to-work state* is a state in which no person can be denied the right to work because of membership or nonmembership in a labor union. Trade unions and employers cannot make membership in a union or payment of union dues or "fees" a condition of employment, either before or after hiring.

Collective bargaining laws differ depending on if the nurses are employed in the private sector in either nonprofit or for-profit organizations or if they are employed in the public sector as city, county, state, or federal employees. Negotiations may be classified as mandatory, prohibited, or permissive. Parties are obligated to negotiate on mandatory subjects of bargaining.

In the private sector, wages, hours, and other terms and conditions of work are considered mandatory subjects for negotiation. In the public sector, the scope of mandatory subjects of bargaining is often far narrower.

The Civil Service Reform Act of 1978 gave certain federal employees the right to organize, bargain collectively, and participate through labor organizations of their choice in decisions affecting their work environment, although it depends on what federal agency is their employer. Wages—a mandatory item in the private sector—is a prohibited subject.

State or local employees, however, fall under state regulations, which vary greatly from state to state. Nurses in state hospitals, for example, would be governed by their state laws. Some states don't allow employees to strike or form collective bargaining units; other states don't allow wages or overtime pay to be part of a union contract.

# Process of Unionization

The process of establishing a union in any setting begins when at least 30 percent of eligible employees sign a card to indicate interest in a union. Then the union petitions the National Labor Relations Board (NLRB) to conduct an election. The NLRB meets with both the union and the employer. At the conclusion of this meeting, the NLRB will determine who is eligible to participate in the union, establish that the signers are employees of the organization, and set a date for the union election.

The process of selecting a bargaining agent produces a tense, emotional climate that affects everyone in the organization. Both nurse managers and staff nurses need to remember that during this period, the rules of unfair labor practice apply. Managers must refrain from any action that could be seen as interfering with the employees' right to determine their collective bargaining representative. Such actions include individually questioning staff nurses about their knowledge of collective bargaining activities and making promises or threats to individual staff members based on the outcome of the election.

Staff nurses also must be careful that their discussions regarding collective bargaining take place away from the work site and not on work time. Nor may employees use their employer's e-mail system to communicate about unionizing activities.

Certification by the NLRB of a union to be the bargaining agent does not automatically mean employees have a contract. The contract is considered to be in effect when both management of the organization and employees agree on its content. The final agreement is subject to a ratification vote by a simple majority of eligible members who vote.

The role of administering the contract then falls to an individual designated as the union representative. This individual may be an employee of the union or a member of the nursing staff.

## The Grievance Process

The grievance procedure will be specified in the agreement and will contain a series of progressive steps and time limits for submission/resolution of grievances. **Grievances** are formal complaints that may be caused by misunderstandings, a lack of familiarity with the contract, or an inadequate labor agreement.

To ensure that there is a balance between the rights of employees and the rights of the public to health care, Congress passed a special set of dispute-settling procedures to be applied in the health care industry:

1.  Before changing or terminating a contract, one party must notify the other of its intent to do so 90 days prior to the contract expiration date. This is 30 days more than specified for other industries.

2.  If after 30 days of this notification both sides cannot agree, then the Federal Mediation and Conciliation Service (FMCS) must be notified.

3.  The FMCS will appoint either a mediator or an inquiry board within 30 days.

4.  The mediator or board must make recommendations within 15 days.

5.  If after 15 more days both sides cannot agree, then a strike vote can be conducted and a **strike**, the organized stoppage of work by employees, can be scheduled.

If a strike vote is affirmed, then a 10-day written notice must be given to management indicating the date, time, and place of the strike. This is to ensure that a hospital has adequate time to provide for continuity of patient care in the event of a strike.

## The Nurse Manager's Role

The nurse manager in a health care organization where nurses are organized into a collective bargaining unit needs to be aware of the five categories of unfair labor practices described by labor law (National Labor Relations Act [NLRA], Sec. 9[e]2).

1.  Interference with the right to organize

2.  Domination

3.  Encouraging or discouraging union membership

4.  Discharging an employee for giving testimony or filing a charge with the NLRB

5.  Refusal to bargain collectively

Another responsibility of the manager is to participate in resolving grievances, using the agreed-upon grievance procedure. Grievances can usually be classified as:

1.  Contract violations

2.  Violations of federal or state law

3.  Failure of management to meet its responsibilities

4.  Violation of agency rules

## CASE STUDY 24-1

### DISCIPLINE PROCEDURE IN A HOSPITAL WITH COLLECTIVE BARGAINING UNIT

Maria Sanchez is the nurse manager for 4 south pediatrics in a university medical center hospital, where the nurses established a collective bargaining agreement with the hospital several years ago. Maria has a disciplinary problem with Tia, a staff nurse, about not completing intake and output documentation or vital sign documentation on her patients during her last shift. Maria notes that Tia had a friendly reminder about failing to complete documentation last month. Per hospital policy, Susan, as Tia's manager, must complete verbal counseling with Tia.

During recent union negotiations between the hospital and the nursing union, it was agreed that when a verbal counseling is needed, the manager must formally say to the staff member, "I am providing you with verbal counseling today about your performance. This is official, will be documented in your file, and if you fail to meet the expectation, the next step in this process is a written notice of warning about failure to meet your job expectations. Do you have any questions about the verbal counseling process before we proceed?" The manager then continues with the verbal counseling about the unmet specific performance issue and policies.

Maria follows the guidelines established in the current agreement in her meeting with Tia, and Tia agrees that she has not been consistent in completing documentation. Tia agrees that Maria should monitor her performance for a week, when they will meet again to determine if Tia has been completing documentation appropriately and consistently.

### Manager's Checklist

The nurse manager is responsible for:

- Preparing notes about the verbal counseling session
- Meeting with employee for verbal counseling session
- Discussing expectations that were not met
- Reviewing policies and guidelines relating to unmet expectations
- Answering employee questions
- Providing coaching as needed

See how one nurse manager handled discipline in a hospital with a collective bargaining agreement in Case Study 24-1.

# Status of Collective Bargaining for Nurses

The majority of American nurses do not work under a collective bargaining agreement, but those that do have higher salaries (Albro, 2008) and are more often satisfied with their wages (Pittman, 2007). Conversely, nurses who do not work in unionized hospitals are more satisfied with their jobs but less satisfied with their pay (Pittman, 2007). Seago and colleagues (2011) posit, however, that union nurses may simply be more willing to voice their dissatisfaction.

The challenge then in a collective bargaining environment is to retain high-performing nurses and help them become more satisfied with their jobs (Lawson et al., 2011). Partnering nursing staff with management personnel is one strategy to improve nurse retention. For example, After a partnership between nursing and management was established at a Magnet-certified institution, turnover decreased and satisfaction improved (Porter, 2010; Porter et al., 2010). Such partnerships are supported by the trend toward labor-management partnerships in other occupational sectors (Hayter, Fashoyin, & Kochan, 2011).

## Legal Status of Nursing Unions

Three areas of supervision over subordinates have been under debate for a number of years. These are:

1.  The responsibility to assign

2.  The responsibility to direct

3.  Independent judgment

The NLRB issued several landmark decisions regarding the supervisory status of nurses (NLRB, 2006). Three cases were considered together and have become known as the *Kentucky River* trilogy. They are *Oakwood Healthcare, Inc.*, *Golden Crest Healthcare Center*, and *Croft Metal, Inc.* These rulings are important to nurses because those employees deemed as supervisors are prohibited from joining a union.

The NLRB clearly defined the supervisory status of nurses in its ruling in 2006, and that ruling stands today (NLRB, 2006). It ruled that:

1. The responsibility to assign includes nurses' responsibility to assign other nurses and assistants to patients.

2. The responsibility to direct includes the responsibility for the actions of those to whom tasks have been assigned.

3. Independent judgment includes the nurse's decision to match staff skills to patient needs.

This ruling has an impact on the eligibility of many nurses who heretofore were not considered supervisors and were thus eligible to be members of a collective bargaining unit. Nurses who are charge nurses either permanently or part-time on a regular basis and who meet the above criteria for assigning, directing, and using independent judgment are considered supervisors and therefore are not eligible to join a union (NLRB, 2006).

Complicating the collective bargaining issue today are numerous other efforts to organize nurses. National Nurses United has affiliate organizations in 12 states plus the District of Columbia, the Virgin Islands, and Veterans Affairs. United American Nurses is an AFL/CIO affiliate. In addition, employees of individual health care organizations often form their own collective bargaining organization and include nurses. Nurses at some health care organizations have formed their own union. So, collective bargaining in nursing runs the gamut from national collaboration of state organizations, to coordination with other employees in health care, to individual units of nurses.

### The Future of Collective Bargaining for Nurses

The use of collective bargaining as a way for nurses to influence the practice environment and to ensure their economic security presents both concerns and promises, especially with the radical changes occurring in health care today. The concerns are that the very processes of collective bargaining separate rather than unite nurses, notably between staff nurses and those in management. What the future holds for collective bargaining in nursing is uncertain and unknown.

## What You Know Now

- Laws governing unions are administered by the National Labor Relations Board.
- Subjects for union negotiations may be mandatory, prohibited, or permissive.
- Private sector subjects differ from public ones, which are generally more restrictive.
- The process of unionization involves selecting a bargaining agent, developing a contract and administering the contract.
- The nurse manager may not interfere in union organizing, but may be involved in resolving grievances.
- Most nurses do not work under collective bargaining agreements.
- The future of collective bargaining for nurses is uncertain and unknown.

## Tools for Handling Collective Bargaining Issues

1. Determine if your organization has a collective bargaining arrangement with its registered nurse employees.
2. If so, become familiar with provisions of the policy and grievance procedure.
3. Contact administration for any questions you may have with contract policies.

4. If your organization does not have a union contract, be aware of the possibility that efforts to establish a collective bargaining unit may be initiated.
5. If attempts are made to unionize your workplace, obtain information on the legal obligations you have as an employee and/or manager.
6. Remember, collective bargaining is an agreement between an employer and its employees; it does not need to be adversarial.

## Questions to Challenge You

1. Are you a member of a collective bargaining unit? Do you know anyone who is?
2. Have you been involved in union organizing? What happened during and after the process?
3. If you have not been involved in union organizing, find someone who has been and ask what happened.
4. What is your opinion of unions for nurses? Name the pros and cons.
5. You are negotiating a union contract on behalf of the nurses. List your demands in priority order.
6. You are negotiating a union contract on behalf of administration. Respond to the demands on your list generated in question 5.

### Pearson Nursing Student Resources
Find additional review materials at
**www.nursing.pearsonhighered.com**
Prepare for success with additional NCLEX®-style practice questions, interactive assignments and activities, Web links, animations and videos, and more!

## References

Albro, A. (2008). "Rubbing salt in the wound": As nurses battle with a nationwide staffing shortage, an NLRB decision threaten to limit the ability of nurses to unionize. *Northwestern Journal of Law and Social Policy, 3*(1), 103–130.

Hayter, S., Fashoyin, T., & Kochan, T. A. (2011). Collective bargaining for the 21st century. *Journal of Industrial Relations, 53*(2), 225–247.

Lawson, L. D., Miles, K. S., Vallish, R. O., & Jenkins, S. A. (2011). Recognizing nursing professional growth and development in a collective bargaining environment. *Journal of Nursing Administration, 41*(5), 197–200.

National Labor Relations Board (NLRB). (2006). Annual report of the National Labor Relations Board. Retrieved August 29, 2011 from http://www.nlrb.gov/sites/default/files/documents/119/nlrb2006.pdf

Pittman, J. (2007). Registered nurse job satisfaction and collective bargaining unit membership status. *Journal of Nursing Administration, 37*(10), 471–476.

Porter, C. (2010). A nursing labor management partnership model. *Journal of Nursing Administration, 40*(6), 272–276.

Porter, C. A., Kolcaba, K., McNulty, S. R., & Fitzpatrick, J. J. (2010). The effect of a nursing labor management partnership on nurse turnover and satisfaction. *Journal of Nursing Administration, 40*(5), 205–210.

Seago, J. A., Spetz, J., Ash, M., Herrara, C. N., & Keane, D. (2011). Hospital RN job satisfaction and nurse unions. *Journal of Nursing Administration, 41*(3), 109–114.

**The Nature of Stress**

**Causes of Stress**

    ORGANIZATIONAL FACTORS

    INTERPERSONAL FACTORS

    INDIVIDUAL FACTORS

**Consequences of Stress**

**Managing Stress**

    PERSONAL METHODS

    ORGANIZATIONAL METHODS

## Learning Outcomes

*After completing this chapter, you will be able to:*

1. Explain why stress is necessary.
2. Describe the organizational, interpersonal, and individual factors that cause stress.
3. Explain the consequences that result from stress, including burnout and compassion fatigue.

4. Discuss how individuals can manage stress.
5. Discuss how managers can help themselves and their staff manage stress.
6. Explain how organizations can help reduce stress in the workplace.

## Key Terms

Burnout

Compassion fatigue

Reality shock

Role ambiguity

Role conflict

Role redefinition

Stress

Consider the following scenario:

*Keandra is a medical nurse with 10 years' experience. She is married and has two children under the age of 6 who attend preschool while she is at work. As a nurse manager, Keandra has 24-hour responsibility for supervision of two 30-bed medical units. She frequently receives calls from the unit nurses during the evenings and nights, and approximately once a week she has to return to the unit to intervene in a situation or replace nurses who are absent. Keandra is responsible for scheduling all the nurses on her unit and has no approval to use agency nurses, in spite of a 20 percent vacancy rate. In addition, Keandra serves on four departmental committees and the hospital task force on consumer relations. She consistently takes work home, including performance appraisals, quality assessment reports, and professional journals. Although Keandra has an office, she has little opportunity to use it because of constant interruptions from nurses, physicians, other departmental leaders, and her clinical director. Recently, Keandra saw her family physician, complaining of persistent headaches, weight loss, and a feeling of constant fatigue. After a complete diagnostic workup, she was found to have a slightly elevated blood pressure, with a resting pulse of 100. Her physician prescribed an exercise program, and she was advised to lighten her workload, take a vacation, and reduce her stress level.*

**Stress** is the nonspecific reaction that people have to demands from the environment that pose a threat. Stress results when two or more incompatible demands on the body cause a conflict. Recognized as the pioneer of stress research, Selye (1978) suggests that the body's wear and tear results from its response to normal stressors. The rate and intensity of damage increase when an organism experiences greater stress than it is capable of accommodating.

Selye maintains that the physiological response to stress is the same whether the stressor is positive, *eustress*, or negative, *distress*. It is easy to see how negative events, such as job loss, can cause stress. However, positive events also may cause stress.

*Anthony was the director of nursing for critical care in a 400-bed hospital. He was offered the opportunity to develop a hyperbaric unit. In assuming the additional responsibility, Anthony began putting in long hours and working weekends. As the project progressed, Anthony became unable to sleep and gained 10 pounds. After the unit opened, Anthony's sleep pattern and weight returned to normal. Clearly, Anthony displayed emotional and physical signs of stress although he was experiencing a "positive" promotion and career opportunity.*

A certain amount of stress is essential to sustain life, and moderate amounts serve as stimuli to performance; however, overpowering stress can cause a person to respond in a maladaptive physiological or psychological manner.

## The Nature of Stress

A balance must exist between stress and the capability to handle it. When the degree of stress is equal to the degree of ability to accommodate it, the organism is in a state of equilibrium. Normal wear and tear occur, but sustained damage does not. When the degree of stress is greater than the available coping mechanism, the individual experiences negative aspects of stress. The situation is often described metaphorically through such statements as "carrying a load on one's shoulders" or "bearing a heavy burden." This often leads to physiological and psychological problems for the person and poor performance for the organization. When the degree of stress is not stimulating enough, lack of interest, apathy, boredom, low motivation, and even poor performance can result.

The experience of stress is subjective and individualized. One person's stressful event is another's challenge. One individual can experience an event, positive or negative, that would prove overwhelming for someone else. Even a minor change in organizational policy may cause some individuals to experience stress, whereas others welcome it. Some nurses seem to thrive on the demands of work, family, school, and community involvement, whereas others find even minimal changes in their expectations a source of great discomfort.

For nurses, stress in the workplace can develop from several sources and may be due to organizational, interpersonal, or individual (intrapersonal) factors.

# Causes of Stress

## Organizational Factors

Stress can result from job-related factors, such as task overload, conflicting tasks, inability to do the tasks assigned because of lack of preparation or experience, and unclear or insufficient information regarding the assignment. Nurses' jobs are often performed in life-or-death situations; emergencies may cause periods of extreme overload.

The physical environment may also be stressful. Consider the intensive care unit with its constant alarms, beeps, and other noises. Studying the effect of environmental factors (e.g., odor, noise, light, and color) on nurses' stress, Applebaum and colleagues found that noise, in particular, correlated with stress, job dissatisfaction, and intent to leave (Applebaum et al., 2010). Besides noise levels, lighting and other comfort factors may increase stress within the environment. Tight quarters, poorly organized work environments, and lack of equipment also augment stress levels.

Nurse managers' stress was studied by Shirey and associates (Shirey et al., 2010). They found that experienced nurse managers used a combination of emotion-focused and problem-centered coping strategies to handle stress and had fewer negative outcomes from stress than novice managers. Furthermore, novice managers reported experiencing more physical exhaustion, sleep problems, and hypertension than their more experienced colleagues.

Other organizational factors that can lead to stress include organizational norms and expectations that conflict with an individual's needs. Managers trying to do more with less, overworked staff, and more acutely ill patients can lead to an organizational environment that by its very nature is stressful. New technology, increased expectations from patients and their families, liability concerns, and increased pressures for efficiency, in addition to the dramatic changes in health care proposed by health care reform legislation, promise to increase stress in nursing and make the role of nurses and nurse managers more difficult, conflicting, and stressful.

## Interpersonal Factors

To add to the pressures created by organizational changes, nurses must contend with strained interpersonal relationships with other health care professionals and administrators. Interprofessional difficulties may precipitate tension. As resources in health care continue to shrink, nurses are being asked or told to assume responsibility for tasks that had been performed by other departments (e.g., phlebotomy, electrocardiography, respiratory therapy).

*In a rehabilitation setting, therapists expect the patients to be bathed, to have eaten breakfast, and to be dressed and ready to start therapy by 8:30 A.M. This expectation places undue stress on rehabilitation nurses, who must motivate patients who complain that they have had far too little sleep. Here is another example of stress due to interprofessional conflict: a radiology technician responds to a 9:00 P.M. page for a chest X-ray examination and informs the registered nurse that the patient will have to be brought back down because the radiology department is understaffed.*

Interactions between physicians and nurses are often strained. Most nurses have experienced an irate response from a physician who is awakened during the night for something the physician thinks should have been handled earlier or might have waited until morning.

*An internist in a small community hospital was well known for his outbursts during middle-of-the-night calls. One experienced nurse dealt with necessary calls to him by directly stating when he answered the phone, "This is Jane Jones from St. Matthew's. I have two important things to tell you about Mrs. Smith. . . ." This helped the internist focus on the problem at hand and eliminated his outbursts.*

The need to fulfill multiple roles is another source of stress. A role is a set of expectations about behavior ascribed to a specific position in society (e.g., nurse, spouse, parent). Conflict between family and professional roles results in stress. Adding to stress is the shift and weekend work required in nursing jobs in hospitals that must be staffed 24 hours a day, seven days a week.

Nurses who work on evening or night shifts may experience family problems if their spouse and children are on different schedules, especially if the nurse rotates shifts. It takes several weeks to adjust physiologically to a change in shifts; however, rotation patterns often require nurses to change shifts several times a month. Managers can reduce the physiological pressure by ensuring that nurses receive adequate rest and work breaks, rotating staff only between two shifts, and never scheduling "double backs" (working eight hours, off eight hours, working eight hours).

## Individual Factors

Stress can result from personal factors as well. One of these factors is the rate of life change. Changes throughout life, such as marriage, pregnancy, or purchasing a new home, generate stress. Each individual responds to stress differently, but the cumulative effects of stress often lead to the onset of disease or illness. The ways people interpret events ultimately determine whether the person sees the event as stressful or as a positive challenge.

New graduates, for example, often do not recognize that they have demonstrated a definitive set of skills and knowledge in having passed all the requirements to become a registered nurse. The stress they experience when changing from the student role to the professional practitioner role has been explained by Kramer (1974) as **reality shock**. When students move from a familiar school culture to a work culture—where values, rewards, and sanctions are different and often seem illogical—they experience surprise and disequilibrium.

Moving from a staff nurse position to management also creates surprise and disequilibrium. New managers often experience a sense of isolation from the peer group of staff nurses who previously provided support. Doing a job and directing others to do a job are different. Directing others is stressful, and a person may be tempted to believe that it will be faster to complete a task by doing it herself or himself.

**Role ambiguity** results from unclear expectations for one's performance. Individuals with high tolerances for ambiguity can deal better with the strains that come from uncertainties and, therefore, are likely to be able to cope with role ambiguity. *Role underload* and *underutilization* can also occur. Being underutilized or not having much responsibility may be seen as stressful by a person who is a high achiever or who has high self-esteem.

**Role conflict** is the result of incompatibility between the individual's perception of the role and its actual requirements. Novice nurse managers experience this type of conflict when they find that administration expects primary loyalty to the organization and its goals, whereas the staff expects the nurse manager's first loyalty to be to their needs.

Role conflicts also occur when an individual has two competing roles, such as when a nurse manager both assumes a patient care assignment and needs to attend a leadership meeting. Another example is the conflict between nurses' personal roles as parents or spouses versus their roles as professional nurses.

## Consequences of Stress

What happens to a person when he or she experiences stress overload? Both physiological and psychological responses can cause structural or functional changes, or both. The warning signs of too much stress include:

- Undue, prolonged anxiety; phobias; or a persistent state of fear or free-floating anxiety that seems to have many alternating causes
- Depression, which causes people to withdraw from family and friends; an inability to experience emotions; a feeling of helplessness to change the situation
- Abrupt changes in mood and behavior, which may be exhibited as erratic behavior
- Perfectionism, which is the setting of unreasonably high standards for oneself and leads to a feeling of constant stress
- Physical illnesses, such as an ulcer, arthritis, colitis, hypertension, myocardial infarction, and migraine headaches

Ineffective coping methods for reducing stress include excessive use of alcohol and other mood-altering substances, which can result in substance abuse or dependence (Epstein, 2010). Some people become workaholics in an attempt to cope with real or imagined demands.

The term **burnout** refers to the perception that an individual has used up all of his or her available energy to perform the job and feels that he or she doesn't have enough energy to complete the task (Epstein, 2010). Burnout is a combination of physical fatigue, emotional exhaustion, and cognitive weariness. As a result, the individual may reduce hours worked or change to another profession.

**Compassion fatigue** is secondary traumatic stress experienced by caregivers (Newsom, 2010). Similar to posttraumatic stress disorder, the term includes those involved in caring for others who are suffering from physical or emotional pain (Yoder, 2010). Symptoms are similar to those of burnout, but may be more severe if the caregiver is providing care to those traumatized by crime, war, and war-related traumatic stress or are emergency workers or first responders.

Additionally, nurses themselves may experience posttraumatic stress disorders (PTSD). Gates, Gillespie, and Succop (2011) found that 17 percent of emergency room nurses who had been involved in a violent incidence were symptomatic for PTSD.

Job performance suffers during times of high stress; so much energy and attention are needed to manage the stress that little energy is available for performance. In addition, increased absenteeism and turnover may result. Although there are various causes of absenteeism and turnover (see Chapter 20), both may occur when the individual attempts to withdraw from a stressful situation. Such a situation is financially costly in industry but even more costly in human health and well-being.

*A director of nursing at a 120-bed nursing home stated that she could no longer handle the overwhelming needs of the patients; the ever-present shortage of qualified, caring nurses; and the consistently dwindling resources. When a for-profit chain purchased the home and further reduced economic resources, the director of nursing left to become a real estate agent.*

## Managing Stress

We will always have factors in our lives that create stress. To manage those factors effectively and keep stress at levels that enhance one's performance rather than deplete energy, the key is to develop some resiliency. To accomplish this requires a comprehensive approach to managing stress, which involves planning, time, and energy.

### Personal Methods

One of the first steps in managing stress is to recognize stressors in the environment. Nurses tend to think they can be "all things to all people." Therefore, it is important to improve one's self-awareness regarding stressors.

Keeping your life in balance is difficult, but it can be done (Sullivan, 2013). Effective habits include role redefinition, time management, and self-care. Development of interpersonal skills and identifying and nurturing social supports can also facilitate stress management.

**Role redefinition** involves clarifying roles and attempting to integrate or tie together the various roles that individuals play. If there is role conflict or ambiguity, it is important to confront others by pointing out conflicting messages. Role redefinition may also involve renegotiation of roles in an attempt to lessen overload.

Much of the stress that nurses and nurse managers experience results from the perception that staff, patient, and work-group needs must be met immediately and simultaneously. A notable method of coping with and reducing this stress of time is through time management. We determine how, where, and when our time is used. Time is the essence of living, and it is the scarcest resource. One lost hour a day every day for a year results in 260 hours of waste, or 6.5 weeks of missed opportunity, annually. (Strategies for time management are included in Chapter 13.)

Caring for yourself physically (e.g., eating a well-balanced diet, exercising regularly, getting adequate sleep) and developing effective mental habits are important self-care strategies for coping with stress. To be able to care for others, nurses need to replenish themselves and practice relaxation techniques. This is not easy, especially for an individual with a high-stress job. Some relaxation methods are listening to music, reading, and socializing with friends. Developing outside interests, such as hobbies and recreational activities, can provide diversion and enjoyment and can also be a source of relaxation. Taking regular vacations, regardless of job pressures, is important for renewal and revitalization.

More personal strategies for keeping a balance in your life can be found in Chapter 14, "Balancing Your Life," in Eleanor Sullivan's book *Becoming Influential: A Guide for Nurses*, 2nd ed. (Prentice Hall, 2013).

## Organizational Methods

Nurse managers are often in the position of helping others identify their level of stress and stressors. If staff appear to be under a great deal of stress, the manager must help identify the source and decide how these can be reduced or eliminated. In addition to suggesting the techniques previously delineated, the manager should explore work-related sources of stress.

The manager must ask these questions:

- Is role ambiguity or conflict creating the stress?
- Can the manager help clarify individual staff members' roles, thereby reducing the conflict or ambiguity?
- Is the manager using an appropriate leadership style? (See Chapter 4.)
- Does the manager need to clarify a staff member's goals and eliminate barriers that are interfering with goal attainment? Involving staff in decision making is one way to identify and reduce such stress.
- Is the stress due to feelings of low self-worth?
- Would additional training or education help reduce the stress?
- Would recognizing and reinforcing positive behaviors and accomplishments reduce stress?
- Can other sources of support, such as the work group, help the individual deal with stress?
- Is an employee assistance program with counseling services available in the organization?

When stress is job related, several strategies can be used. First, proper matching of the job with the applicant during the selection and hiring process is an important step in reducing stress (see Chapter 15). Adequate orientation about what to expect on the job and using more experienced nurses as preceptors can reduce stress in novice nurses (Epstein, 2010). Skills training also reduces stress and promotes better performance and less turnover (see Chapter 17).

In addition, the organization can provide employee assistance programs (EAPs). Organizations that not only provide EAPs but promote their use in the organization report greater use of the service than organizations that promoted wellness and prevention instead of EAPs (Azzone et al., 2009).

Nurse managers can learn to recognize symptoms of stress-related problems among their staff and initiate referrals to EAPs. It is essential, however, to help remove the stigma about using such services (Epstein, 2010).

Communication and social support are additional factors in reducing stress. Both upward and downward communication channels should be open. Keeping personnel informed about what is going on in an organization helps reduce suspicion and rumor. Team building encourages staff to build a network of support with each other (see Chapter 11).

Policies that reduce the stress of shift work are also important. The number of hours in the night shift, weekend, and holiday work assignments also affects the level of stress. Providing adequate opportunities for breaks and meals is an important function of the organization.

Nurse managers are also vulnerable to stress. Shirey and colleagues found lower stress among nurse managers with more experience, those with a greater span of control, and those empowered by their chief nurse (Shirey et al., 2010). Thus, in addition to individual coping strategies, organizations can provide support for nurse managers and make them more likely to remain in their positions.

See Case Study 25-1 for an example of how one nurse managed her own stress and helped her staff manage theirs.

## CASE STUDY 25-1

### MANAGING STRESS

Madeline Mears, RN, is nurse manager of emergency services and critical care units at two corporately owned suburban hospitals. The corporation recently purchased three not-for-profit hospitals located in the urban center of the metropolitan area. Madeline and several other nurse managers at the suburban hospitals have been informed by the vice president for patient care services that they will now be responsible for managing the same service lines at the newly acquired hospitals. Managers at the urban hospitals will move into charge nurse roles on their respective units.

Madeline has the challenge of effectively and efficiently managing emergency services and critical care units at five separate facilities, all located within a 60-mile metropolitan radius. Her past experience in merging the management responsibilities at the two suburban hospitals will be extremely useful as she works to transition the new hospitals into the health care system.

Madeline anticipates that staff at the hospitals will be concerned over the changes in ownership and management. Some staff may be fearful of the unknown and worried about their jobs, while others may be excited at the opportunity for increased pay and job mobility in the health care system. Former managers at the hospitals may be angry about their demotion. Human resources representatives have indicated that they will offer former managers the opportunity to apply for open management positions in the health care system.

Myriad reactions among the staff members are expected as well as the potential for increased stress. Madeline and the other nurse managers meet and develop a transition plan. The transition plan defines the tasks, time frames, and expectations for merging the patient care units. Additionally, the plan helps decrease the stress Madeline and her fellow managers experience by organizing and delineating roles and responsibilities. Consistency in implementing change will help decrease stress among the staff at the urban hospitals. Each manager is committed to meeting with staff on each unit to address questions, concerns, and morale issues. Madeline plans to schedule a lunch meeting with each former manager to discuss the unit's strengths and weaknesses as well as her goals for the unit.

Three months into the transition, Madeline's units have had low turnover, and staff members report they are satisfied with the new management structure. In particular, staff nurses enthusiastically have accepted the clinical ladder promotion program and evidence-based practice implementation. Two of the former managers have moved into management roles in the health care system. The transition has been stressful, but Madeline has enjoyed the opportunity to stretch her leadership skills.

### Manager's Checklist

The nurse manager is responsible for:

- Recognizing the impact of stress, both positive and negative, on themselves and their staff
- Utilizing personal and professional strategies to identify stressors and develop a plan to manage stress
- Communicating openly and honestly with employees who are stressed in their work environment
- Using creative solutions to address stress so employees are able to effectively perform their jobs
- Assessing the effectiveness of solutions and adjust as necessary

Regardless of the work or life situation, everyone experiences stress, both positive and negative. It is how stress is handled that makes life interesting or excessively difficult. Stress-management strategies enable nurses to improve job performance and professional satisfaction.

## What You Know Now

- Stress is a person's reaction to demands from the environment.
- Stress can be both positive and negative; regardless, the physiological response is the same.
- Causes of stress come from organizational, interpersonal, and individual factors.
- Stress can cause physical and psychological problems, including burnout and compassion fatigue.
- Individuals can help manage stress by recognizing stressors, redefining roles, time management, and self-care.
- Managers can help their staff and themselves manage stress.
- Organizations can support employees to manage work-related stress by matching applicants to appropriate jobs, providing adequate orientation and skills training, and using experienced nurses to preceptor novice nurses.
- Organizations can provide employee assistance programs and promote their use to staff.

## Tools for Managing Stress

1. Recognize that stress is necessary for life.
2. Acknowledge the impact of stress, both positive and negative, on your professional and personal life.
3. Review your stress-management strategies and evaluate them for effectiveness.
4. Pay attention to your stress levels and try to create opportunities to help deal with stress.
5. If you are experiencing an exceptional amount of stress, consider various ways to care of yourself.

## Questions to Challenge You

1. What causes you the most stress?
2. What methods do you use to cope with stress?
3. Have you seen others respond negatively to stress? Explain what happened.
4. Have you experienced any of the consequences of stress described in the chapter? How did you handle it? Explain.
5. Have you experienced role ambiguity or role conflict? Describe the situation. How did you handle it?
6. What ways do you care for yourself? What other ways might you add to your repertoire of self-care skills?

**Pearson Nursing Student Resources**

Find additional review materials at
**www.nursing.pearsonhighered.com**

Prepare for success with additional NCLEX®-style practice questions, interactive assignments and activities, Web links, animations and videos, and more!

## References

Applebaum, D., Fowler, S., Fiedler, N., Osinubi, O., & Robson, M. (2010). The impact of environmental factors on nursing stress, job satisfaction, and turnover intention. *Journal of Nursing Administration, 40*(7/8), 323–328.

Azzone, V., Hiatt, D., Hodgkin, D., & Horgan, C. (2009). Workplace stress, organizational factors and EAP utilization. *Journal of Workplace Behavioral Health, 24*(3), 344–356.

Epstein, D. G. (2010). Extinguish workplace stress.

*Nursing Management, 41*(10), 34–37.

Gates, D. M., Gillespie, G. L., & Succop, P. (2011). Violence against nurses and its impact on stress and productivity. *Nursing Economics, 29*(2), 59–66.

Kramer, M. (1974). *Reality shock.* St. Louis, MO: Mosby.

Newsom, R. (2010). Compassion fatigue: Nothing left to give. *Nursing Management, 41*(4), 42–45.

Selye, H. (1978). *The stress of life* (2nd ed.). New York: McGraw-Hill.

Shirey, M. R., McDaniel, A. M., Ebright, P. R., Fisher, M. L., & Doebbeling, B. N. (2010). Understanding nurse manager stress and work complexity. *Journal of Nursing Administration, 40*(2), 82–91.

Sullivan, E. J. (2013). *Becoming influential: A guide for nurses* (2nd ed.). Upper Saddle River, NJ: Prentice Hall.

Yoder, E. A. (2010) Compassion fatigue in nurses. *Applied Nursing Research, 23*(4), 191–197.

# Advancing Your Career

**Envisioning Your Future**

**Managing Your Career**

**Acquiring Your First Position**

APPLYING FOR THE POSITION

THE INTERVIEW

ACCEPTING THE POSITION

DECLINING THE POSITION

**Building a Résumé**

TRACKING YOUR PROGRESS

IDENTIFYING YOUR LEARNING NEEDS

**Finding and Using Mentors**

**Considering Your Next Position**

FINDING YOUR NEXT POSITION

LEAVING YOUR PRESENT POSITION

**When Your Plans Fail**

TAKING THE WRONG JOB

ADAPTING TO CHANGE

## Learning Outcomes

*After completing this chapter, you will be able to:*

1. Describe how to envision your future.
2. Explain why your career requires planning.
3. Discuss how to obtain your first job.
4. Build a résumé.

5. Explain how to find and use mentors.
6. Explain how to find your next job.
7. Discuss what to do when your plans fail.

## Key Terms

Activity log
Certification

Mentor

Résumé

## Envisioning Your Future

The future is always uncertain, which leads many to believe they cannot do anything about it. The future, however, is shaped by human decisions and actions, including our own, made daily. What any one person cannot do is control the future. Nonetheless, we are affecting the future by what we do today or what we fail to do.

The future seems like something over which we have so little control that it isn't realistic to plan for it. Wait to see what happens, try to handle the circumstances, and hope for the best, are as much planning as most people do.

Instead, imagine yourself in one year, creating in your mind the life you most desire. What are you doing? What have you done over the course of the past year?

Now imagine what you are doing in five years. How about what you are doing in 10 years? Finally, what will you be doing right before you retire? Will you be satisfied with what you've done? What will you wish you had done?

> *A nurse met with the advisor in a baccalaureate program designed for RNs. After talking about the requirements of the program, the classes she needed, and her own schedule, they concluded that by taking one course a semester, it would take the nurse five years to complete the program. The RN looked discouraged. The advisor asked her what was wrong.*
>
> *"If I enroll in this program I'll be 35 in five years," she said.*
>
> *The advisor smiled. "Yes, and you'll be 35 in five years if you don't."*

## Managing Your Career

Finishing school and searching for your first job is a priority. Worrying about your career can wait. Or so you think. Shirey (2009) advises otherwise. She divides a nursing career into three stages:

- Phase 1: Promise (first 10 years). Initial experiences in the promise phase are essential building blocks for a long-term, successful career.
- Phase 2: Momentum (11 to 29 years). Continuing to learn and grow, choosing multiple experiences, and becoming visible in the profession are all important for continued success.
- Phase 3: Harvest (last years of career). While continuing to grow and learn, nurses also share their experiences and expertise with younger nurses and leave a legacy for the next generation. Shirey (2009) further posits that a career doesn't just happen: it is planned and cultivated.

## Acquiring Your First Position

The first step, after you've completed your basic nursing education, is to select your first job. The purpose of this job is to learn as much as you can and to perfect your clinical skills. Additionally, you will make contacts among your colleagues and supervisors.

Here are some criteria for choosing your first job.

- You will have opportunities to hone your skills in a clinical area of interest.
- You will learn from more experienced clinicians who are willing to teach you.
- The culture of the organization and, especially, the administration are supportive of nursing.
- The organization's mission fits your values (e.g., a teaching hospital that serves the poor).
- There are opportunities for advancement.

No job is perfect, just as no relationship, home, career, or family is perfect. Use the above criteria to assess the position and the organization. If the position and the organization fit most of them, especially the criteria most important to you, consider the following additional criteria.

- The schedule fits your lifestyle.
- The institution is near your home.

The least important criteria for selecting your first job is the salary. A small amount more in your hourly pay is worth much less than opportunities to help meet your future goals. Remember, you have a long time to be in your career; don't sacrifice opportunities in the future for a slight difference in salary now.

## Applying for the Position

Some organizations ask you to fill out an application, either online, by mail, or in person; others request a résumé. A **résumé** is a written record of your educational achievements, employment, and accomplishments. (See Box 26-1 for a sample.) Your résumé might also include your

---

**BOX 26-1 Sample Résumé**

### Chloe R. Stevenson, RN, BSN
5625 Summit Lane
Overland Park, KS 66222
913.555.2222
chloestevenson@anyprovider.net

### Objective
To obtain a position as a professional registered nurse in a dynamic intensive care unit that will utilize my strong clinical skills, work ethic, problem-solving ability, and passion for providing superior patient care.

### Work Experience

***Registered Nurse***

May 2009–Present

Telemetry Unit, Memorial Hospital, Overland Park, KS

- Currently provide direct patient care to a variety of cardiac and postoperative cardiac patients on a 30-bed telemetry unit.
- Clinical duties include assessment, medication administration (as well as titration of cardiac IV medications), cardiac monitoring, and all other aspects of nursing care.
- Actively develop, implement, and monitor individualized patient plans of care as well as document patient response and outcomes.
- Became ACLS-certified and serves as leader of unit's critical response team.
- Participates as a member of an evidence-based practice committee for cardiology services.

***Patient Care Technician***

January 2008–May 2009

Telemetry Unit, Memorial Hospital, Overland Park, KS

- Worked under the supervision of an RN to provide direct patient care, including taking vital signs, dressing changes, bathing, ambulation of patients, and assisting with the admission and discharge process.
- Was responsible for appropriate clinical documentation.
- Was trained to perform 12-lead EKGs as well as cardiac monitoring.
- Served on unit's quality improvement team.

### Education
- Bachelor of science in nursing, May 2009, University of Kansas, GPA: 3.7/4.0
- Registered nurse, state of Kansas, June 2009
- Advanced Cardiac Life Support (ACLS) certified, August 2009

### Awards
- Jane Smith Award for Excellence in Clinical Nursing, May 2009; awarded by faculty to the senior nursing student who demonstrates excellence in clinical skills and academic coursework.

References available upon request.

immediate professional goal, such as "gain clinical experience" and/or your long-term goal, such as "become a manager."

Education includes:

- Degrees, institutions, years attended, graduation date (actual or expected)
- Specialty training
- Continuing education

Employment includes:

- Positions held
- Names of employers
- Dates of employment

Accomplishments might include:

- Volunteer service, such as helping in a homeless shelter
- Organizational service, such as serving as student body president
- Awards won, such as Outstanding Junior Student

Once you have applied for a position and the organization contacts you to say a representative is interested in meeting you, you will agree on a time and place for an interview. The interview is your chance (sometimes your only chance) to sell yourself to a potential employer. Make no mistake: if you can't sell yourself, no one can. You need to prepare for your interview just as you would for any other important meeting. That includes knowing who you are meeting, learning as much as you can about the organization, and anticipating questions you might be asked.

## The Interview

### Preparing for the Interview

The purpose of an interview is twofold: for a potential employer to learn about you and for you to learn about the organization (Krischke, 2010). Ideally, the two of you will discover if there is a role for you in the organization, what is known as a good "fit."

To prepare, identify:

- What you want to know about the position and the organization
- What questions you might be asked about your education or past experiences. Be prepared to describe briefly your achievements.
- What you think your strengths and weaknesses are and how those fit with your potential employer's needs
- What you want to know about the organization and the job

Find out who will be interviewing you and ask for the person's position and role in the organization. You may interview with someone in the human resources office as well as the person who would be your supervisor.

Be especially courteous to office staff; they have the power to smooth your way or report your behavior to their boss. Try to schedule your interview for a time when you can be rested and unhurried, not right after a long day at work or when you must be somewhere else immediately afterward.

You will probably be sent some information about the organization (or you can request it). A position description is essential—you can compare it with your qualifications. The materials you receive may include the organization's mission statement, its vision for the future, and its goals. (See Chapter 2 for examples.)

An organizational chart also is helpful, but not always available. The important information for you is where this position fits in the organizational structure. That will tell you to whom you would report and also explain that person's reporting relationship. The most direct line to top administration is the most powerful.

### What to Wear to the Interview

Most people anguish over what to wear to an interview. With good reason. The way you dress creates your first impression and can enhance or detract from your words. Keep it simple and conservative. You want the interviewer to focus on your qualifications, not your clothing.

Clean, pressed slacks, and a tie and jacket for men is appropriate. Women can wear pants or a skirt with a jacket in neutral colors, low-heeled shoes, simple jewelry, and carry a handbag or briefcase. Wear something you feel comfortable in. Resist the urge to buy a new outfit unless you don't have anything suitable in your wardrobe.

### At the Interview

Take along a copy of your résumé even if you filled out an application. (You can refer to it if you are asked to explain an item.) Ask for explicit directions to the building and office where you will go, and plan to arrive a few minutes early. Prepare mentally by reminding yourself of the qualifications you bring to the position, noting items on the position description that fit you. Enter the office with confidence, smile, and shake hands firmly.

To consider what questions you might be asked in an interview, see examples of general questions in Table 26-1 and review Table 15-1 for examples of behavioral interview questions. In addition, you will be asked questions about your education and work history. Answer questions honestly, but don't feel you must explain anything you are not asked. You will have an opportunity to ask your questions about the position and the organization. Be sure you are prepared to do so. A candidate who has no questions suggests a lack of interest or expertise.

Most interviewers today understand what questions are legal to ask and what are not. You are not required to answer questions about how many children you have, their ages, or your marital status, for example. (See Table 15-2 for a list of illegal questions.) Simply being asked

---

**TABLE 26-1    Examples of Interview Questions**

**YOUR CURRENT JOB**

What do you do in your present job?
What do you like best about your present job?
What do you like least?
Why do you want to leave your present job?

**YOUR ACHIEVEMENTS AND GOALS**

What are you most proud of accomplishing?
What do you think you do especially well?
What are your areas of weakness?
What are your long-term goals?
What do you plan to do to meet your goals?

**YOUR INTEREST IN THE POSITION**

Why are you interested in this position?
What do you see yourself doing next?
Why do you think you are right for this position?
Is there anything you would like to add about your qualifications that we haven't already discussed?

From Sullivan, E. J. (2013). *Becoming influential: A guide for nurses* (2nd ed.). Upper Saddle River, NJ: Prentice Hall Health. Used with permission.

such questions indicates an organizational bias, and if you are asked such questions, you might want to reconsider your interest in the organization. Chapter 15 also includes information about interviewing from the employer's position.

To practice for an interview, role-play using the interview script in Box 26-2.

### After the Interview

Send a thank-you letter within 24 hours of the interview to everyone who interviewed you. Your letter can be handwritten on nice quality notepaper or typed on letter-sized stationery. It should be brief, thanking the interviewer for interest in you and saying that you enjoyed the meeting. Include a few words summing up your qualifications that fit the position. Close the letter by saying that you are looking forward to hearing from her or him soon.

---

### BOX 26-2 | Interview Script

**MANAGER:** Hi, I'm Paula Green. I'm the nurse manager for the surgical care unit. Thank you for coming in today! I'd like to start by telling you a little about the surgical care unit and then we'll talk about you and why you would like to work here.

The unit is a 32-bed patient care unit that is open 24 hours a day, seven days a week. We provide care to patients who have most typically had abdominal surgeries or orthopedic surgeries. The average length of stay for a patient here is three days. All rooms are private, with one patient to a room. We encourage a family member to stay overnight in the sleeper chair if desired. We work hard to create a good experience for every patient.

Now, tell me about you and why you've chosen to consider working with us.

**INTERVIEWEE:** I'm Samuel Jones. I've been a nurse for three years. I went to school at Upstate University. I worked in the community hospital surgical unit after I graduated from nursing school; I had clinicals there during my studies.

Now, I would like to move on to a larger facility that has a greater variety of patients. I've read a lot about your hospital and was very excited to see the job posting. I think this organization would be an excellent place for me to work.

**MANAGER:** Tell me more about why you think our hospital is a good fit for you.

**INTERVIEWEE:** Well, I know you keep adding more floors and services, and I want to be part of a growing place. I also know your Web site says you have just received Magnet designation. I want to be at a hospital where nursing is valued and growth is encouraged. A member of my family came here for care and loved it. He said everybody was very warm and professional.

**MANAGER:** That is very good to hear! So, let's talk about your work experience at the community hospital. Tell me about your role there.

**INTERVIEWEE:** Well, I'm a staff nurse in the surgical unit. I work the night shift. After working there about a year and a half, I took a preceptor class and began helping train new nurses. I am also the charge nurse there. I lead the shift, help my coworkers with their patients, get patients placed in a room when they're admitted, and talk to patients who have concerns about their care.

**MANAGER:** It sounds like you've done well in the last three years. Tell me about being the charge nurse leader. That's a large responsibility. Why do you like that responsibility, and how you think your peers would describe you in that role?

**INTERVIEWEE:** I like working hard and being a role model to encourage the other staff members to work hard. I also think that most issues can be fixed with good communication, so I try to always get people to talk and to share information. I think my coworkers would say I'm always asking them if they need help with their patients. I want them to know I'm there for them.

**MANAGER:** Tell me about your strengths as a nurse.

**INTERVIEWEE:** I try to keep myself and everybody focused on the patient. I'm also very dependable. This is the third year in a row that I've had a perfect record of attendance at work.

**MANAGER:** Tell me about your weaknesses.

**INTERVIEWEE:** I think sometimes I don't ask for help and then I get overwhelmed with my work. I always try to help others but get embarrassed when I need to ask for help. I need to learn to give and take better.

**MANAGER:** We all have strengths and weaknesses. We can build on your strengths and help you learn to deal with your weaknesses. Would you like to tour the unit now?

### A Second Interview

It is not unusual to have a second interview if you have passed initial scrutiny and appear to be an appropriate candidate for the position. The second interview usually includes colleagues and managers with whom you would work. You will probably tour the unit and meet potential co-workers, giving you an opportunity to assess the environment.

Situational questions are often asked at this time. For example, you are given a scenario and asked how you would handle the situation. Take your time to think through an answer. Obviously they think you can handle such situations because you have been asked back. Keep your answer short and to the point. Your goal is to show you are a competent, confident professional.

Interviewing with potential coworkers is also your opportunity to find out what you want to know about the specific responsibilities and challenges of the position. You might ask, "What are the most pressing problems facing the unit?" or "What do you need most from a nurse practitioner in this clinic?"

You will probably be asked if you are still interested in the position. If you are, ask when a hiring decision will be made. Following this interview, again send thank-you letters, but only to the new people who have interviewed you.

## Accepting the Position

When you are offered the position, you have an opportunity to negotiate. Don't ignore this opportunity in your excitement of getting the job.

Salary is usually the main topic for negotiation. Most employers have some flexibility with salary if they have a justifiable reason for it, but they will seldom tell you that. It is much more common for an organization to offer the lowest salary in its range and see if the candidate asks for more. Ask for a number higher than your lowest acceptable figure, but don't get carried away. Asking for a salary that is a great deal higher than the offer is not only unprofessional, but it makes you appear to be more interested in the money than the job.

Follow up your verbal agreement with a formal letter of acceptance to the administrator who hired you. Thank the individual for having confidence in you and your potential, and state again how pleased you are to be joining the organization.

## Declining the Position

Sometimes you will decide not to accept a position offered to you. It might not be the right job, at the right time, or in the right organization. Be sure to let the appropriate person know your intention as soon as possible. Thank him or her for the offer and the confidence the organization has in you. Explain briefly why you cannot accept the job at this time and state that you hope the organization will keep you in mind in the future. Follow up with a letter as well. Even if you are not interested in this position or this organization, someone there might prove valuable in referring another organization to you in the future, for example. Your career will be long; never alienate potential connections.

# Building a Résumé

Once you have accepted your first position, it is time to think about what you will need to advance in your career.

*The first step is to assess yourself.* Identify:

- Your personality, values, beliefs, likes, and dislikes
- Your lifestyle
- Your family
- Your friends and social life
- Your hobbies and personal activities
- Your vision of your future

- Your skills
- Your knowledge
- Your nursing preferences

The last item refers to the areas of nursing that suit you best. This may take some time and experience in practice. Then ask yourself:

- Do you like a fast-paced environment, such as an ER, OR, or trauma care?
- Do you prefer to have time with your patients? Rehabilitation nursing, a medical floor, or long-term care might suit you better.
- Which patient conditions and treatments do you prefer?
- Which patient conditions intrigue you the most? Cardiac problems, psychiatric conditions, or diagnostics (e.g., GI lab)?
- Would you like to work in a clinic, medical office, in home care, or in public health?
- Would you enjoy school nursing or occupational health?

This assessment is not done quickly; it involves a period of time in practice, introspection, asking friends and family members for their thoughts about you, and learning from reading or attending programs. It is also flexible and responsive to ways in which you grow and change. Your family and social life change also, sometimes making adjustments in your plan necessary.

*The next step is to assess the environment.*

Consider what might change in the health care system (today, changes occur rapidly). How will changes proposed in health care reform legislation affect your future? Are any new medications or vaccines pending that might eliminate current jobs or create new opportunities for you? Are any new educational programs being proposed?

The clinical nurse leader, as explained in Chapter 4, is an example. As advances in transplant technology proliferate, new specialties of nurses and physicians are created. Today's non-invasive technology for monitoring and treating patients for a variety of ills and from a distance suggests that many changes in clinical care may be on the horizon.

There are many ways to learn about the environment. Certainly, paying attention to popular media reports on scientific breakthroughs and advances in technology is one way. Reading your professional literature, checking certain professional Web sites for updates, or attending programs in your interest area is another. Joining a professional or specialty organization and receiving its newsletters and journals is especially useful because those target your interests.

Observing others may prove worthwhile. Many people chose their career path after watching more experienced members of the profession. Nurses who pursue teaching and administration often do so after working with an especially competent role model.

Talking with experts, colleagues, and administrators is also valuable. Keep alert to what you hear, evaluate its credibility, and assess its usefulness to you. Gathering information is an ongoing process. Your plan will not be fixed; it will change in response to changes in your life, your goals, and the environment.

Once you have assessed yourself and the environment, determine what your options are. Include legal constraints or possibilities (e.g., is the nurse practice law in your state going to be changed to allow more privileges for nurse practitioners?), new programs proposed (e.g., a local university is starting an acute care nurse practitioner program), your own desires (e.g., doctoral education to become a nurse researcher), and how willing you are or might become to relocate, go into debt, or sacrifice the time to reach your goal. The latter issues are likely to change over time as your family life or lifestyle changes.

Evaluate what experiences you need and where you might get those from a continuing education program, on-the-job training, a certificate offered by your institution's education department, or a graduate degree. Is there a license or certification you need? What organizations, such as working at a trauma center or accepting a leadership position in your chapter of Sigma Theta Tau International, could help you achieve your goals? Are there publications or online resources that would help?

Nursing offers an incredible array of opportunities in clinical areas as diverse as cardiac surgery and trauma care to home health and rehabilitation nursing. You can be a clinician or a specialist, a teacher, administrator, or researcher. You can become an entrepreneur, an information systems specialist, you can branch into pharmaceutical sales, or, for that matter, you can write books about nursing—all the while being a nurse. See how one nurse advanced his career in Case Study 26-1.

Create a plan that is long term and flexible. No one knows what will happen in his or her own life or in the environment over time, or what opportunities may emerge. Keep an open mind; talk to other professionals; explore your interests. What we do know is that we are contributing to our own future by what we do or fail to do today.

## Tracking Your Progress

Keep an **activity log** to track everything you are doing so that when the time comes to apply for a new position, you are not frantically trying to remember your accomplishments, what continuing education programs you took, or when you completed a course at your hospital. Note the name of the program, activity, certification, or accomplishments, add the dates, who sponsored it and where, and note anything special you received or learned. Include a list of accomplishments on your job, such as teaching a class or preceptoring students, or skills you've acquired. Include any cross-training as well. Table 26-2 shows an example of a format you could use.

Every item on your activity log will not go on every résumé. A résumé must be crafted to meet the purpose you have for submitting it. For example, the résumé you submit to an

## CASE STUDY 26-1

### ADVANCING YOUR CAREER

Trevor Briggs, RN, BSN, has worked as the operating room supervisor for the past four years. The department has used a stand-alone clinical information system for the past two years, and Trevor has been an integral part of the successful implementation of technology in the OR. In addition to training staff to use the system, Trevor has worked with the IT vendor to enhance the system's capabilities. Recently, Trevor was appointed by his nurse manager to serve on a hospital-wide clinical information system selection committee. Administration has initiated the process of selecting an integrated clinical information system and is seeking input from each service line.

Trevor enjoys working with the committee and learning about the implementation processes. The chief information officer met with the committee and announced the creation of a new role: clinical systems team leader. Team leaders will be nurses who are specially trained to work with the IT department in implementing the new clinical information system. Trevor's background with the OR system makes him an excellent candidate for the team leader position. After interviewing with the IT department manager, Trevor is selected as a clinical systems team leader. Trevor also learns that the hospital is willing to pay for specialized training, including tuition reimbursement for graduate classes.

To increase his knowledge of information systems, Trevor enrolls in a master of information management

systems program at the city university. After completing the initial 12 hours of the master's program, Trevor must decide whether to pursue a specialty track in software development or project management. Trevor reviews market trends to determine the best option and also considers his personal preferences. He also takes the time to meet with an instructor in the masters program, who is an informatics nurse specialist and has worked in the IT field for 10 years. Trevor decides to pursue a track in project management, which will allow him to utilize his strong leadership and people management skills. After completing his master's degree, Trevor is promoted to clinical systems nurse manager and is now pursuing certification in nursing informatics.

### Manager's Checklist

The nurse manager is responsible for:

- Determining what career track best suits individual skills, talents, and interests.
- Looking for opportunities to enhance skills and knowledge outside of your current career.
- Analyzing market trends for emerging roles.
- Networking with experts and mentors in the field that may present opportunities.

| TABLE 26-2 | Activity Log for Career Progress |
|---|---|
| **Activity** | **Content** |
| Education earned | Include names of schools, location, dates attended, degrees |
| Employment | Include all positions, including summer jobs and part-time or full-time work while in school |
| Licenses | Include license number and state |
| Certificates/Credentials | Include name, date earned, sponsoring organization |
| Professional Organizations | Include name, date joined, any committees or offices held with dates |
| Publications | Include title, name of publication, date |
| Volunteer Activities | Include name of organization and your participation |
| Accomplishments | Include accomplishments from your job, professional activities, volunteer experiences |

From Sullivan, E. J. (2003). *Becoming influential: A guide for nurses* (2nd ed.). Upper Saddle River, NJ: Prentice Hall Health. Used with permission.

organization to be considered for membership differs from one you would use to apply to graduate school. Having a comprehensive list of all your activities and accomplishments helps ensure that when you put together an application or submit your résumé, you will be less likely to forget some of your achievements.

Keep track of your expenses as well. Note them in your activity log or in a separate file organized by year; this information comes in handy at tax time. You can use a document on your computer or in a notebook. It is helpful to keep continuing education (CE) certificates and receipts in a file as well.

### Identifying Your Learning Needs

Pursuing a career involves lifelong learning. You can learn in many ways. Online courses, specialty certification, graduate school, books, journals, Web sites, and professional meetings are just a few of the ways you can acquire the knowledge you need. To develop skills, however, you need experience. Several options are possible.

#### Baccalaureate Education for RNs

Today, many RNs have added a baccalaureate degree in nursing to their basic education from a hospital diploma program or an associate degree from a community college. In addition, the Institute of Medicine (2010) recommends that 80 percent of nurses be prepared at the baccalaureate or higher level by 2020. Most baccalaureate programs in nursing have an option for RNs to complete their degrees without repeating content from their basic program, and many offer programs online.

#### Certification

Certification is growing in nursing as clinical care becomes more specialized. **Certification** is a formal recognition that a nurse has acquired specialized knowledge, skills, and experience that meet identified standards (Miller & Boyle, 2008). Nursing certification programs are accredited by either the National Commission for Certifying Agencies (NCCA) or the American Board of Nursing Specialties (ABNS). Nursing certifications are available in a wide range of clinical specialties, including nurse practitioner, clinical nurse specialist, and clinical specialties, such as cardiac rehabilitation, gerontological nursing, informatics, and primary care.

Nurses may be reluctant to pursue certification for several reasons (Watts, 2010), including the costs of the examination and study guides, lack of employer support, or absence of on-the-job rewards. However, the benefits to your long-term career may offset the immediate disadvantages.

### Graduate Education

Graduate school, in either a master's or doctoral program, offers both didactic content and experience, which might be clinical for a practitioner program or research in a doctoral program, depending on your goals. If you want to be a nurse practitioner, teach nursing, become a nurse researcher, or advance as an administrator, you need graduate preparation.

Choosing a graduate program is a difficult and time-consuming endeavor. You must learn as much as you can about the program, its requirements, and its graduates' success to determine if the program will meet your needs. Gather literature, meet with admissions staff and faculty, and talk to students and colleagues. Compare national rankings of the schools that interest you. Request the names of recent graduates to contact for references and interview them. Ask your teachers, supervisors, and preceptors for advice.

This is one of the most important decisions you will make in your career. It can also be the most valuable. Take your time, consider your options, and be fully committed before you enroll.

Many options are available to pay for graduate school education. As with the decision to select a school and a program, finding sources of funding takes perseverance. The school's financial aid office can help you locate loans and scholarships. Service clubs, such as Rotary International, support nursing scholarships.

It is helpful to know your long-term goal, especially if you are interested in an area of need. For example, a nursing faculty shortage is increasing as retirements thin the ranks of today's teachers. Nurse practitioners are needed to work in disadvantaged areas; some scholarships exist for nurses who agree to provide care in these areas for a period of time after graduation. In addition, the military offers scholarships in return for a service commitment.

### Continuing Education

Finding continuing education to further your career is not difficult; determining the quality of the program is not as easy. If you receive information about a program that interests you and fits with your career goals, evaluate the information using the following:

- Is the program sponsored by a known organization, such as a college or professional association?
- Who are the speakers? Are their credentials appropriate to their presentations?
- Is the content appropriate to you at this stage in your development—neither too advanced nor too elementary?
- Can you obtain financial assistance to attend? If you do, what will you owe the organization? Bringing back a report of a program you've attended is an excellent way to reinforce your own learning. This will give you an opportunity to speak in public as well.
- Consider attending, even if you must pay your own way. You may be able to deduct the expense on your taxes and, after all, you and your career are the beneficiary.
- Can you arrange to be off work, if necessary, and afford the time and expense?

### Professional Associations

Membership in professional associations offers many opportunities for learning. Journals, newsletters, Web sites, blogs, listservs, meetings, conventions, and programs are just the beginning. The opportunity to meet and network with your colleagues and senior people in the profession and to learn by serving on committees, task forces, and boards is immense. Many successful nurses began their career by participating in a professional association.

Nursing associations cover every specialty and interest. Membership in the American Nurses Association is open to all registered nurses through its constituent member associations. Sigma Theta Tau International has more than 400 chapters affiliated with schools of nursing around the world. Specialty organizations exist for nurses who work in many clinical areas, such as the American Association of Critical Care Nurses or the American Psychiatric Nurses Association. Each of these organizations has divisions, committees, and boards where your time and talents are welcomed.

## Finding and Using Mentors

One of the most important tasks in your career is to identify and cultivate mentor relationships. A **mentor** is a person who has more experience than you and is willing to help you progress in your career. A mentor introduces you to key people and tells you what you need to know and do to move ahead. A mentor provides opportunities for learning, counsels you on mistakes, and takes pride in your successes.

A mentor may be a senior nurse or someone in another closely aligned profession, mostly because the mentor must have contacts that can be useful to your career. Often you work for the same organization, but that is not a requirement. You can have more than one mentor, but usually not at one time.

You might identify someone you would like to be your mentor, or the mentor might select you. The arrangement of mentor and mentee, however, is rarely named as such. Usually, you find yourself relying more and more on one or two people for advice, or a mentor singles you out for special opportunities or assignments. If any of those do not work out especially well, or if the two of you don't seem to be compatible, nothing is lost. You both go on your way without any bad feelings. A person becomes a mentor when positive experiences accumulate, bringing satisfaction to you both.

A number of benefits accrue for both you and your mentor. You gain a sense of accomplishment by working with a mentor, and the mentor acquires fulfillment from contributing to you, and by extension, to your profession. People who are senior in the field have a responsibility to pass along what they've learned and to prepare those who come after them. These are the satisfactions of a career done well.

The time will come, however, when you move away from your mentor. You take a new job or your mentor does. Your relationship changes as a result. You may then become colleagues and friends, and you may acquire a new mentor in the new organization. Sometimes you will move ahead of the mentor, a situation that requires tact and commitment from both of you. Accomplished professionals know that they will always owe a debt to their mentor, and they will continue to show their appreciation in large and small ways.

## Considering Your Next Position

The time to think about your next job is when you accept the first one. Begin to assess how much you can learn in this job and think about your next step. Take every opportunity you can to learn.

*One new grad had already determined that she wanted to teach nursing and knew that she needed clinical experience before she went on to graduate school. She used each clinical experience as a learning opportunity. She made notes on the patients she cared for and looked up their conditions, treatments, and meds on her time off from work. In less than a year, she had compiled a study guide of her own notes. She began graduate school full-time and continued to work part-time, continuing to add notes throughout her graduate school experience. By the time she graduated, she was an experienced clinician, although the actual hours she spent in clinical work were fewer than most of the other new nurse faculty.*

### Finding Your Next Position

When jobs are plentiful, you have many opportunities for finding the next job in your career. This move must not be taken lightly, however, no matter how many jobs are available. This is where self-assessment is essential. You want to be certain you are ready to leave your current job, that you have learned and accomplished what you came there to do, that you will not be leaving at a crucial time (e.g., an imminent Joint Commission visit), and that you have selected the job that fits your needs now.

When you are ready, there are many ways to find potential positions. Online sources abound; Nurse.com is one example (www.nurse.com/jobs). Professional associations offer job search services. These include Sigma Theta Tau International at http://stti.monster.com, and the American Nurses Association at www.nursecareercenter.com. (See the Web Resources at the end of this chapter.)

Career fairs, ads in newspapers and nursing publications, and faculty from the school where you graduated are additional ways to inquire about opportunities and to let others know you are interested in considering future options.

### Leaving Your Present Position

Just as there is a way to find a job, there is also a way to leave a job. First, check to see how much notice your employer requires. Tell your supervisor as soon as you have accepted the new position, and follow up with a formal letter of resignation. Add some friendly comments, regardless of how you feel about the organization, your coworkers, or the supervisor. Your goal is to leave on good terms.

Resist the urge to just walk out, regardless of the situation. The only reason for doing this would be that you are in physical danger, and the organization is not providing adequately for your safety. This is a rare, though not unknown, situation.

Always be polite in your interactions with your coworkers and your supervisor. Resist, also, the urge to belittle the organization or the administration. Negative comments about others reflect mostly on you. Of course, don't say anything that is untrue. If the situation is difficult, the other employees know it as well. You needn't say anything at all, even if you're asked. You never know what the future will bring, and ending relationships politely is best for your future.

## When Your Plans Fail

Be assured that the future you envision will not work exactly as you hope (it might work out better), and you will make mistakes. All successful people take risks, and all have failed at some point in their careers. What makes their career progress significant, however, is that they learn from their mistakes and are willing to go on when external events affect their plans.

### Taking the Wrong Job

Sometimes you will take a job that is not the right one for you. Maybe you thought you were ready for a management job, but are now overwhelmed by the responsibility. No job turns out exactly the way we thought it would, but sometimes the disconnect between our expectations and what actually happens is so far apart that we cannot continue.

Maybe you took the right job, but for the wrong reason. You wanted a faster-paced environment and accepted a position in a busy surgical ICU, working nights. You soon discover that the pressure, loss of sleep, and the acuity of your patients is more than you can handle.

When you think you may have made a mistake, try to get some advice from someone you trust. An advisor, teacher, or a mentor may be able to help you sort out what's wrong. It may not be the job. Maybe you need a brief period of counseling or to learn better ways to handle stress. (See Chapter 25, "Managing Stress.")

If you decide you must leave this job, do so with as much care as you can. You will undoubtedly be leaving your employer in a difficult position, so you want to do everything you can to help. Also, having a short-term employment on your résumé is generally seen as negative, so you want to be able to explain this experience in the future and ensure that your employer will report that you did all you could to help the organization once you realized you did not fit the job.

### Adapting to Change

Change occurs every day in health care, and the pace of change seems to come faster and faster. In order to pursue the career you want and to find satisfaction in that career, you must be able to adjust and respond to change. The most important attribute you can bring to this effort is to remain flexible. The courage to change direction is essential for nurses, according to Shaffer (2006).

> *Marika, experienced in psychiatric nursing and home care, entered a master's program, intending to work as a mental health clinical specialist for a home health care agency. While she was in graduate school, she learned that the agency would no longer be reimbused by insurers for the services of a mental health specialist, and they had eliminated the position.*
>
> *Fortunately, Marika had a backup plan. She changed course, continued on in graduate school, and obtained her doctorate. She became a nursing faculty member and now researches mental health problems in patients with home care needs.*

Other events can change your future. Your spouse is offered a job in another part of the country. You find you're going to become a parent. Your parents need more care than you have been providing. When events intrude on your plan, you may need to adjust your time schedule, taking graduate classes more slowly, for example.

Life is a work in progress. We never know what our future will bring. Allow for unplanned events, such as illness, pregnancy, or the closing of your hospital. Plan for contingencies, but keep your eye on your vision. Remain flexible. You might discover that new opportunities await you, bringing a better future than one you had imagined.

*Note:* This chapter was adapted from content in Sullivan, E. J. (2013). *Becoming influential: A guide for nurses* (2nd ed.). Upper Saddle River, NJ: Prentice Hall.

## What You Know Now

- You have learned how to envision your future.
- You recognize that your career consists of three phases: promise, momentum, and harvest phase.
- You have learned how to select your first position, and how to apply, interview, and accept or decline the position.
- You have learned how to create and build a résumé.
- You have learned how to track your progress and identify your learning needs.
- You have learned how to find and use mentors.
- You have learned how to find your next position and leave your current one.
- You have learned that flexibility is needed to adapt to change.

## Tools for Advancing Your Career

1. Select positions and professional activities that further your short- and long-term goals.
2. Keep a log of your activities and accomplishments.
3. Keep abreast of the health care and policy environment, noting possibilities for your future.
4. Evaluate educational opportunities for their appropriateness for your learning needs and career advancement.
5. Identify and cultivate mentor relationships.
6. Evaluate your progress periodically and update with new information or interests.

## Questions to Challenge You

1. Answer the questions posed in the chapter about how you envision your future. Is the study or work you are currently doing helping you progress toward that future? If not, what do you need to do to help yourself?

2. Role-play the interview with a colleague in Box 26-2 and then reverse roles. How is the experience different if you are the interviewer versus the candidate being interviewed?

3. Create or review your résumé. Is it up to date? If not, add all the missing information. Take a few moments to ponder your accomplishments.

4. Begin an activity log. Periodically review your accomplishments.

5. Do you have a mentor? Evaluate that relationship. What more might you want from your interactions with your mentor? How might that occur?

6. What educational needs do you have? Investigate potential opportunities to acquire the necessary education or certification.

7. Have you ever had your professional plans fail? What, if anything, would you do differently in the future?

**Pearson Nursing Student Resources**

Find additional review materials at
**www.nursing.pearsonhighered.com**

Prepare for success with additional NCLEX®-style practice questions, interactive assignments and activities, Web links, animations and videos, and more!

## Web Resources

Nurse.com: www.nurse.com/jobs
Sigma Theta Tau International: http://stti.monster.com
American Nurses Association: www.nursecareercenter.com

## References

Institute of Medicine (2010). *The future of nursing: Leading change, advancing health.* Retrieved April 26, 2011 from http://www.thefutureofnursing.org/IOM-Report

Krischke, M. M. (2010). Nursing interview guide, Part II: Asking the right questions at the right time. Retrieved December 16, 2010 at www.NurseConnect.com

Miller, P. A. & Boyle, D. K. (2008). Nursing specialty certification: A measure of expertise. *Nursing Management, 39*(10), 10–16.

Shaffer, J. (2006). Cultivating personal courage. *American Nurse Today, 1*(10), 52–53.

Shirey, M. R. (2009). Building an extraordinary career in nursing: Promise, momentum, and harvest. *The Journal of Continuing Education, 40*(9), 394–400.

Sullivan, E. J. (2013). *Becoming influential: A guide for nurses* (2nd ed.). Upper Saddle River, NJ: Prentice Hall.

Watts, M. D. (2010). Certification and clinical ladder as the impetus for professional development. *Critical Care Nursing Quarterly, 33*(1), 52–59.

**4 Ps of marketing** Four strategies included in marketing plans: product, place, price, and promotion.

## A

**Absence culture** The informal norms within a work unit that determine how employees of that unit view absenteeism.

**Absence frequency** The total number of distinct absence periods, regardless of their duration.

**Accommodating** An unassertive, cooperative tactic used in conflict management when individuals neglect their own concerns in favor of others' concerns.

**Accountable care organization** A group of health care providers that provide care to a specified group of patients.

**Accountability** The act of accepting ownership for the results or lack thereof.

**Activity log** An ongoing record of professional progress, including educational programs, training, certifications, and accomplishments.

**Adaptive decisions** The type of decisions made when problems and alternative solutions are somewhat unusual and only partially understood.

**Additive task** A task in which group performance depends on the sum of individual performance.

**Adjourning** The final stage of group development, in which a group dissolves after achieving its objectives.

**Age Discrimination Act** A law prohibiting discrimination against applicants and employees over the age of 40.

**Ambiguous evaluation standards problem** The tendency of evaluators to place differing connotations on rating scale words.

**Americans with Disabilities Act** A law prohibiting discrimination against qualified individuals who have physical or mental impairments that substantially limit one or more of the major life activities.

**Artificial intelligence** Computer technology that can diagnose problems and make limited decisions.

**Assignment** Allocating tasks appropriate to the individual's job description.

**Attendance barriers** The events that affect an employee's ability to attend (e.g., illness, family responsibilities).

**Authority** The right to act or empower.

**Avoiding** A conflict management technique in which the participants deny that conflict exists.

## B

**Baylor plan** A staffing plan developed at Baylor University Medical Center whereby nurses work 12-hour shifts on the weekend and are paid for a standard work week.

**Behavioral interviewing** Interview questions that use the candidates' past performance and behaviors to predict behavior on the job.

**Behavior-oriented rating scales** A type of scale, used in evaluations, that focuses on specific behaviors and uses critical incidents grouped into performance dimensions.

**Benchmarking** A method of comparing performance using identified quality indicators across institutions or disciplines.

**Benefit time** Paid time, such as vacation, holidays, and sick days, for which there is no work output.

**Block staffing** Scheduling a set staff mix for every shift so that adequate staff is available at all times.

**Bona fide occupational qualification (BFOQ)** A characteristic that excludes certain groups from consideration for employment.

**Brainstorming** A decision-making method in which group members meet and generate diverse ideas about the nature, cause, definition, or solution to a problem.

**Budget** A quantitative statement, usually in monetary terms, of the expectations of a defined area of an organization over a specified period of time in order to manage its financial performance.

**Budgeting** The process of planning and controlling future operations by comparing actual results with planned expectations.

**Bureaucracy** A term proposed by Max Weber to define the ideal, intentionally rational, most efficient form of organization.

**Burnout** The perception that an individual has used up all available energy to perform the job and feels that he or she doesn't have enough energy to complete the task.

**Business necessity** Discrimination or exclusion that is allowed if it is necessary to ensure the safety of workers or customers.

## C

**Capital budget** A component of the budget plan that includes equipment and renovations needed by an organization in order to meet long-term goals.

**Capitation** A fixed monthly fee for providing services to enrollees.

**Certification** Formal recognition that the nurse has acquired specialized knowledge, skills, and experience that meet identified standards.

**Chain of command** The hierarchy of authority and responsibility within an organization.

**Change** The process of making something different from what it was.

**Change agent** One who works to bring about change.

**Charge nurse** An expanded staff nurse role with increased responsibility and the function of liaison to the nurse manager.

**Chronic care model** A system-wide, proactive model designed to provide daily care to patients by clinical teams.

**Clinical ladder** A system of using performance indicators to advance an employee within an organization.

**Clinical microsystems** A small unit of care that maintains itself over time.

**Clinical nurse leader**   A lateral integrator of care responsible for a specified group of clients within a microsystem of the health care setting.

**Coaching**   The day-to-day process of helping employees improve their performance.

**Cohesiveness**   The degree to which the members are attracted to the group and wish to retain membership in it.

**Collaboration**   All parties working together to solve a problem.

**Collective bargaining**   Collective action taken by workers to secure better wages or working conditions.

**Committees or task forces**   Groups that deal with specific issues involving several service areas.

**Communication**   A complex, ongoing, dynamic process in which the participants simultaneously create shared meaning in an interaction.

**Compassion fatigue**   Secondary traumatic stress experienced by caregivers.

**Competing**   An all-out effort to win, regardless of the cost.

**Competing groups**   Groups in which members compete for resources or recognition.

**Competitive conflict**   A type of conflict that is resolved through competition, in which victory for one side and loss for the other side is determined by a set of rules.

**Compromise**   A conflict management technique in which the rewards are divided between both parties.

**Conflict**   The consequence of real or perceived differences in mutually exclusive goals, values, ideas, attitudes, beliefs, feelings, or actions.

**Confrontation**   The most effective means of resolving conflict, in which the conflict is brought out in the open and attempts are made to resolve it through knowledge and reason.

**Conjunctive task**   A task in which the group succeeds only if all members succeed.

**Connection power**   Power based on an individual's formal and informal links to influential or prestigious persons within and outside an organization.

**Consensus**   A conflict strategy in which a solution that meets everyone's needs is agreed upon.

**Content theories**   Motivational theories that emphasize individual needs or the rewards that may satisfy those needs.

**Continuous quality improvement (CQI)**   The process used to improve quality and performance.

**Controlling**   The process of comparing actual results with projected results.

**Cost center**   The smallest area of activity within an organization for which costs are accumulated.

**Creativity**   The ability to develop and implement new and better solutions.

**Critical incidents**   Reports of employee behaviors that are out of the ordinary, either positive or negative.

**Critical pathways**   Tools or guidelines that direct care by identifying expected outcomes.

**Critical thinking**   A process of examining underlying assumptions, interpreting and evaluating arguments, imagining and exploring alternatives, and developing reflective criticism for the purpose of reaching a reasoned, justifiable conclusion.

# D

**Dashboards**   Electronic tools that can provide real-time data or retrospective data, known as a scorecard.

**Decision making**   A process whereby appropriate alternatives are weighed and one is ultimately selected.

**Delegation**   The process by which responsibility and authority are transferred to another individual.

**Demand management**   A system that uses best-practices protocols to predict the demand for nursing expertise several days in advance.

**Democratic leadership**   A leadership style that assumes individuals are motivated by internal forces; leader uses participation and majority rule to get work done.

**Descriptive rationality model**   A decision-making process that emphasizes the limitations of the rationality of the decision maker and the situation.

**Diagonal communication**   Communication involving individuals at different hierarchical levels.

**Direct costs**   Expenses that directly affect patient care.

**Directing**   The process of getting the work within an organization done.

**Discipline**   The action taken when a regulation has been violated.

**Disjunctive task**   A task in which the group succeeds if one member succeeds.

**Disruptive conflict**   A type of conflict in which winning is not emphasized and there is no mutually acceptable set of rules; parties involved are engaged in activities to reduce, defeat, or eliminate the opponent.

**Diversification**   The expansion of an organization into new arenas of service.

**Divisible task**   Tasks that can be broken down into subtasks with division of labor.

**Downward communication**   Communication, generally directive, given from an authority figure or manager to staff.

**DMAIC**   A Six-Sigma process improvement method.

**Driving forces**   Behaviors that facilitate change by pushing participants in the desired direction.

# E

**Efficiency variance**   The difference between budgeted and actual nursing care hours provided.

**Electronic health records (EHRs)**   Integrated records that include information from all medical sources and can be accessed from multiple locations by sanctioned providers.

**Emergency operations plan (EOP)**   The EOP includes preparation, education and training, and implementation of the hospital's response to emergency situations.

**Emotional intelligence**   Personal competence (self-awareness and self-management) and social competence (social awareness and relationship management) that begin with authenticity.

**Empirical-rational model**   A change agent strategy based on the assumption that people are rational and follow self-interest if that self-interest is made clear.

**Engagement**   When an employee is inspired by an organization, willing to invest effort, likely to recommend the organization, and planning to remain in the organization.

**Equity theory** The motivational theory that suggests effort and job satisfaction depend on the degree of equity or perceived fairness in the work situation.

**Evidence-based practice** Applying the best scientific evidence to a patient's unique diagnosis, condition, and situation to make clinical decisions.

**Expectancy theory** The motivational theory that emphasizes the role of rewards and their relationship to the performance of desired behaviors.

**Expense budget** A comprehensive budget that lists salary and nonsalary items that reflect patient care objectives and activity parameters for the nursing unit.

**Experimentation** A type of problem solving in which a theory is tested to enhance knowledge, understanding, or prediction.

**Expert power** Power based on the manager's possession of unique skills, knowledge, and competence.

**Expert systems** Computer programs that provide complex data processing, reasoning, and decision making.

**Extinction** The technique used to eliminate negative behavior, in which a positive reinforcer is removed and the undesired behavior is extinguished.

## F

**Family and Medical Leave Act (FMLA)** A federal law stating that employers must provide employees with leave when serious illness or family issues arise, while maintaining insurance and an equal position within an organization.

**Felt conflict** The negative feelings between two or more parties.

**First-level manager** The manager responsible for supervising nonmanagerial personnel and day-to-day activities of specific work units.

**Fiscal year** A specified 12-month period during which operational and financial performance is measured.

**Fixed budget** A budget in which amounts are set regardless of changes that occur during the year.

**Fixed costs** Expenses that remain the same for the budget period regardless of the activity level of the organization.

**Fogging** A communication technique in which one agrees with part of what was said.

**Followership** An interactive and complementary relationship to leadership.

**Forcing** A conflict management technique that forces an immediate end to conflict but leaves the cause unresolved.

**Formal committees** Committees in an organization with authority and a specific role.

**Formal groups** Clusters of individuals designated by an organization to perform specified organizational tasks.

**Formal leadership** Leadership that is exercised by an individual with legitimate authority conferred by position within an organization.

**Forming** The initial stage of group development, in which individuals assemble into a well-defined cluster.

**Full-time equivalent (FTE)** The percentage of time an employee works that is based on a 40-hour workweek.

## G

**Goal setting** The relating of current behavior, activities, or operations to an organization's or individual's long-range goals.

**Goals** Specific statements of outcomes that are to be achieved.

**Goal-setting theory** The motivational theory that suggests that the goal itself is the motivating force.

**Grievances** Formal expressions of complaints, generally classified as misunderstandings, contract violations, or an inadequate labor agreement.

**Group** An aggregate of individuals who interact and mutually influence each other.

**Group evaluation** An evaluation process whereby managers compare individual and group performance to organizational standards.

**Groupthink** A negative phenomenon occurring in highly cohesive, isolated groups in which group members come to think alike, which interferes with critical thinking.

## H

**Halo error** The failure to differentiate among the various performance dimensions when evaluating.

**Hawthorne effect** The tendency for people to perform as expected because of special attention.

**Hidden agendas** A group member's individual, unspoken objectives that interfere with commitment or enthusiasm.

**Horizontal integration** Arrangements between or among organizations that provide the same or similar services.

**Horizontal promotion** A program to reward a high-performing employee without promoting the employee to a management position.

## I

**Incident reports** Accurate and comprehensive reports on unplanned or unexpected occurrences that could potentially affect a patient, family member, or staff.

**Incremental (line-by-line) budget** A budget worksheet listing expense items on separate lines that is usually divided into salary and nonsalary expenses.

**Indicator** A tool used to measure the performance of structure, process, and outcome standards.

**Indirect costs** Necessary expenditures that do not affect patient care directly.

**Informal committees** Committees with no delegated authority that are organized for discussion.

**Informal groups** Groups that evolve from social interactions that are not defined by an organizational structure.

**Informal leadership** Leadership that is exercised by an individual who does not have a specified management role.

**Information power** Power based on an individual's access to valued data.

**Innovation** A strategy to bridge the gap between an existing state and a desired state

**Innovative decisions** The type of decisions made when problems are unusual and unclear and creative solutions are necessary.

**Integrated health care networks** Organizational health care structures that deliver a continuum of care, provide coverage for a group of individuals, and accept fixed payments for that group.

**Integrative decision making**  A conflict strategy that focuses on the means of solving a problem rather than the ends.

**Interrater reliability**  An agreement between two measures by several interviewers.

**Interruption log**  A journal of specific information regarding interruptions, analysis of which may help identify ways to reduce interruptions.

**Intersender conflict**  Difficulty in interpreting the intended meaning of a message due to two conflicting messages received from differing sources.

**Interview guide**  A written document containing questions, interviewer directions, and other pertinent information so that the same process is followed and the same basic information is gathered from each applicant.

**Intrarater reliability**  An agreement between two measures by the same interviewer.

**Intrasender conflict**  Difficulty in interpreting the intended meaning of a message due to incongruity between verbal and nonverbal communication.

**Involuntary absenteeism**  Absenteeism that is not under the employee's control.

**Involuntary turnover**  When an employee is terminated by his or her employers.

**J**

**Job enlargement**  A flatter organizational structure that causes positions to be combined and results in managers having more employees to supervise.

**Just culture**  An environment for reporting of errors without fear of undue retribution.

**L**

**Lateral communication**  Communication that occurs between individuals at the same hierarchical level.

**Lateral violence**  Harassment between employees of equal rank.

**Leader**  Someone who uses interpersonal skills to influence others to accomplish specific goals.

**Lean Six Sigma**  A quality program that focuses on improving process flow and eliminating waste.

**Leapfrog Group**  A coalition of public and private employers organized to bring attention to consumers about quality indicators in health care and mobilize employers to reward health care organizations that demonstrate quality outcome measures.

**Legitimate power**  A manager's right to make requests because of authority within an organizational hierarchy.

**Leniency error**  The tendency of a manager to overrate staff performance.

**Line authority**  The linear hierarchy of supervisory responsibility and authority.

**Logic model**  A practice-based research network (PBRN) that provides a framework for planning and evaluation of primary care

**Lose-lose strategy**  A conflict strategy in which neither side wins; the settlement reached is unsatisfactory to both sides.

**M**

**Magnet® recognition program**  Recognition by the American Nurses Credentialing Center that an organization provides quality nursing care.

**Manager**  An individual employed by an organization who is responsible for efficiently accomplishing its goals.

**Marginal employees**  Employees who never reach the expected level of competence.

**Medical home**  A patient-centered model where all services are provided by a group of health care professionals.

**Mediation**  Use of a third-party mediator to help settle disputes.

**Mentor**  A more experienced person who guides, supports, and nurtures a less experienced person.

**Metacommunications**  Nonverbal messages in communication, including body language and environmental factors.

**Mission**  A general statement of the purpose of an organization.

**Motivation**  The factors that initiate and direct behavior.

**N**

**Negative assertion**  A communication technique in which one accepts some blame for what was said.

**Negative inquiry**  A communication technique used to clarify objections and feelings (e.g., I don't understand . . .).

**Negligent hiring**  Failure of an organization, responsible for the character and actions of all employees, to ascertain the background of an employee.

**Negotiation**  A conflict management technique in which the conflicting parties give and take on various issues.

**Nonsalary expenditure variances**  Deviation from the budget as a result of changes in patient volume, supply quantities, or prices paid.

**Normative-reeducative strategy**  A change agent strategy based on the assumption that people act in accordance with social norms and values.

**Norming**  The third stage of group development, in which group members define goals and rules of behavior.

**Norms**  Informal rules of behavior shared and enforced by group members.

**Nursing care hours (NCHs)**  The number of hours of patient care provided per unit of time.

**O**

**Objective probability**  The likelihood that an event will or will not occur based on facts and reliable information.

**Objectives**  Statements of specific outcomes within a component of an organization.

**On-the-job instruction**  An educational method using observation and practice by which employees learn new skills after being employed.

**Operant conditioning**  A process by which a behavior becomes associated with a particular consequence.

**Operating budget**  An organization's statement of expected revenues and expenses for the upcoming year.

**Ordinary interacting groups**  Common types of groups; generally have a formal leader and are run according to an informal structure with the purpose of solving a problem or making a decision.

**Organization**   A collection of people working together under a defined structure to achieve predetermined outcomes.

**Organizational culture**   The basic assumptions and values held by members of an organization.

**Organizational environment**   The system-wide conditions that contribute to a positive or negative work setting.

**Organizing**   The process of coordinating the work to be done within an organization.

**Orientation**   A process by which staff development personnel and managers ease a new employee into an organization by providing relevant information.

**Outcome standards**   Standards that reflect the desired result or outcome of care.

**Overdelegation**   A common form of ineffective delegation that occurs when the delegator loses control over a situation by giving too much authority or responsibility to the delegate.

## P

**Patient classification systems (PCSs)**   Systems developed to objectively determine workload requirements and staffing needs.

**Patient-centered care**   A nursing care delivery system that is unit based and consists of patient care coordinators, patient care associates, unit support assistants, administrative support personnel, and a nurse manager.

**Patient Protection and Affordable Care Act (PPACA)**   The health care reform bill signed into law in 2010 designed to expand American's access to health care that awaits court decisions for implementation

**Peer review**   A process by which other employees assess and judge the performance of professional peers against predetermined standards.

**Perceived conflict**   One's perception of another's position in a conflict.

**Performance appraisal**   The process of interaction, written documentation, formal interview, and follow-up that occurs

between managers and their employees to give feedback, make decisions, and cover fair employment practice law.

**Performing**   The fourth stage of group development, in which group members agree on basic purposes and activities and carry out the work.

**Personal power**   Power based on an individual's credibility, reputation, expertise, experience, control of resources or information, and ability to build trust.

**Personnel decision**   A decision that affect the terms, conditions, and privileges of employment.

**Philosophy**   The mission, values, and vision of an organization.

**Planning**   A four-stage process to establish goals, evaluate the present situation and predict future trends and events, formulate a planning statement, and convert the plan into an action statement.

**Policy**   Decisions that govern action and determine an organization's relationships, activities, and goals.

**Political decision-making model**   A decision-making process in which the particular interests and objectives of powerful stakeholders influence how problems and objectives are defined.

**Politics**   A means of influencing the allocation of scarce resources, events, and the decisions of others.

**Pooled interdependence**   A type of interdependence in which each individual contributes to the group but no one contribution is dependent on any other.

**Pools**   Internal or external groups of workers that are used as supplemental staff by an organization.

**Position control**   A monitoring tool used to compare actual numbers of employees to the number of budgeted FTEs for the nursing unit.

**Position description**   Describes the skills, abilities, and knowledge required to perform the job.

**Position power**   Power of an individual that is determined by the job description, assigned responsibilities, recognition, advancement, authority, the ability to withhold money, and decision making.

**Power**   The potential ability to influence in order to achieve goals.

**Power-coercive strategies**   Change agent strategies based on the application

of power by legitimate authority, economic sanctions, or political clout.

**Power plays**   Attempts by others to diminish or demolish their opponents.

**Practice partnership**   A nursing care delivery system in which senior and junior staff members share patient care responsibilities.

**Preceptor**   An experienced individual who assists new employees in acquiring the necessary knowledge and skills to function effectively in a new environment.

**Presenteeism**   When an employee is at work but disabled by physical or mental illness.

**Probability**   The likelihood that an event will or will not occur.

**Probability analysis**   A calculation of the expected risk made to accurately determine the probabilities of each alternative.

**Problem solving**   A process whereby a dilemma is identified and corrected.

**Process standards**   Standards connected with the actual delivery of care.

**Process theories**   Motivational theories that emphasize how the motivation process works to direct an individual's effort into performance.

**Productivity**   A measure of how well the work group or team uses the resources available to achieve its goals and produce its services.

**Profit**   The difference between revenues and expenses.

**Progressive discipline**   The process of increasingly severe warnings for repeated violations that can result in termination.

**Punishment**   A process used to inhibit an undesired behavior by applying a negative reinforcer.

**Punishment (coercive) power**   Power based on penalties that a manager might impose if the individual or group does not comply with authority.

## Q

**Quality initiatives**   Various initiatives designed to reduce medical errors.

**Quality management**   A preventive approach designed to address problems efficiently and quickly.

**Quantum leadership**   A leadership style based on the concepts of chaos theory.

# R

**Rate variances** The difference between budgeted and actual hourly rates paid.

**Rational decision-making model** A decision-making process based on logical, well-grounded, rational choices that maximize the achievement of objectives.

**Real (command) groups** Groups that accomplish tasks in an organization and are recognized as legitimate organizational entities.

**Reality shock** The stress, surprise, and disequilibrium experienced when shifting from a familiar culture into one whose values, rewards, and sanctions are different (e.g., from a school culture to a work culture).

**Recency error** The tendency of a manager to rate an employee based on recent events, rather than over the entire evaluation period.

**Reciprocal interdependence** A type of interdependence in which members must coordinate their activities with every other individual in the group.

**Redesign** A technique that examines the tasks within each job with the goal of combining appropriate tasks to improve efficiency.

**Referent power** Power based on admiration and respect for an individual.

**Re-forming** A stage of group development in which the group reassembles after a major change in the environment or in the goals of the group that requires the group to refocus its activities.

**Reinforcement theory (behavior modification)** The motivational theory that views motivation as learning and proposes that behavior is learned through a process called operant conditioning.

**Reportable incident** Any unexpected or unplanned occurrence that affects or could potentially affect a patient, family member, or staff.

**Resistance** A behavior that can be positive or negative and may mean a resistance to change or disobedience, or at times an effective approach to handling power differences.

**Resolution** The stage of conflict that occurs when a mutually agreed-upon solution is arrived at and both parties commit themselves to carrying out the agreement.

**Responsibility** An obligation to accomplish a task.

**Restraining forces** Behaviors that impede change by discouraging participants from making specified changes.

**Retail medicine** Walk-in clinics that provide convenient services for low-acuity illnesses without scheduled appointments.

**Résumé** A written record of an individual's educational achievements, employment, and accomplishments.

**Revenue budget** A projection of expected income for a budget period based on volume and mix of patients, rates, and discounts.

**Reverse delegation** A common form of ineffective delegation that occurs when someone with a lower rank delegates to someone with more authority.

**Reward power** Power based on inducements offered by the manager in exchange for contributions that advance the manager's objectives.

**Risk management** A program directed toward identifying, evaluating, and taking corrective action against potential risks that could lead to injury.

**Robotics** Using robots to deliver supplies and remote care.

**Role** A set of expectations about behavior ascribed to a specific position.

**Role ambiguity** The frustrations that result from unclear expectations for one's performance.

**Role conflict** The incompatibility between an individual's perception of the role and its actual requirements.

**Role redefinition** The clarification of roles and an attempt to integrate or tie together the various roles that individuals play.

**Root cause analysis** A method to work backwards through an event to examine every action that led to the error or event that occurred.

**Routine decisions** The type of decisions made when problems are relatively well defined and common and when established rules, policies, and procedures can be used to solve them.

# S

**Salary (personnel) budget** A budget that projects salary costs to be paid and charged to the cost center during the budget period.

**Salary compression** The effect of a higher starting pay for new nurses or rewarding those with fewer years of experience with higher increases that results in the salaries of long-term employees being at or below those of less-experienced nurses.

**Satisficing** A decision-making strategy whereby the individual chooses a less-than-ideal alternative that meets minimum standards of acceptance.

**Self-scheduling** A staffing model in which managers and their staff completely manage staffing and schedules.

**Sequential interdependence** A type of interdependence in which members must coordinate their activities with others in some designated order.

**Servant leadership** The premise that leadership originates from a desire to serve; a leader emerges when others' needs take priority.

**Service-line structures** Organizational structures in which clinical services are organized around patients with specific conditions.

**Shaping** The selective reinforcement of behaviors that are successively closer approximations to the desired behavior.

**Shared governance** An organizational paradigm based on the values of interdependence and accountability that allows nurses to make decisions in a decentralized environment.

**Shared leadership** An organizational structure in which several individuals share the responsibility for achieving an organization's goals.

**Shared visioning** An interactive process in which both leaders and followers commit to an organization's goals.

**Six Sigma** A quality management program that uses measures, goals, and management involvement to monitor performance and ensure progress.

**Smoothing** Managing conflict by complimenting one's opponent, downplaying differences, and focusing on minor areas of agreement.

**Social media** Connects diverse populations and encourages collaboration and the exchange of images, ideas, opinions, and preferences through various interactive online methods.

**Span of control** The number of employees that can be effectively supervised by a single manager.

**Staff authority** The advisory relationship in which responsibility for actual work is assigned to others.

**Staffing** The process of balancing the quantity of staff available with the quantity and mix of staff needed by an organization.

**Staffing mix** The type of staff necessary to perform the work of an organization.

**Stakeholders** People or groups with a direct interest in the work of an organization.

**Standards** Written statements that define a level of performance or a set of conditions determined to be acceptable by some authority.

**Status** The social ranking of individuals relative to others in a group based on the position they occupy.

**Status incongruence** The disruptive impact that occurs when factors associated with group status are not congruent.

**Storming** The second stage of group development, in which group members develop roles and relationships; competition and conflict generally occur.

**Strategic planning** A process of continual assessment, planning, and evaluation to guide the future.

**Strategies** Actions by which objectives are to be achieved.

**Stress** The nonspecific reaction that people have to threatening demands from the environment.

**Strike** The organized stoppage of work by employees within the union.

**Structure standards** Standards that relate to the physical environment, organization, and management of an organization.

**Subjective probability** The likelihood that an event will or will not occur based on a manager's personal judgment and beliefs.

**Suppression** The stage of conflict that occurs when one person or group defeats the other.

**Synergy model of care** An organizational model that matches patients' needs to nurses' competencies.

## T

**Task forces** Ad hoc committees appointed for a specific purpose and a limited time.

**Task group** Several individuals who work together to accomplish specific time-limited assignments.

**Team building** A group development technique that focuses on the task and relationship aspects of a group's functioning in order to build team cohesiveness.

**Teams** Real groups in which people work cooperatively with each other in order to achieve some goal.

**Terminate** To fire an employee.

**Throughput** A performance measure related to moving patients into and out of the health care system.

**Time logs** Journals of activities that are useful in analyzing actual time spent on specific activities.

**Time waster** Something that prevents a person from accomplishing a job or achieving a goal.

**To-do list** A list of responsibilities to be accomplished within a specific time frame.

**Total quality management (TQM)** A management philosophy that emphasizes a commitment to excellence throughout an organization.

**Total time lost** The number of scheduled days an employee misses.

**Transactional leadership** A leadership style based on principles of social exchange theory in which social interaction between leaders and followers is essentially economic, and success is achieved when needs are met, loyalty is enhanced, and work performance is enhanced.

**Transformational leadership** A leadership style focused on effecting revolutionary change in an organization through a commitment its vision.

**Transitions** The periods of time between the current situation and when change is implemented.

**Trial-and-error method** A method whereby one solution after another is tried until the problem is solved or appears to be improving.

**Turnover** The number of staff members who vacate a position.

## U

**Underdelegation** A common form of ineffective delegation that occurs when full authority is not transferred, responsibility is taken back, or there is a failure to equip and direct the delegate.

**Upward communication** Communication that occurs from staff to management.

## V

**Validity** The ability to predict outcomes with some accuracy.

**Values** The beliefs or attitudes one has about people, ideas, objects, or actions that form a basis for behavior.

**Variable budget** A budget developed with the understanding that adjustments to the budget may be made during the year.

**Variable costs** Expenses that depend on and change in direct proportion to patient volume and acuity.

**Variance** The difference between the amount that was budgeted for a specific cost and the actual cost.

**Vertical integration** An arrangement between or among dissimilar but related organizations to provide a continuum of services.

**Virtual care** Technologies used to assess, intervene, and monitor patients from remote locations.

**Vision** A mental model of a possible future.

**Vision statement** A description of the goal to which an organization aspires.

**Volume variances** Differences in the budget as a result of increases or decreases in patient volume.

**Voluntary absenteeism** Absenteeism that is under the employee's control.

**Voluntary turnover** When an employee chooses to leave an organization.

# W

**Win–lose strategy** A strategy used during conflict in which one party exerts dominance and the other submits and loses.

**Win–win strategy** A conflict strategy that focuses on goals and attempts to meet the needs of both parties.

**Withdrawal** The removal of at least one party from the conflict, making it impossible to resolve the situation.

**Work sample questions** Questions that are asked to determine an applicant's knowledge about work tasks and the ability to perform a job.

**Workplace violence** Any violent act, including physical assaults and threats of assault, directed toward persons at work or on duty.

**Written comments problem** The tendency of evaluators not to include written comments on appraisal forms.

# Z

**Zero-based budget** A budgetary approach that assumes the base for projecting next year's budget is zero; managers are required to justify all activities and every proposed expenditure.

# INDEX

Page numbers followed by *f* indicate figures and those followed by *t* indicate tables or boxes.